W9-CTD-568

COUNSELING & PSYCH
SERVICES
WILLARD 134 CU-BOULDER
303 492 6766

WOMEN'S SEXUAL EXPERIENCE

Explorations of the *Dark Continent*

WOMEN IN CONTEXT: Development and Stresses

Editorial
Board:

Matina Horner, *Redcliffe College*
Martha Kirkpatrick, *University of California at Los Angeles*
Claire B. Kopp, *University of California at Los Angeles*
Carol C. Nadelson, *Tufts—New England Medical Center*
Malkah T. Notman, *Tufts—New England Medical Center*
Carolyn B. Robinowitz, *American Psychiatric Association*
Jeanne Spurlock, *American Psychiatric Association*

WOMEN'S SEXUAL EXPERIENCE
Explorations of the *Dark Continent*

Edited by
MARTHA KIRKPATRICK, M.D.

PLENUM PRESS • *NEW YORK AND LONDON*

Library of Congress Cataloging in Publication Data

Main entry under title:

Women's sexual experience.

(Women in context)
Includes bibliographical references and index.
1. Women—United States—Sexual behavior—Addresses, essays, lectures. I.
Kirkpatrick, Martha. II. Series.
HQ29.W675   306.7′088042   82-482
ISBN 0-306-40793-0   AACR2

© 1982 Plenum Press, New York
A Division of Plenum Publishing Corporation
233 Spring Street, New York, N.Y. 10013

All rights reserved

No part of this book may be reproduced, stored in a retrieval, system, or transmitted,
in any form or by any means, electronic, mechanical, photocopying, microfilming,
recording, or otherwise, without written permission from the Publisher

Printed in the United States of America

"...after all, the sexual life of adult women is a dark continent of psychology."

FREUD (1926)
The Question of Lay Analysis
Standard Edition XX, p. 212

Contributors

Louise Armstrong • Author: *Kiss Daddy Goodnight: A Speak-out on Incest;* National Women's Health Network, Washington, D.C.

Elissa Benedek, M.D. • Clinical Professor, Director of Training, Center for Forensic Psychiatry, University of Michigan, Ann Arbor, Michigan

Harold P. Blum, M.D. • Clinical Professor, Department of Psychiatry, New York University, New York, New York

J. Robert Bragonier, M.D., Ph.D. • Adjunct Associate Professor, Department of Obstetrics and Gynecology, Harbor–UCLA Medical Center, Torrance, California

Edward M. Brecher • Journalist/Author: *An Analysis of Human Sexual Response, The Sex Researchers,* and *Love, Sex, and Aging,* West Cornwall, Connecticut

June Dobbs Butts, Ed.D. • Assistant Professor, Department of Psychiatry, Howard University College of Medicine, Washington, D.C.

Merle G. Church, M.A. • Legislative Advocate, former President, California Alliance Concerned with School Age Parents, Manhattan Beach, California

Marlene Echohawk, Ph.D. • Assistant Clinical Professor, Pediatric Psychology, Department of Psychiatry and Behavioral Sciences, University of Oklahoma Health Sciences Center, Oklahoma City, Oklahoma

B. Genevay, M.S.W. • Consultant in Aging, Family Services of King County, Seattle, Washington

King K. Holmes, M.D., Ph.D. • Professor, Department of Medicine, Adjunct Professor, Department of Microbiology, Immunology, and Epidemiology; Head, Division of Infectious Diseases, USPHS Hospital, Seattle, Washington

Jennifer James, Ph.D. • Associate Professor, Department of Psychiatry and Behavioral Sciences, University of Washington Medical School, Seattle, Washington

Helen S. Kaplan, M.D., Ph.D. • Clinical Professor, Department of Psychiatry, Cornell University Medical College; Human Sexuality Program, Payne–Whitney Clinic at New York Hospital–Cornell Medical Center, New York, New York

Lois Lee, Ph.D. • Founder, Children of the Night, a social service program for teenage prostitutes, Beverly Hills, California

Lloyd M. Levin • Founder, All Together, Inc., an organization providing resources for participants in alternate life-styles, Suite 3612, 405 North Wabash Avenue, Chicago, Illinois

Del Martin • Commissioner, California Commission on Crime Control and Violence Prevention, Sacramento, California

Rachel Edgarde Pape, M.D. • Assistant Clinical Professor, Department of Psychiatry, University of California at Los Angeles School of Medicine, Los Angeles, California

Lillian B. Rubin, Ph.D., M.F.C. • Research Sociologist, Institute for Scientific Analysis, San Francisco, California

Lidia M. Rubinstein, M.D., F.A.C.O.G. • Associate Professor, Department of Obstetrics and Gynecology and Family Planning Clinic, University of California at Los Angeles School of Medicine, Los Angeles, California

Joann DeLora Sandlin, Ph.D. • Professor, Department of Sociology, San Diego State University, San Diego, California

Leslie R. Schover, Ph.D. • Assistant Professor of Urology (Psychology), Department of Urology, M. D. Anderson Hospital and Tumor Institute, Houston, Texas

Erica Sucher, M.S.W. ● Human Sexuality Program, New York Hospital–Cornell Medical Center, New York, New York

Max Sugar, M.D. ● Clinical Professor, Department of Psychiatry, Louisiana State University Medical Center, New Orleans, Louisiana

Roland Summit, M.D. ● Assistant Clinical Professor, Community Consultation Service, Harbor–UCLA Medical Center, Torrance, California; Department of Psychiatry, University of California at Los Angeles School of Medicine, Los Angeles, California

Miriam Tasini, M.D. ● Assistant Clinical Professor, Department of Psychiatry, University of California at Los Angeles School of Medicine, Los Angeles, California

Richard Vaughn, Ph.D. ● West Shore Mental Health Center, Muskegon County Community Mental Health Board, Muskegon, Michigan

Judith E. Vida, M.D. ● Psychiatrist in private practice, Pasadena, California

Joan Crofut Weibel, Ph.D. ● The Alcohol Research Center, Neuropsychiatric Institute, University of California at Los Angeles; Assistant Professor, Anthropology Department, University of Southern California, Los Angeles, California

Gail Elizabeth Wyatt, Ph.D. ● Clinical Psychologist; Assistant Professor, Department of Psychiatry, Neuropsychiatric Institute, University of California at Los Angeles School of Medicine, Los Angeles, California

Preface

This book, like its companion volume, *Women's Sexual Development,* is a potpourri of ideas, not campaign literature to promote a particular point of view. The editor agrees with some of her authors and strongly disagrees with others. The "facts" are few, the questions many. The intent of both books is to evoke questions, delay convictions, invite controversy, and plead for opening minds. The examination and explanation of women's sexual experience has long been the province of men. The "is" and the "oughts" have been hopelessly confused by the investigators' (or exhorters') biases and limited experience, as well as by the use of the male sexual experience as the model for all human sexual experience. Women, at long last, are talking not only to each other, in personal journals and letters, but also in the more formal worlds of academic and scientific publications.

The papers in this book come from many sources. Some are academic; some are experiential, journalistic, or personal. Several emphasize the lack of adequate research and data but address an issue that is just appearing on the surface of contemporary controversy and concern. Many topics and sources of information are missing. Perhaps another book, at another time, will fill some of the glaring gaps (such as women's reactions to visual sexual stimuli, women's sexual fantasies, the question of adaptable and flexible sexual object choice in women, the role of holding and sensuality in female sexual satisfaction, the sexuality of breast feeding, and Latino women's sexual experience).

It is sometimes said, true or not, that the male's sexual fulfillment takes 2.6 minutes, and the female's takes nine months. Reaching for the even more delayed climactic moment of completing this volume, this editor has felt like an elephant gestating after mating with a whale. I hope timorously that the little Seussian offspring will flipper and gambol into its place in the strange kingdom of the study of human sexual life.

I am grateful for the support and tolerance of family and friends during this prolonged gestation. Most especially, I appreciate the patience and good nature of my secretary and assistant, Elayne Mitchell, who has endured the endless penciling and revising of those pristine pages she thought were final. She has been a healer and a midwife.

Martha Kirkpatrick

Los Angeles, California

Contents

PART I

The General Condition

Chapter 1

Women's Sexual Response

HELEN S. KAPLAN AND ERICA SUCHER

WHAT IS NORMAL SEXUAL DESIRE?

Our concept of what constitutes the normal range of sexual desire is highly subjective, in contrast with our concept of normalcy with respect to genital functioning. Erections and orgasms can be observed objectively and therefore can be accurately described and defined, but our data regarding normalcy of libido in men and women are incomplete and largely anecdotal. However, there is a sense of the normal range of sexual interest, and while there is confusion in borderline situations, professional consensus does exist—at least in a general way—regarding the extreme and clearly pathological deviations from the norm. For example, most clinicians would agree that a married woman of 39 who never feels sexual desire, is attracted neither to her husband nor to anyone else, and never fantasizes or masturbates has an abnormally low libido. A history of significant change in libido also suggests that desire has become pathologically low and is not simply low normal (Kaplan, 1977).

The sexual response of males and females may be divided into three phases: desire, excitement, and orgasm. Desire is an appetite that has its locus in the brain (limbic brain and hypothalamus); excitement and orgasm involve autonomic reflexes of the genitals. Excitement in both males and females is the result of dilation of the blood vessels that invest the genital organs, while orgasm is produced by the contraction of certain genital muscles (Kaplan, 1974b, 1979).

HELEN S. KAPLAN, M.D., PH.D. ● Clinical Professor, Department of Psychiatry, Cornell University Medical College; Human Sexuality Program, Payne–Whitney Clinic at New York Hospital–Cornell Medical Center, New York, New York 10021.   ERICA SUCHER, M.S.W. ● Human Sexuality Program, New York Hospital–Cornell Medical Center, New York, New York 10029.

THE NORMAL SEXUAL EXPERIENCE

Normal sexual development can be described in only the most general terms because of the current incomplete state of our knowledge. But it seems that in the healthy individual some form of sexual appetite is present throughout life. As with any human trait, the intensity of the sex drive varies widely. At the extremes, it may be difficult to determine what is a pathological and what a normal variation. In other words, some normal persons apparently have such a low sex drive that they appear to be suffering from a pathological inhibition of sexual desire (Kaplan, 1977).

Sexual appetite changes in intensity with age and takes a gender-specific course of development. Infants seem to have the capacity for some erotic feelings, and these are evoked when their genitals are stimulated. When tiny clitorises and penes are stimulated in the course of bathing and dressing, infants express pleasure by smiling and cooing. If they are not stopped, children masturbate and later play sexual games that entail looking and touching. We tend to forget or to repress many of these early sexual fantasies and experiences, but some memory is normally retained. And if during a psychosexual evaluation the patient remembers *no* prepubescent erotic feelings, one can assume a certain amount of early sexual inhibition.

There is a substantial increase in sexual desire at puberty. It is correlated both with the maturation of the cerebral circuits that govern sexual expression and also with the increase in testosterone produced by the gonads at this time, which activates these circuits. After puberty, sexual development takes a different course in the two genders. In the male, sexual desire seems to peak at around 17 years and then slowly declines. The normal adolescent male is very interested in sex, is easily aroused, and in the absence of a partner masturbates from several times a week to several times a day while conjuring up erotic fantasies. If there is no sexual outlet, he experiences frustration. So predictable is this phenomenon that if the sexual history reveals no adolescent increase in sexual desire as reflected in masturbation and/or fantasy or actual intercourse, one may suspect a problem in psychosexual development. The intensity of the male sex drive diminishes gradually after adolescence. At middle age, he still desires sex but often can go without sexual outlet for longer and longer periods of time without experiencing frustration. His sexual desire can, however, be aroused under exciting circumstances all during his life.

Females also experience an intense increase in libido at puberty. However, in our culture, currently, it does not decline after adolescence but slowly increases and peaks around the age of 40. Female sexual desire then also slowly declines. In general, female sexual desire is more variable than that of males. While women have a greater orgasmic potential, their sexuality is also more easily suppressed.

Clinically, it seems that female sexual desire is more easily inhibited than that of the male, especially during youth, when the sex drive in the male is so intense. In other words, inhibition of sexual desire can be produced in women of all ages and in aging men by relatively less intense factors. It takes relatively more substantial psychological pressure to produce an inhibition of sexual desire in a young male. Speculations about the relative contributions of biological or cultural determinants to these gender differences in sexual desire are legion and inconclusive at this time.

Thus, the normal person throughout his or her life both experiences spontaneous sexual desire and has the capacity to have desire evoked by an attractive partner. When the sex drive is high, the person experiences spontaneous desire and is aroused by a wide range of stimuli. As desire diminishes, the range of stimuli that evoke the sexual appetite narrows.

Both genders usually experience an increase in sexual appetite when in love, and both genders experience a decrease in sexual desire when they are under stress. Even when a couple have an excellent romantic bond, sexual desire normally fluctuates, but it never remains absent for long (Kaplan, 1974b, 1979).

Normal Asexuality

The asexual state is certainly not universally abnormal. It has already been mentioned that some persons have a constitutionally determined sexual appetite that is on the low side of the normal distribution.

There are also many circumstances in which a person's sexual desire is inhibited on a nonpathological basis. It is not appropriate to find all potential sexual partners or situations attractive. Many persons do not really enjoy sex unless they have an intimate and sensitive relationship with the partner or unless the partner meets some special emotional and physical ideal. Such persons may choose to inhibit their sexual feelings until they can find a desirable partner to whom they can form a gratifying attachment. Celibacy on this basis is a constructive, mature, and dignified choice and should not be classified as pathological. The healthy celibacy in which desire is suppressed until a really satisfying partner becomes available should be differentiated from a neurotic rejection of suitable partners (Kaplan, 1977, 1979).

Thus, the capacity to inhibit as well as to express one's sexuality is a part of normal human functioning.

THE STAGES OF THE SEXUAL RESPONSE

We shall now describe in detail and compare the physiological sexual responses of men and women.

In order for the small, flaccid, urinary penis to be transformed into the erect, reproductive phallus, and in order for the dry, tight potential space of the vagina to be metamorphosed into the succulent, open reproductive receptacle, profound physiological reactions must occur. Masters and Johnson (1966) have described the sequence of events that prepares males and females for sexual union so beautifully and usefully that their descriptive scheme has become incorporated in the vocabulary of the field and now constitutes basic material in the curricula of training programs. Briefly, Masters and Johnson divided the male and female sexual response into four stages: excitement, plateau, orgasm, and resolution. The changes are comprised basically of genital vasocongestion and involuntary smooth as well as striated muscle responses.

In the female, during *excitement*, vasocongestion of labial, bulbar, and perivaginal blood vessels causes vaginal lubrication and swelling of the genitals. In addition, the vagina expands and balloons internally, and the uterus rises. This reaction reaches its extreme expression during *plateau*, when the intense local swelling has been termed the "orgasmic platform" by Masters and Johnson. *Orgasm* in the female does not include an emission phase; it consists of rapid involuntary contractions of the striated muscles surrounding the vagina. The pleasurable orgastic sensations are correlated with these involuntary contractions, as they are in the male. *Resolution* represents a drain of fluid from the genitals and the consequent return to the basal state.

In the male, *excitement* is characterized by erection. This becomes maximal during *plateau*, when erection reaches its limit; the testes, which are now enlarged and congested, rise into apposition with the perineal floor. *Orgasm* in the male consists first of *emission*, or the gathering of seminal fluid in the posterior urethra by the reflex contraction of the smooth muscle of the prostate, the seminal vesicles, and the vasa deferentia. This process is perceived by the man as the sensation of ejaculatory inevitability. It is followed a split second later by *ejaculation*. The latter response consists of rapid involuntary contractions of the striated muscles surrounding the base of the penis, as well as of the smooth muscles of the penile urethra. The pleasurable sensations of orgasm accompany this ejaculatory part of the response.

Resolution consists of an abatement of local vasocongestion and a return to the basal state.

THE TRIPHASIC NATURE OF THE SEXUAL RESPONSE

In both genders, the manifest appearance of the sexual response is a smooth sequence of events: desire leads to excitement and culminates in a climax. It would appear that it is an indivisible, unified event. However, a closer look reveals that the sexual response is actually a well-coordinated sequence of three discrete physiological responses: desire, lubrication-swelling, and orgasm in the female, and desire, erection, and ejaculation in the male (Kaplan, 1979).

There is much evidence for such a triphasic concept. First, in the male, the two genital components are innervated by different parts of the nervous system. Erection is mediated by the parasympathetic, as well as the sympathetic, divisions of the autonomic nervous system, while the emission phase of ejaculation is controlled by the sympathetic and somatic nerves (Kaplan, 1974b).

The erectile response is essentially due to hydraulic pressure against the limits of the tough penile fascia. This pressure occurs when there is dilation of the penile arterioles, a parasympathetically controlled reaction, together with a shutting down of valves (or polsters) in the penile vesicles, which prevents rapid drainage of blood. The polster reflex is probably initiated by sympathetic nerves.

Orgasm in the male consists of the two phases described above. Emission, or contraction of the internal male reproductive viscera, is governed by sympathetic nerves. Ejaculation, which consists mostly of involuntary clonic contraction of striated perineal musculature, is presumably innervated by somatic nerves that flow from a reflex center located in the sacral cord (Kaplan, 1974b).

Moreover, recent studies show discrete cerebral localization of desire, erection, and ejaculation (Kaplan, 1979). Definite loci in the primate brain, if stimulated electrically, produce ejaculation, even in the absence of erection. Electrical stimulation of different but closely related brain areas causes the animal to have an erection, but he does not ejaculate. Clinical observations also show that ejaculation and erection can be impaired separately. In retarded ejaculation, erection is not affected. The man is normally aroused and typically maintains his erection for long periods of time. However, his orgasmic reflex is inhibited, and he may have great difficulty ejaculating. Indeed, there is a rare syndrome that we have termed *partial retardation*, wherein the emission phase is intact, and only the pleasurable ejaculation part of the male orgasmic response is inhibited. On the other hand, many men who suffer from erectile dysfunction and cannot attain or maintain an erection do ejaculate with a limp penis and feel normal orgasmic sensations if they are stimulated sufficiently.

The discreteness of the vasocongestive and orgasmic components of the sexual response has until recently been clinically recognized only for the male. However, an exactly analogous situation exists for the female. In the female, also, the arousal aspect of the sexual response consists of genital vasocongestion. Of course, the dilation of vessels and capillaries occurs diffusely in the perivaginal, labial, and pelvic areas, not in a discrete space, nor are there special caverns or valves in the female genitalia. However, the female genitals are richly supplied with blood vessels. The female genital vasocongestion does not produce an erection. It causes, instead, swelling and transudation. The latter appears on the vaginal wall in the form of vaginal lubrication. The swelling produces what has been described by Masters and Johnson as formation of the "orgastic platform." Thus, female genital lubrication and swelling are analogous to erection in the male.

The orgasmic reflex is also analogous in the two genders. Of course, there is no emission of ejaculate in the female. However, the female orgasm is triggered by similar stimuli and is expressed by motor discharge similar to that of the ejaculation phase of the male climax. In the male, orgasm is elicited by rhythmic stimulation of the skin of the glans and the shaft of the penis. Similarly, in the female, orgasm is brought about by sensory input provided by stimulation of the skin of the clitoris, which is embryologically derived from the same tissues that produce the penile shaft and glans. In the male, the motor expression of orgasm consists of rapid, rhythmic contractions of the muscles at the base of the penis: the bulbocavernosus, the ischiocavernosus, and some perineal floor muscles. These same muscles are involved in the orgasmic expression in women. These muscles contract against the thickened, engorged perivaginal tissues to produce the female orgasm.

The neurophysiology of the female sexual response has not yet been studied. However, by analogy, one can speculate that a similar discrete but related nervous-system organization of the two aspects of the sexual response exists in both genders. Clinically, also, one sees two separate dysfunctional syndromes in women that are produced by the discrete inhibition of the two components of the female sexual response. The more severe disorder is general sexual unresponsiveness, which is analogous to impotence, and the other is orgasmic dysfunction, which is in many respects similar to retarded ejaculation in males (Kaplan, 1974a).

THE FEMALE ORGASM

There is much confusion about the nature of the female orgasm, much of which is inherited from the old vaginal–clitoral orgasm dichotomy. According to psychoanalytic theory, there are two kinds of orgasm: "clitoral" and "vaginal." The clitoral orgasm is supposed to be neurotic, while the vaginal orgasm is supposedly the healthy expression of female sexuality. A little girl first feels erotic sensations in her clitoris. Clitoral eroticism is considered a normal but immature stage of psychosexual development appropriate to early infancy and childhood only. The normal woman "advances" to vaginal eroticism after latency, in early adolescence. Classic psychoanalytic theory contends that the normal mature woman feels erotic sensations chiefly in the vagina and has only vaginal orgasms during coitus, solely in response to the penis inside the vagina. If a woman feels erotic sensations in the clitoris only and has only clitoral orgasms, she is neurotic. According to this view, such women harbor either unconscious penis envy or are the victims of unresolved oedipal conflicts. Accordingly, the aim of psychoanalytic therapy is to resolve these alleged unconscious conflicts and thereby foster vaginal orgasms in the woman.

There is much evidence against the psychoanalytic positions that (1) there are two kinds of female orgasm and (2) orgasm achieved by clitoral stimulation is a manifestation of pathology. Masters and Johnson (1966), who observed and studied thousands of women while they were having orgasms, found that all female orgasms, those resulting from coitus and those evoked by direct stimulation of the clitoris, are physiologically identical. Moreover, the female orgasm is never clitoral or vaginal. It always has *both* components (Kaplan, 1974b).

Perhaps the confusion surrounding the nature of the female orgasm can be dispelled a bit by a consideration of the orgasm as a *reflex*. Like all other reflexes—the blink reflex, the patellar reflex, the startle reflex, and so on—it has a sensory and a motor component. There is no real controversy about the *motor* component of the female orgasm. There is now no doubt that the involuntary, rapid, rhythmic spasms of the perivaginal muscles are accompanied by exquisitely pleasurable sensations and constitute the motor expression of all female orgasms. This is true whether orgasm is triggered by direct stimulation of the clitoris or whether it is elicited by coitus.

The major controversy centers on the sensory component of the female orgasm. Such a controversy exists over no other reflex. For instance, it would never occur to anyone to question whether the blink reflex, which consists of an involuntary contraction of the muscles of the eyelid when the cornea is touched, has a motor component that is distinct from its sensory component. The muscles of the eyelid are innervated by the eighth cranial nerve, while the cornea receives its nerve supply from the ophthalmic division of the fifth nerve. No one is distraught because the sensory trigger spot for the eye blink is not located in the muscles of the eyelid. But many clinicians get intensely upset when faced with evidence that suggests that while the female orgasm consists of rhythmic spasms of the muscles surrounding the *vagina* and is therefore felt as emanating from the vagina and deep in the pelvis, it is characteristically triggered by stimulation of the sensory endings of the *clitoris*, which, incidentally, yield a distinctly different, but also highly pleasurable, erotic sensation. Moreover, it is not surprising that women differ in their orgasmic thresholds. As for any other reflex, there is a normal range. All physicians who have conducted neurological examinations know that there is a substantial range in the ease or difficulty with which the patellar reflex can be elicited. Some patients respond with a hefty kick at the slightest tap of the hammer, while others, whose neurological apparatus is entirely intact and normal, require the physician to hammer away with considerable force at the patient's knee, and sometimes to distract the patient before the knee "jerk" can be elicited. Moreover, it is difficult, if not impossible, to tell whether such a difficult patient merely has a high and physiologically normal threshold, or whether the threshold is raised by psychogenic inhibition. The patient may be so overcontrolled and tense that she or he is involuntarily inhibiting the reflex.

Similarly, various levels of female orgasmic thresholds are encountered in clinical practice, and current evidence is insufficient to make it clear where normalcy ends and inhibition begins. Clearly, the orgasmic reflex is subject to psychogenic inhibition, but we have not yet defined the normal range of the female orgasm.

At the lower end of the continuum of orgasmic response are women (about 8% of the female population of the United States) who have never experienced an orgasm. Presumably, all physically normal women are capable of orgasm, and the totally anorgastic state represents inhibition. Thereafter, the distinctions between normal and pathological are less certain. Next in the spectrum of orgasmic threshold are women who can climax only if they are alone, employ fantasy, and use the intense clitoral stimulation produced by a vibrator. Less severely inhibited women may not be able to climax in the presence of a partner but can do so without mechanical stimulation by manual masturbation, with the additional stimulation of their erotic fantasies. Next in the continuum of orgasmic threshold are the women who can climax in the presence of a lover, but only if he directly stimulates the clitoris—orally, manually, or mechanically. Further along on the continuum are women who can reach orgasm with the stimulation provided by coitus alone. This group includes those who are able to reach orgasm by clitoral stimulation as well and those who are able to climax only during intercourse (Kaplan, 1974a, 1974b).

Implicit in this description of the distribution of the thresholds of the female orgasmic reflex is the contention that intercourse does *not* provide as strong a stimulus for orgasmic release as does direct clitoral stimulation. Many find this view objectionable, and the relationship between coitus and orgasm is a highly controversial subject. Paradoxically, coitus produces only the mild physical stimulus provided by traction on the clitoral hood and, in some positions, the additional stimulus of the pressure of the partner's pubic bone against the clitoral area. Of course, the relatively mild mechanical stimulation that is produced by coitus is offset, to some degree, by the psychic stimulus provided by penile containment and closeness to the partner and by the partner's rising excitement and pleasure. However, the fact remains—and it must be faced—that coitus does not produce as intense physical stimulation as does direct clitoral manipulation, and only women blessed with a relatively low orgasmic threshold seem to be able to climax on coitus alone.

There is currently a great deal of controversy over the question of precisely where in this distribution of female orgasmic thresholds normalcy ends and pathology begins. Psychoanalysts tend to define any woman who does not achieve coital orgasm as inhibited and neurotic and in need of treatment, even if she is otherwise responsive. An alternate viewpoint, to which we subscribe, attributes no particular significance to coital orgasm. In our view, some cases of "coital frigidity" are a product of inhibition and are correctable with treatment; for many other healthy women, orgasm achieved by direct clitoral stimulation while the woman is engaged with her partner falls within the normal range of the female sexual response and is not a reflection of pathology.

At this time, there are not enough fundamental data available to determine with certainty what constitutes normalcy and pathology of the female orgasmic reflex. However, in the admitted absence of the necessary hard facts, and on the basis of our experience with sex therapy, we have developed the following working scheme, which of course is subject to modification as data accumulate. We feel that all physically normal women can have an orgasm if they receive effective stimulation. However, we do not yet know if every normal woman can climax on intercourse because we do not have data on the normal physiological range of the female orgasmic thresholds. Therefore, we are guided by the following therapeutic philosophy with regard to the treatment of orgasmically dysfunctional women. We accept all orgasmically dysfunctional women, including those suffering from coital orgasmic difficulty, for treatment. Virtually all totally anorgasmic women can be taught to have masturbatory orgasms. Similarly, most orgasmically inhibited women can eventually come to climax in the presence of their partners if the sexual ambience becomes more reassuring and free. However, only approximately one-half of our patients who compain of coital anorgasmy are able to climax in intercourse after treatment. We do not regard those who do not as treatment failures. Instead, we counsel such couples that reliance on clitoral stimulation may be a normal variant of female sexuality. Lovemaking can be exquisitely pleasurable and satisfying for both partners, providing that neither considers this a "second-best" mode of sexual experience.

It should also be noted that women who are coitally orgasmic, but who are not able to reach orgasm with clitoral stimulation, while not generally regarded as suffering from sexual inhibition, find themselves at a disadvantage when there is a decrease in their partners' coital capacity as a result of aging. These women, if they are able to accept the changes necessary in the couple's sexual pattern, can usually learn to reach orgasm on clitoral stimulation. The same is true for women who can have orgasm with a partner but are inhibited with respect to masturbation. They can learn to masturbate to orgasm, if this is seen as an acceptable sexual outlet for the time when no suitable partner is available.

AGE-RELATED CHANGES IN FEMALE SEXUAL FUNCTIONING

Female sexuality appears to be subject to far greater individual variations than is male sexuality, although direct comparison is impossible. This variability makes it more difficult to generalize, and statements about female sexuality are less reliable than those about males with respect to age-related sexual changes.

Girls, like boys, experience diffuse sexual pleasure during early childhood. They too masturbate, have sexual fantasies, and enjoy sex play if it is not prevented. Gender differences in the pattern of sexual development first begin to appear during adolescence.

Girls also undergo marked physical development and a sudden increase in sexual interest at this time. However, they tend to be more preoccupied with attracting boys or with being in love with one boy than with the purely physical aspects of sex. Girls are, on the whole, slower to awaken to sexuality, and their orgasmic urge is apparently less intense. While virtually all normal boys masturbate, approximately 30%–40% of women report that they either do not masturbate at all or that they did not start to masturbate until after they had had a sexual experience that had led to orgasm or to intense arousal. In contrast to men, where the absence of adolescent masturbation raises a suspicion of psychiatric disturbance, women who have never masturbated are not necessarily pathological. Even so, absence of masturbation is a frequent finding in the histories of women who later complain of orgasmic difficulties.

The initial sexual experiences of boys and girls—at least, in our culture—tend to differ significantly. A boy may be shy and clumsy and may ejaculate more rapidly than he would like to the first time he attempts intercourse. Nevertheless, initial attempts at intercourse usually result in an orgasm for him. This is not so for the girl. If the initial sexual experiences consist of petting and manipulation without intercourse, and if they include stimulation of the breasts and the clitoris, they may be the most arousing experiences in the girl's sexual life—and yet she may not experience orgasm. Frequently, the initial coital experiences of young girls are disappointing and do not produce orgasm or even pleasurable vaginal sensations. In fact, intercourse may be physically uncomfortable, and the girl may become alarmed at her failure to enjoy the experience.

During the early years of marriage in the 20s, frequency of intercourse is at its peak. Kinsey et al. (1948) reported two to five times per week to be the normal range. However, this frequency is likely to be the result primarily of the young husband's intense sexual desire. During this time, he wants sex often, is rapidly aroused, and frequently enters and reaches orgasm quickly, often leaving his wife unsatisfied.

In our culture, women tend to reach the peak of their responsiveness in their late 30s and early 40s. During this time, Kinsey et al. (1953) reported the greatest prevalence of female extramarital sexual involvement. Masters and Johnson (1966) observed rapid and intense responsiveness during this period, especially after the birth of several children. They attributed this heightened responsiveness, at least in part, to the increased vascularity of the pelvic viscera that occurs after childbirth. Vaginal lubrication, the equivalent of male erection, occurs instantly, and multiple orgasms are frequently reported in this age group. In our experience also, many but not all women in this age group report that they experience more interest in sexuality and a greater ease in orgasmic responsiveness than during their earlier years. It may be speculated that this greater sexual responsiveness of the middle years is not primarily biologically determined. It may be produced by a combination of gradual loss of inhibitions and greater security about being accepted by and pleasing to the partner.

Over the years, these women have developed a degree of sexual autonomy and have learned to ask their partners for the type of stimulation that arouses them with less shame and fear than was present earlier.

Female sexual functioning during the menopausal years is extremely variable and depends on the woman's general psychic state and on her relationship with her partner. The abrupt cessation of ovarian functioning produces a drastic drop in the circulating estrogen and progesterone. These endocrine changes are accompanied in some— but by no means all—women by the familiar irritability, depression, emotional instability, and aggressive behavior of the menopause. A similar emotional crisis or period of "tension"—accompanied by a striking increase in the incidence of psychotic episodes, crimes of violence, accidents, and medical illness—is experienced by a small number of women during their monthly "minimenopause," that is, the eight-day period around menstruation, which is characterized by a temporary drop in circulating estrogen and progesterone.

The effect on libido of the withdrawal of the female sex steroids is again quite variable. Clearly, if a woman is depressed, irritable, and insecure, she is not likely to be very interested in sex. Yet while some women report a decrease in sexual desire, many women actually feel an increase in erotic appetite during the menopausal years. Again, the fate of libido seems to depend on a constellation of factors during this period, including physiological changes, sexual opportunity, and diminution of inhibition. From a purely physiological standpoint, libido should theoretically increase at menopause, because the action of the woman's androgens, which is not materially affected by menopause, is not opposed by estrogen. Indeed, some women do seem to behave in this manner, especially if they are not depressed and can find interested and interesting partners. However, if the middle-aged husband is avoiding sex, and if the insecure, depressed, and angry woman attributes this avoidance to her declining physical attractiveness, she too may avoid sexuality in order to spare herself the pain of frustration or rejection.

After the 50s, the postmenopausal years of female sexual responsiveness also show great individual variation. Women of this age group depend for their sexual expression on a dwindling supply of men, whose sexual needs have declined markedly. A woman who has regular sexual opportunity tends to maintain her sexual responsiveness; without such opportunity, sexuality declines markedly. Apart from the effect of opportunity, a slow gradual physical decline in sexual drive seems to occur in women, as in men. After age 65, a woman tends to be less preoccupied with sex than she was at 40, but she may still seek out and certainly can respond to sexual opportunities. Erotic involvements with men and masturbation are not unusual at these ages, and erotic dreams are often reported by women over 65. Physiologically, there is a decline. Masters and Johnson (1970) have reported that vaginal lubrication tends to occur more slowly, and that clonic contractions of the pelvic platform during orgasm are less vigorous and frequent, declining from five or six at 30, to two or three at 70. There is a lessening of the general myotonia that accompanies sexual excitement, and erotic sensations are reported to be less intense.

In sharp contrast to men, elderly women remain capable of enjoying multiple orgasms. In fact, studies indicate that 25% of 70-year-old women still masturbate. Nevertheless, many women cease having intercourse during their 50s and 60s. This abstinence is not primarily biologically determined; it is more influenced by social and psychological factors. When elderly women lose their partners, they do not tend to seek replacements actively unless they are unusually active and secure and possess exceptional personal assets.

Actually, age-related trophic changes of the body, and specifically of the genitalia and the breasts, are more profound in women than in men and are caused by the abrupt decline of estrogen and progesterone after menopause. Paradoxically, these relatively severe physical changes are accompanied by comparatively minimal changes in the libidinous aspects of women's sexuality.

How can these gender differences be accounted for? It is the biological component that declines with age, while the psychic aspects of sexuality remain relatively unaffected, and perhaps the physical determinants of sex are relatively more important for male than for female sexuality. This seems especially true during youth, when the physical substrate of sexuality in males is a powerful force. In females, the physical determinants of sexuality seem less pressing than the psychic and learned contributions, and therefore age erodes females' sexuality far less than males'. According to this concept, as the biological urge lessens with age, older males become more like women in their sexual behavior in that fantasy and ambience become more important in lovemaking, and there is relatively less preoccupation with orgasm. In older men, as the physical factors that motivate sexuality decline, psychic determinants become heavier contributors to the final sexual response.

Learning seems to be an extremely important determinant in female sexuality, while it is of relatively less importance in males. It has been speculated that the middle-age peaking of female sexuality, which is usually seen in women who have a history of successful sex and secure relationships with men, can be accounted for in terms of the accumulated reinforcement derived from repeated pleasurable sexual experiences, which increase in gratification as sexual techniques are accommodated to the special needs of women, as well as to the gradual diminution of the inhibitions and insecurities of youth.

We have described the normal sexual development and responses of women as far as these are currently understood. The advances in our knowledge of the physical aspects of women's sexual functioning, accomplished in recent decades, have helped both men and women toward a greater acceptance and appreciation of female sexuality. It is to be hoped that future research will further increase our knowledge in this area and will help an even greater number of women reach optimal sexual functioning.

REFERENCES

Kaplan, H. S. The classification of the female sexual dysfunctions. *Journal of Sex and Marital Therapy*, 1974, *1*(2), 124–138. (a)

Kaplan, H. S. *The new sex therapy*. New York: Brunner/Mazel, 1974. (b)

Kaplan, H. S. Hypoactive sexual desire. *Journal of Sex and Marital Therapy*, 1977, *3*(1), 3–9.

Kaplan, H. S. *Disorders of sexual desire*. New York: Brunner/Mazel, 1979.

Kinsey, A. C., Pomeroy, W. B., & Martin, ·C. E. *Sexual behavior in the human male*. Philadelphia: Saunders, 1948.

Kinsey, A. C., Pomeroy, W. B., Martin, C. E., & Gebhard, P. H. *Sexual behavior in the human female*. Philadelphia: Saunders, 1953.

Masters, W., & Johnson, V. *Human sexual response*. Boston: Little, Brown, 1966.

Masters, W., & Johnson, V. *Human sexual inadequacy*. Boston: Little, Brown, 1970.

Chapter 2

The Sexual Experience of Afro-American Women

A Middle-Income Sample

GAIL ELIZABETH WYATT

HISTORY OF RESEARCH ON AFRO-AMERICAN SEXUALITY

Documentation of sexual behavior in America was left to personal accounts, fantasy, and imagination until 25 years ago, when Kinsey and his research group published the shocking findings that 1 out of 2 married women in their sample of 6,000 reported having had intercourse before marriage (1953). These studies supported other evidence that premarital sex had been established as a trend in sexual behavior since the 1920s (Terman, 1938; Burgess & Wallin, 1953). Masters and Johnson (1966, 1970) pioneered a more in-depth examination of the physiology of human sexuality and the incidence of sexual dysfunctions. More contemporary research has documented the variety of female sexual behaviors (Hite, 1976). However, most of these studies are limited to white, highly educated samples from the urban northeastern part of the United States. With the exception of some data by the Kinsey research group, minority groups, teenagers, and geriatric populations were excluded from these landmark studies of sexual behavior.

The literature regarding the sexual behavior of Afro-Americans has been limited in scope. A nationwide sampling of 1,200 single high school and college students was conducted in the 1960s by Ira Reiss

GAIL ELIZABETH WYATT, PH.D. ● Clinical Psychologist; Assistant Professor, Department of Psychiatry, Neuropsychiatric Institute, University of California at Los Angeles School of Medicine, Los Angeles, California 90024.

(1967) to examine attitudes about sexual permissiveness as it related to social and cultural characteristics. He found blacks and males to be more permissive than whites and females. Reiss explained that males tended to be more permissive because of the double sexual standard and that blacks included in the study were more frequently of lower socioeconomic status, which may have accounted for more permissive sexual attitudes. In his study of premarital sexual standards, Reiss (1964) also found Afro-Americans to have a more permissive premarital sexual code than whites, with Afro-American males being most permissive and white females most inhibited.

In 1966, Rainwater observed that lower-class Afro-Americans' attitudes toward sexual relations were highly competitive among their same-sex peers and exploitative toward the opposite sex. However, these studies, based on attitudinal research or the investigators' observations, suffer from limitations placed on them by the investigators' own preconceived definitions of the white, middle-class standards on which Afro-American sex life was evaluated (Staples, 1973).

Studies of the influence of social class on sexual behavior eventuated mainly in studies of Afro-Americans because they constitute a greater concentration of the lower socioeconomic class than do whites. Accordingly, Afro-American females were found to have sexual relations about two years earlier than the average white, middle-class female. The Kinsey group (Gebhard, Pomeroy, Martin, & Christenson, 1958) also found that the level of exposure to premarital sexual relations for black female teenagers was three to four times higher than for their white female peers. On the other hand, the same study revealed that college-educated Afro-American women were closer in their attitudes to white peers than to lesser-educated white females. These studies illustrate the influence of socioeconomic level on exposure to and attitudes toward sexuality.

Other studies have compared aspects of Afro-American anatomy to that of whites. For example, information gathered by the Kinsey group on the penis length of Afro-American and white males revealed no significant differences in the length of the erect penis (Bell, 1968).

A number of more recent studies have examined rates of conception among adolescent and adult Afro-American populations (Brunswick, 1971; Teele, Robinson, Schmidt, & Rice, 1967; Graves & Bradshaw, 1975; Johnson, 1974), the incidence of premarital sex (Zelnick & Kantner, 1972b), sexual permissiveness (Gispert & Falk, 1976), contraceptive knowledge (Delcampo, Sporakowski, & Delcampo, 1976), and health care for disadvantaged adolescents (Fielding & Nelson, 1973). However, these studies focused on populations that utilize public health clinics or hospitals and were frequently experiencing pregnancy-related health problems at the time that the data were collected.

The selection of Afro-Americans as subjects in these studies of premarital sexual behavior, pregnancy, knowledge of health, and sexual issues creates the assumption that these problems pertain exclusively to Afro-Americans of lower socioeconomic status and raises questions as to the availability of similar white populations. One investigator admitted that nonminority females carrying pregnancies to term were difficult to find for research purposes. However, another researcher purposely selected Afro-American teenagers to study because one out of four American births is to a teenage mother, and there is a high incidence of illegitimacy among lower socioeconomic groups, especially nonwhite populations.

There are a few studies that extend beyond the economic and educational factors that influence pregnancy and health care in Afro-American adolescents and adults (Billingsley, 1968; Gutman, 1976; Ladner, 1971; Staples, 1973). These studies have as their focus dynamic aspects of sociocultural factors that historically and currently influence sexual codes and behaviors. These studies offer a dimension to understanding male–female relationships and family life that has been previously lacking in the literature. However, information regarding actual sexual behavior and identification of some of the influential factors that result in individual or group differences is minimal to nonexistent and fails to offset or clarify the nature of Afro-American sexuality (Wyatt, Strayer, & Lobitz, 1976).

MYTHS OF AFRO-AMERICAN SEXUALITY

Myths and stereotypes regarding Afro-American sexual patterns continue to serve as substitutes for factual reports of behavior because of the lack of more accurate information. A very few of the myths of Afro-American sexuality have been reported in the literature and dispelled as erroneous (Hill, 1976; Wyatt et al., 1976).

Myths of Afro-American sexuality, which developed from this country's history of sexual exploitation during the slavery era, are perpetuated as stereotypes in the minds of whites and some Afro-Americans today (Poussaint, 1971). Descriptions of Afro-American sexual behavior can be found in contemporary magazines (Young, 1974) and are often not accompanied by research data. Unfortunately, the media also contribute to the perpetuation of a myriad of myths of sexual behavior. These myths have a specific focus. For Afro-American men, there are some early written descriptions of hyposexuality (Kardiner & Ovesey, 1951). The portrayal of the passive, ignorant, asexual man whom few would find sexually threatening supports the myth of Afro-American male hyposexuality most popular in the 1920–1930 motion-picture era (Bogle, 1973). On the other hand, today, the myth of the "superstud" pervades the minds of most when the sexuality of Afro-American males comes to mind.

The reports of the bestiality and the potency of males began when Christian missionaries observed sexual practices in Africa. The early descriptions of sexual behavior may have piqued interest in the physical aspects of Afro-Americans, though their morality was perceived as barbaric and permissive as compared with Christian doctrine. During slavery, the myth of Afro-American hypersexuality was intended to discourage early sexual experimentation between male slaves and white women (Thomas & Sillen, 1972), but it also served as a rationale for maintaining political, educational, and economic oppression. However, the "superstud" image has continued to create a mystique around Afro-American, Caribbean, and African men, often making them the most sought-after of sexual partners in order for women to "test the myth" (Hernton, 1965). It has, in fact, created an area of achievement for Afro-American males that some of their white peers now wish to emulate. The once-negative connotation of being a "sexual superachiever" now carries a positive valence in this society, where "super" feats are valued over average performance. However, many Afro-American men internalize the expectation that they have extraordinary genitalia and sexual prowess. This situation can create sexual dysfunction problems when an individual does not live up to these stereotypes (Wyatt et al., 1976). The image of supersexuality has also been ascribed to Afro-American women, but the positive valence has not generalized to them. The myth of their sexuality also stems from the slave era and was intended to serve the same oppressive ends, but the impact of these myths is far more negative and pervasive than the impact of the myths describing the superhuman feats of Afro-American men.

RIGHTS OF SEXUAL OWNERSHIP. African women brought to this country in slavery and their Afro-American descendants have been subjected to premeditated sexual abuse unequal to that of any other ethnic minority group. As recently as the 1970s, Afro-American women are just beginning to experience "sexual ownership": the right to decide how, when, and with whom their sexuality is to be expressed. The Afro-American woman has never been held in as high esteem as the American white woman, the woman on whom the standard for acceptable feminine behavior—and sexual behavior, in particular—is based.

Thus, myths about the sexual morality of many Afro-American women were defined in slavery and remained unaltered, particularly for poverty-stricken Afro-American women through the post–Civil War and Reconstruction period. Economic survival of the lower-class Afro-

American family often bore the price of the woman's becoming a "domestic prostitute" or servant for white families, children, and businesses (Staples, 1973). Employment was often contingent on her compliance with the sexual advances of her superiors. Afro-American men were often unable to protect their women from sexual abuse and were forced to accept this new form of slavery because of very limited educational and occupational advancement during that time.

As a result of more economic security, Afro-American middle-class women were better able to minimize the unwanted sexual advances of men, particularly those in control of employment, and to approximate the position of the "protected one" in male–female relationships (Dollard, 1957). However, middle-class Afro-American women often had to defer sexual gratification for educational or occupational goals. This deferment process often separated middle-class women from those who were less economically advantaged, and it served as the basis for the description of middle-class Afro-American women as hyposexual or cold and uninterested in sexual relationships.

The historical descriptions of some of the consequences of slavery, which has affected the sexual expression of Afro-American women, strongly indicate that some factors may be more influential in their lives than in the lives of women of other ethnic groups.

PURPOSE

The purpose of this chapter is to identify sociocultural factors that influence Afro-American women's sexual experiences from early childhood to adulthood. Included among these factors are the myths of hypo- or hypersexuality and the extent to which Afro-American women have regained their rights to sexual ownership. It is important to emphasize that the majority of sex research has been limited to low-income Afro-American women, who tend to utilize public health clinics rather than private physicians and frequently experience problems around the termination of a pregnancy. For this chapter, there was an attempt to interview a sample of Afro-American women who are seldom selected for sex research: healthy women, some of whom may have been raised in low-income families but, because of their educational and occupational goals, are currently aspiring to or have achieved middle-income status and health care.

THE FORMAT

This study focused on obtaining reports of sexual behavior, values, and attitudes through chronological histories beginning in early childhood and extending through adolescence and adulthood. The intent was not only to identify variables that influence early and present-day values and behaviors of this group of Afro-American women, but to give the participating women an opportunity to discuss these issues with one another.

Two discussion groups were held in Los Angeles. In an effort to reach as many women as possible, participants were invited or brought by friends. They volunteered to meet in private homes for three to four hours with the author to discuss a number of topics regarding the sexual experience of Afro-American women. Each group was asked to respond to the same questions and issues, and the confidentiality of individual comments was assured. Though most of the women were eager to clarify some of the factors influencing Afro-American sexuality, each group was told that divulgence of personal and intimate experience was not a prerequisite for participation. The women had prior knowledge of the topics to be discussed and offered many rich personal vignettes to illustrate their experiences. Not all of the women volunteered information: some chose to listen with interest. Because of the scarcity of accurate information regarding Afro-American women, we learned from one another.

THE SAMPLE

The two discussion groups consisted of 43 Afro-American women who interacted with the author. Though attempts were made to obtain a range in age, socioeconomic and experiential background, marital status, and education, the participants were not selected by random sampling methods, and consequently, they do not represent the population of Afro-American women in the United States nor in the Los Angeles area. Most of the participants agreed to fill out individual demographic sheets that would describe them as a group, but some chose not to respond to every question.

The 43 women identified themselves as Afro-American and ranged in age from 25 to 58, with a median age of 32. Of these 43 women, 40% were single, 25% were married, 25% were divorced, and 7% were separated. For those 26 women who were either currently married or had been married at one time, the length of the marriage ranged from four months to 12 or more years. The median length of marriage was 7 years. Of the 26 women who had been or were currently married, 20 had married only once; thus, permanence and stability in their marital relationship or a failure to remarry was evident.

There are many factors that influence the experiences of Afro-Americans in the United States in terms of cultural exposure, religious education, and economics. Of the participants, 45% were reared in the West, 14% in the South, 16% in the New England and Mid-Atlantic states, 16% in the Midwest, and 4% on the East Coast. Though there was a range in education from completion of high school to professional degrees, half (51%) of the women held master's degrees. Their income levels ranged from $5,000 to more than $25,000, with the modal income being $15,000–$25,000. In spite of their income levels, only one person perceived herself as within the upper class, while 51% of the women identified themselves as middle-class, 26% as lower-middle class, and 14% as working but poor.

In general, this was a population of young, articulate, and highly educated women who had experienced sexual relationships and were involved in male–female relationships in the present or had been in the past.

The results of the discussion groups are divided chronologically and by issue.

RESULTS OF DISCUSSION GROUPS

EARLY-CHILDHOOD SEXUAL EDUCATION

Question: What were the factors found to influence your early sexual education? There were a number of factors that the women reported as influential in their early education. The first were verbal messages: "All boys want to do is get in your pants"; "Be a good girl and don't get pregnant"; "Keep your legs crossed and your dress down"; "They [men] will leave you afterwards." In other words, the message in early childhood regarding sexuality was generally prohibitive.

The nonverbal messages communicated in some homes were also very clear: "They didn't tell us anything about sex; you silently knew that you did not ask: sex was secretive; you were told to keep your hands off yourself and other people." None of the women's parents discussed sex with them before the age of 10.

Question: How was nudity handled in the home? There were a range of responses. On one extreme, it was reported that it was quite normal to see people seminude around the house, but it was understood that you did not ask about body parts or ask questions relating to sexual behavior. However, nudity decreased around the time of adolescence, and many women reported that they never saw their fathers without clothes. On the other extreme, some girls were required to clothe themselves fully as soon as they got up in the morning. One woman reported that her grandparents were extremely strict about nudity, while others grew up in households where nudity was permitted because of the extremely hot weather in Baltimore, and there was no prohibitive message communicated about it.

Question: How was sex explained to you during early childhood? One woman reported that sex was described by using the mating of dogs as an example. While her mother reported that sex was beautiful, she could not appreciate its beauty mainly because of the example given. Another woman reported that when she became an adolescent, each time she commented about a boy, a sexual interpretation would be made that was not necessarily intended. Another woman was told by her parents that they had "prayed" for her, and she grew up with the understanding that if you prayed, a child would be born.

Siblings were also found to contribute to sex education. Some exploration took place with older brothers, while "playing doctor" or other sexual games in the closet. Though some children were often punished, there was no consequence for this behavior for others. Peers were influential in "playing doctor" until age 5 or 6. This sex play taught some women about sex differences. Playing "post office" and other kissing games during early adolescence helped the participants identify sexual feelings. The peer group communicated that being pregnant had a negative connotation. "Bad" girls often disclosed their sexual activities to others, and while their peers lived vicariously, they did not dare to participate in sexual exploration.

Finally, the church had a powerful influence on sex education. The message was that good Christian girls don't have premarital sex. The minister would often state from the pulpit that "Christian women don't do certain [sexual] things." In some Baptist churches, when a young girl had a baby, she was asked to stand in front of the congregation and apologize for her "sinful" behavior. Only one woman reported that a sex education course was offered by her church. Another woman shared a very colorful vignette of her experiences attending a church-related college, which included a large parlor for the purpose of entertaining company on Sunday. The house mother wore soft-soled shoes and frequently would sneak up on a couple who were "petting" and place the young woman on a six-week punishment for such behavior. Another woman confirmed this attitude of *in loco parentis* at Afro-American church-affiliated prep schools and colleges. A friend had been found kissing her boyfriend and had to live in the infirmary for one month. In another example, she reported that each month, girls were to report to the infirmary and to "sign their name in red ink," documenting the dates of their menstrual cycles. The women noted the differences between the predominantly Afro-American universities, where there was far more supervision regarding sexual behavior, and the majority of white colleges, where there were fewer curfews and restrictions placed on the residents. However, it was noted that the Afro-American as well as the predominantly white schools seem to have a far more liberal attitude today regarding sexuality, in that birth control clinics are now available, and information regarding contraception is offered.

MENSTRUATION

Question: How did you learn about menstruation? To quote one woman, "I learned about menstruation when it happened. I thought I had hurt myself and hid any evidence that I was bleeding from my mother because I thought that she would become angry." Another woman's experience was expressed this way: "Not only did I learn about menstruation at school at around eleven years of age, but I also finally understood the process of conception. However, my peers misinformed me quite a bit. I learned such things as 'If you kiss, you'll get pregnant.' " The general opinion about sexuality and menstruation was that they were "nasty." Many women reported shame or embarrassment about menstruating and having to purchase the necessary articles. They also learned many taboos that were evidences of more misinformation about menstruation. For example, "Do not get your feet wet, do not wash your hair, and do not bathe." For some women, these taboos were often difficult to unlearn.

HOMOSEXUALITY

Question: What were your parents' attitudes about homosexuality that shaped your opinions? Most women felt that Afro-Americans were not "naturally" homosexual, but that when homosexuality is present, it is a result of acculturation of Afro-Americans into the mainstream society. Other women reported that in their parents' homes, homosexuality was treated as a "pathetic joke," and that gay people were the butt of the joke. Female homosexuals were called "bull-daggers" and males were called "sissies." The threat of women dating or befriending homosexual men did not appear to be a problem, but to bring home a homosexual female friend appeared to be more threatening to parents, and these friendships were openly discouraged. Many women reported that they did not understand the sexual aspect of homosexuality until age 17 or 18 and assumed that homosexuals had a romantic relationship that was essentially asexual. In college, most of the participants became aware of homosexuality, but no one really talked about it. When homosexuality within the black community was discussed, one woman reported that she recalled a gay church in Harlem where all of the members dressed in white each Sunday. Some participants felt that black male homosexuality was increasing because of pressure to provide sexual satisfaction and to be the breadwinner of the family as well.

Some women perceived the Afro-American church as encouraging gay life because of its positive reinforcement of emotionalism. Others disagreed and felt that homosexuality in general is more open, and that the church is more accepting of nonaggressive men who do not wish to emulate the supermacho image. Most women remarked that it's more difficult today to label men or women as homosexual because they "don't look it," and these women were learning to tolerate and to accept this alternative style of sexuality.

Some women who were over 30 and not married remarked that they had been labeled as lesbians. Their mothers had warned them that people would "talk about you" because "if you hadn't married by the age of thirty, people thought something must be wrong with your sexual preference."

PREMARITAL SEX

Question: What was the message communicated to you about premarital sex from your parents that shaped your attitudes and behavior? The women said the following: "Good girls keep themselves nice and don't do it"; "Keep your pants up and your dress down"; "It's dangerous, and you're asking for trouble"; "Boys won't respect you if you give up your body"; and "You'll be a fallen woman." The biggest disgrace was reportedly to have an illegitimate child, because some women were taught that it would taint the family and that their lives would be destroyed. Some mothers recognized their daughters' sexuality with instructions to protect themselves if they had to do "something." One woman was told by her mother, "If you can't help yourself, cover it [the penis] up." We remarked on the ambiguity of such a statement and how easily it would be misunderstood by a young, preadolescent girl. On the other hand, there was also recognition and acceptance of extended-family members coming to live with the family from another city because they had become pregnant.

The parents of these women usually communicated a mixed message about sex and failed to accept the participants as sexually active in spite of their age and marital status. For example, one woman reported that in order to defuse intense relationships when she was young, she was encouraged by her parents to "see a lot of guys," but when she became older, to avoid seeming promiscuous, she was encouraged to settle down to one man.

Question: What was the role of the father in sex education? Fathers were seen as protective, as were older brothers, who often expected to chaperone their sisters to parties during the evening. One woman's brother was told, "Remember the girl you take out is someone else's sister"—the implication being that he should treat her with respect. The strongest message communicated was "Make sure I'm a father-in-law before I'm a grandfather." One father taught his daughter sex education, even though others reported that their parents generally felt that teaching a child about sex would give them permission to act out.

Most women resented the double standard for men when they were growing up, even though they learned that "Men are dogs"; or "Men can't help themselves; sex is in their nature." They failed to see how men's "nature" differed from that of women.

EXTRAMARITAL SEX

Question: What were you told about extramarital sex? The message communicated was that it is taboo, and the women in the group agreed. One woman remarked that it was different if a woman was living with a man. It was difficult for her grandparents to accept this kind of behavior because they generally perceived her as promiscuous because of her living arrangement. Another mother of a participant had always taught her daughter about the taboos of extramarital sex but, as she grew older, seemed to develop a more liberal attitude about sex. She stated that if she were young again, she would experience sexual relations with another man at some time in her life.

The expression of sexuality was obviously a very serious matter to the parents of these women, which prompted the question, "Why was sex taken so seriously?" These were the reasons: The stereotype regarding hypersexuality in Afro-American women is based on white propaganda. Contrary to the literature, these women perceived Afro-American women as marching at a slower pace, and as more sexually conservative. Most Afro-American women require more "wining and dining" and a stable relationship before they agree to become a sexual partner. Many mothers want their daughters to attain certain goals and to avoid falling into the same trap that so many other Afro-American girls have fallen into. Consequently, the women in this group were often encouraged to pursue higher degrees and were protected by their families, and overt sexual expression was minimized. Pregnancy appeared to carry tremendous consequences because once an Afro-American girl "fell," she was more likely to lose the opportunity for a "good life." While other girls were getting pregnant, parents would comment, "Don't have sex. You'll get pregnant, and Afro-American people have it harder, anyway. Your chances for success will be over." Some women felt that this message to defer sexual gratification was too strongly communicated, resulting in sexual hang-ups for some women in the group. Women reported that their grandparents' opinions about sex had very strong moral overtones: Sex was "to make babies" and not for pleasure. One woman was told to conduct herself differently from the other impoverished girls, even though she was also poor. The attitude communicated by her mother was to conduct herself with dignity and respect: "You can be poor, but you don't have to be lower class [defined in terms of behavior and attitude toward sexuality]."

One group participant said that her mother had come from a small Southern town, where she was considered a "lady" by their standards, and had moved into the Los Angeles area, where it was assumed that she was "loose." She was very concerned that her daughter's body posture and sexual behavior would be perceived by others as "ladylike."

In summary, one participant offered an astute interpretation of why parents are so concerned about the sexuality of Afro-American women. She considered parental attitudes an overreaction to the mass rape of Afro-American women by white men in earlier periods of this country's history. In an effort to restore the dignity and semblance of African values and behavior prior to those disgraceful times, parents became overly concerned about Afro-American sexuality. One great-grandmother of a participant who had lived on the tip of slavery frequently told stories of Afro-American parents' having no control over sexual relationships. Many times their daughters were simply snatched away and raped, and they had absolutely no ability to protect their children. After the Civil War, many Afro-American parents became overly protective so that whites would no longer continue to believe that they were sexually "free."

However, many women reported experiences of still being perceived as hypersexual. They told of childhood incidents of standing at bus stops where white men would drive by and make sexual (insulting) comments to them, and how their fathers, on hearing about these experiences, had to protect them. One woman reported that while standing on a corner, she saw a white man driving through the community, looking for what she termed "black meat." When she attempted to copy down his license plate numbers, she found that they were covered up. Some women felt that since the riots and the civil rights movement of the 1960s, the open seduction of Afro-American girls and women still exists but is more subtle than it was before.

INTERCOURSE. The age range of initial intercourse for these women was between age 9 or 10 and the mid-20s. One participant who reported having intercourse between the ages of 18 and 20 had selected a partner because she felt it was time to experience sex. Another woman who, in her late teens, felt that she was ready to experience sex was not asked because everyone "respected her too much."

Fears were expressed about being able to achieve intercourse. Some women had been afraid to use tampons because they thought that the vaginal opening would be too small but were quite relieved to find that they had no difficulty having intercourse. Along with these fears came some myths about the relationship of intercourse and cancer.

Some women felt pressured by men to experience sex and finally grew tired of "beating them off." However, one woman had been rejected by several boys who did not want to experiment with her sexually because she was a virgin. This vignette was offered to illustrate the influence of peer pressure against virginity and the value of being sexually sophisticated. One woman at age 16½ and two female friends made a bet that none of them would be a virgin by Christmas. When she asked a young boy to have sex with her, she found that he was also a virgin, and the experience was catastrophic for both of them.

Some women felt that the message to inhibit sex was too strong and that the guilt feelings and the fear of pregnancy were extreme. Questions such as "Do I look any different?" and "Did I let anybody down by having intercourse?" remained in many women's minds and plagued them throughout adulthood. Others believed that a woman should marry the man with whom she had sex, but entered into relationships that were based only on sex, not love. One woman described herself as very adventurous, experiencing sexual relationships at the age of 10 and having a "very good time," but not realizing the consequences of her behavior until she became pregnant at age 16. On the other hand, one woman at age 20 planned her first sexual experience with a man 10 years older, who was quite sexually sophisticated, but for whom she had no emotional feelings. She chose an older man because of his experience, and because of being rejected by younger men due to her virginity.

The relationship between religion and sex was again noted in one woman's report of praying every month that she would not become pregnant. After her menstrual period was over, she would "try her luck" again. Some women expected that intercourse was an initiation into adulthood and that they would suddenly feel grown-up or mature but then found adulthood to be far more complex than experiencing sex.

MASTURBATION. One woman reported that she had an orgasm by "accident." She had read in *Playboy* magazine about the location of the clitoris, an area of her body that she knew nothing about. Now she reported that she wouldn't settle for anything less than having orgasms during intercourse. Another woman stated that masturbation is practical for women alone, as well as for married women whose partners are not available. Many women who felt disappointed with intercourse were relieved to learn to masturbate and not to accept being "shortchanged." One woman admitted that she didn't masturbate but did know her own body. She felt that sex is for mutual pleasure, and that it is important to communicate with one's partner in order to direct him to the pleasurable body areas.

ISSUES

PREGNANCY WITHOUT MARRIAGE. Several issues emerged from the discussions to which the participants responded in interesting and diverse ways. The first issue asked the question, "Why do young Afro-American teenagers have babies outside of marriage?" There were five reasons cited:

1. Because of economic factors, very poor people are less likely to be exposed to sex education.

2. The lack of the middle-class morality or the lack of independence from men is accompanied by certain attitudes that many Afro-American parents ingrain in their daughters: "Don't let anybody put you down," and "Don't stoop to anyone." Before the riots, one woman felt that middle-class values were perpetuated in most homes, and many parents wanted their daughters to achieve certain goals and to defer others. Since the riots, people have been espousing the philosophy to "do your own thing," and many groups are reinforcing having babies outside of marriage. It appears that the values regarding having children outside of marriage are more relaxed, and this relaxation has resulted in the increase in unwed mothers.

3. Another woman raised the issue of having children for a very different reason—to justify identity: "I'm somebody because I have a baby." In some communities, there is much peer pressure to have a baby or a baby shower because it initiates a woman into adulthood. However, these young women often fail to evaluate the consequences of pregnancy and the physical, financial, and emotional investment required to raise a child. One woman asked about the role of parents in counseling their children about having babies out of wedlock. The response from others was that parents often have little knowledge themselves and, even though it is available, may be illiterate or uninformed about contraceptive information.

4. Some parents had babies early in adolescence themselves, and their children perpetuate this pattern. In spite of the ease of obtaining abortion or contraceptive information, they do not ascribe a negative valence to early parenting. It becomes a way of life to some, and many Afro-American parents don't believe in abortion. They find that they can incorporate a child into the extended family. They may also tend to rely on older relatives to raise children and for this reason may not hastily place the elderly in nursing homes.

5. Consider the role models of today: Afro-American heroes like Muhammad Ali have had children outside of marriage, and the "Hollywood" image of cohabiting with a partner and having children appears to reinforce the young people's attitudes and behaviors.

The general consensus was that many young people do not accept and express their sexuality in a responsible way. It seems to be not a lack of education, but misinformation, some confusion, and the denial of one's sexuality that are the problem underlying teenage pregnancy. Going to the doctor and being fitted for an IUD or a diaphragm suggests that you are sexually active and are ready to accept the responsibility that sexual maturity requires. Most young people simply are not ready for that level of responsibility. Additionally, parents communicate a mixed message because they do not know how to talk to their children about sex but will help the daughter to raise a baby once it is born.

SEXUAL RELATIONSHIPS BETWEEN AFRO-AMERICAN MEN AND WOMEN. Many women felt that their sense of racial consciousness increased during college and the civil rights movement of the 1960s because racial heritage and pride were stressed. They became more aware that "black was beautiful" and also became increasingly concerned about some issues influencing male–female relationships.

Their first concern was the "superstud" image that many Afro-American men believe they must emulate. Some men are reportedly very egotistically involved in being able to generate pleasure and need to know that their performance is highly rated. However, some of the participants described feeling reluctant to reveal that they were often more sexually experienced than their partners and that they did not achieve satisfaction during intercourse. Their fear was that their partners might interpret this feedback as a failure to "do their job" as superstuds. Contrary to the stereotype, some of the group participants perceived Afro-American men as sexually conservative or less willing to experience more exotic approaches to sexual expression, such as anal sex and the use of mechanical devices, though other women disagreed. Generally, there was a consensus among the group that Afro-American men are tender and sensitive partners. Some women found white men to be harsh and cold and more likely to believe the myth of Afro-American women as "hot and ready" sexual partners. Consequently, these women did not perceive white men as potential sexual partners. On the other hand, one woman had been involved in an unsuccessful marriage and had a low opinion of Afro-American men in general. This woman found white men to be more sympathetic. We were impressed with how personal experiences bias attitudes about men and how ethnicity becomes associated with these negative experiences.

The women who perceived their ethnic mates as sexually conservative went a step further. They also described them as more reluctant to engage in oral sex. To quote one participant, "Most men have a negative opinion about oral sex and express this in public, though they might engage in it in private. If word got around that a man engaged in oral sex, he would be ostracized socially by other Afro-American men." Many of these women had been told by men that oral sex is a demeaning sexual act. However, their opinion was that oral sex is becoming more acceptable within the Afro-American community.

EMOTIONAL DISTANCE BETWEEN AFRO-AMERICAN MEN AND WOMEN. One woman commented that the reported relationship conflicts between Afro-American men and women began with the frequent physical separation of the family during slavery. Today, many relationship problems are myths that are perpetuated by the media. However, other interpersonal conflicts are real. These Afro-American women felt that one problem contributing to emotional distance is that they have not been appreciated for their contribution to maintaining stability and survival in the Afro-American family and within their interpersonal relationships. Their physical appearance and language are often not accepted as equal to the white standard for beauty. They felt that their men frequently do not give them the respect that they deserve. One woman asked the question, "Who is going to defend the Afro-American woman if the Afro-American man isn't going to appreciate her as she is? If her man says that she is not beautiful, then who will think that she is?" This is one of the reasons that these participants felt that Afro-American women have to be strong and assertive and to validate their own beauty. For example, one woman reported that she joined the Nation of Islam because they were the only group at the time that acknowledged the beauty of Afro-American women. She felt a very strong need to have her beauty and importance validated by Afro-American men.

This group expressed anger toward certain interracial relationships, because they perceived them as further distancing Afro-American women and men. Most women felt that relationships of Afro-

American women with white males are acceptable because they acknowledged that the selection pool of educated Afro-American men is much smaller than that of white men. However, they expressed very hostile feelings toward relationships between Afro-American men and white females. Many women perceived the white female in these relationships as frequently not on the same educational level as the man and sometimes lacking concern about her physical appearance. One woman reported that if an Afro-American man is seen with a white female, he is considered "lost" and not worth anything by his ethnic group.

The groups attempted to find reasons for the reported increase in interracial coupling, particularly the Afro-American man–white woman dyads. The women pointed out that within the ethnic group, Afro-American men can select a partner from those ranging in skin color and hair textures. Physical appearance could not be the only factor attracting Afro-American men to women of other ethnic groups. They agreed that it is the role of the woman to be supportive of Afro-American men because they continue to be subjected to educational and occupational oppression and are denied opportunities to gain the status of their white peers. The women stressed the importance of clarifying for Afro-American men how they can attain status in this society without overlooking Afro-American women to seek instead white women, who, society dictates, meet the acceptable standard of beauty and with whom status may seem more easily attainable.

MYTHS OF AFRO-AMERICAN SEXUALITY

The groups were asked to reflect on their personal experiences and to corroborate or refute myths of Afro-American sexuality that the author had collected from the literature and from discussions with other professional and lay groups.

MYTH NUMBER 1: WHAT DOES THE SOCIETY CONVEY ABOUT YOUNG AFRO-AMERICAN GIRLS? Stories were shared describing young Afro-American girls becoming pregnant as early as the seventh grade because they are more "provocative, sexy, and seductive" and are exposed to more sex in their homes and neighborhoods than white girls. However, this is a stereotype that appears to be assigned to young Afro-American girls regardless of economic status and this permissive image is not perpetuated for girls of other ethnic groups. For example, one woman overheard a joke that "You have to go to the second grade in the inner city (black neighborhood) to find a virgin." There were, however, some girls that these women had worked with, particularly those in foster homes or juvenile halls, who were familiar with

sexual vernacular and had some exposure to sex, including intercourse, at an early age.

MYTH NUMBER 2: AFRO-AMERICAN GIRLS GROW UP SEXUALLY
FASTER THAN WHITE GIRLS. Most women disagreed. On the contrary,
they felt that some Afro-American girls are frequently ashamed of their
physical maturity and are concerned about their body carriage for fear
that they may be perceived as sex objects. This concern may be expressed in the tendency to overeat, thereby making oneself sexually
unattractive. As mentioned earlier, men often perceive Afro-American
women as sexually permissive, and assume that they are "easy and
unconcerned about pregnancy." This assumption appears to be based
on the fact that Afro-American women reportedly become sexually active early in their teens. Those who become pregnant often choose not
to obtain abortions, either because they are unable to afford them or
because they value human life, regardless of the consequences. Consequently, their children are more visible evidence of sexual activity,
and these women frequently are perceived as sexually permissive. The
group participants felt that white women tend to have more abortions,
though they are frequently not reported in the statistics. Some women
felt that Afro-American girls tend to be sexually inhibited and distance
themselves from black and white men alike, because of the fear of
being labeled sex objects. On the other hand, they felt that white girls
frequently do not have to deal with the consequences of their sexual
activity because their parents can afford to help them maintain the
image of being cherished and respectable by obtaining abortions for
them, often through private sources, where one's personal experiences
are kept confidential.

MYTH NUMBER 3: AFRO-AMERICAN PEOPLE ENGAGE IN WIFE SWAP-
PING, GROUP SEX, OR "SWINGING." The group felt that Afro-American
morality does not disappear with adulthood. Wife swapping and other
behaviors are not acceptable within the community. They reiterated
their feelings that promiscuity in Afro-Americans, in general, is an
inappropriate stereotype. While some individuals or couples within
the community may engage in these alternative sexual practices, Afro-
Americans, for the most part, participate much less than the white
community in these activities. They also agreed that Afro-Americans
perceive sex as a natural act and do not appreciate the need for mechanical or excessive stimulation in order to achieve sexual gratification.

MYTH NUMBER 4: AFRO-AMERICAN WOMEN ARE MORE CLOSELY
ATTACHED TO THEIR MOTHERS THAN TO THEIR HUSBANDS. Some women
felt that this is a myth that developed from the matriarchy theory of a
domineering mother controlling her married daughter's life and belittling men. However, most women felt that mothers are happy when

their daughters marry because of the limited selection of available and suitable Afro-American men. One woman reported that "Your mother is always in your corner and somewhere down the line is always available to come to your rescue, but this does not suggest that her relationship is closer than that of the relationship with the husband." Another woman stated that if there is truth to the myth that women are closer to their mothers, it may be that relationships don't last as long as they once did, and women find themselves with more than one partner during their lives. The relationship with the mother, girlfriend, or extended family may be more stable than the male–female relationship in some women's lives.

MYTH NUMBER 5: AFRO-AMERICAN FEMALES DEVALUE SEX FOR PLEASURE AND EMPHASIZE PERFORMANCE. Some women stated that this myth may be true for older people because they were often taught to enjoy sex for the purpose of childbearing alone. Adolescents may also overrate performance because of peer pressure to become sexually active, without being mature enough to appreciate what is to be expected from sex. Most of the women disagreed with this myth and felt that it could not be generalized to all Afro-American women.

MYTH NUMBER 6: AFRO-AMERICAN MEN ARE MORE SEXUALLY CONSERVATIVE AND PRUDISH THAN WHITE MEN. The women agreed that Afro-American men may be less likely to engage in exotic forms of sexual behavior because their values have been heavily influenced by their mothers, who are "the keepers of morality." This conservatism is also reinforced by fathers, even though the double standard is practiced in the Afro-American community. Consequently, Afro-American men may grow up to be more conservative in their sexual relationships, but this conservatism was perceived as an aspect of morality and family training, rather than as the men's being rigid and unloving.

MYTH NUMBER 7: AFRO-AMERICAN FEMALES USE SEX TO GET WHAT THEY WANT MATERIALLY. The participants had often heard Afro-American women described as negative, hostile, and rejecting. One woman stated that women, regardless of color, sometimes use sex to get what they want, and she cited several famous women in the media as examples. There was, however, more of a consensus that Afro-American women make more demands on their men, not for material gains, but for a stable relationship.

MYTH NUMBER 8: AFRO-AMERICAN MEN ARE SUPERSTUDS. The groups agreed that though this is not true, Afro-American men are generally good sexual partners. The women described them as warmer, more understanding, and more "beautiful" because of their rich brown skin tone.

MYTH NUMBER 9: AFRO-AMERICAN WOMEN ARE BETTER LOVERS

THAN WHITE WOMEN. Most of the participating women replied "yes" to this question because they felt that the Afro-American culture and family encourage the expression of emotions. Therefore, if the woman who decides to become sexually active does so at a time in her life that is condoned by her family and the subculture, she is likely to have no difficulty in being a warm and demonstrative lover.

A final question was asked: Does ethnicity influence your choice of a sexual partner? Ethnicity appears to be a strong factor in the selection of sexual partners for these women. However, the availability of partners was also important. The group appeared to prefer Afro-American men because they perceived them as more "beautiful and sexy." However, many women modified their selection criteria to value any man who could satisfy and appreciate them.

DISCUSSION

This chapter on Afro-American sexuality differs considerably from other descriptions of attitudes and sexual behaviors of Afro-Americans in that it includes reports of attitudes toward a wide range of sexual behaviors and factors that influence sexual expression from early childhood through adulthood.

These participants, members of an economic and ethnic group not often reported, were highly articulate women, and were well educated and skilled enough to receive an income that assured them of at least a middle-class lifestyle. Their responses to the issues demonstrated their insight into some influences on their sexuality from early childhood to adulthood. Their reactions to some of the myths discussed strongly suggested that regardless of whether the myths were fact or fantasy, they were perpetuated throughout society and were known to the young as well as to the older group members.

Generally, sex education during childhood for these women was minimal, but it included verbal and nonverbal prohibitive messages. Peers and siblings appeared to be somewhat influential, but the parents and the church were most influential in communicating deferment of sexual activity. However, the prohibitive message was accompanied by a well-articulated rationale: "Carry yourself in such a way as not to be considered a sex object, as many Afro-American women are." Second, an even stronger message was to defer sexual activity until marriage. Becoming pregnant before marriage might mean being perceived as hypersexual and lacking in self-control. The results of becoming a parent at an early age could also minimize chances to transcend economic and educational barriers that Afro-Americans face daily.

Though few women disclosed that they had become pregnant as teenagers, those who did admitted lacking accurate information regarding conception. However, the group felt that lack of information was not the reason for teenage pregnancy today. They listed several contributing factors, including misinformation about conception, emulation of models, inability to talk to parents, and lack of acceptance of one's own sexuality.

Regardless of the prohibition on premarital sex, the few women who were teenage mothers in this sample kept their babies and were accepted back into their families. They also received support and encouragement to continue to seek their educational and occupational goals.

Contrary to myths about middle-class Afro-American women, these women did perceived themselves not as hyposexual but as preferring to defer sexual gratification until a stable relationship could be attained or a definite decision could be made to raise the child as a single parent.

Contrary to myths of Afro-American hypersexuality, most of these women experienced sexual intercourse around age 19, the time of adolescence at which most American girls have been found to become sexually active (Zelnick & Kantner, 1972a).

The groups' contradictory statements about resenting white men's perceptions and treatment of them as "hypersexual objects," while at the same time admitting that Afro-American woman–white man relationships would be satisfactory, were striking. Some of the women were able to move beyond their own ethnocentrism toward whites and to evaluate the qualities of a partner without allowing skin color to interfere. Other women clearly preferred Afro-American, African, or Caribbean men. Even though there was less likelihood of finding a partner of similar educational and occupational level, they preferred to limit their male–female relationships to their own ethnic group. These groups felt that their sexual behavior identified Afro-American men and women as highly moral, because of the influence of moral training in early childhood and the emphasis on the value of human life communicated within the Afro-American family. They did not attribute deferment of sexual activity or participation in exotic sexual behaviors to being inhibited. They also did not subscribe to the myth of the Afro-American male's being "hypersexual." In fact, they rated Afro-American men highly more for their warmth and sensitivity than for their superhuman sexual feats. As one woman stated, "Afro-Americans don't need a lot of gimmicks to enjoy sex. They see sex as natural." For that reason, some of the women felt that if there is an increase in homosexuality, wife swapping, and other alternatives to

sexual expression among Afro-Americans today, it is due to the acculturation process and the lessening of some Afro-American people's
sense of morality. There were many issues relating to Afro-American
sexuality and male–female relationships that these women felt were
perpetuated by the media, that many whites believe and some Afro-
Americans appear to emulate.

Finally, being perceived as sexually active or having visible evidence of sexual activity (children) appeared to be critical to these
women, because it is frequently associated with myths of hypersexuality. Fewer options for success in life appeared to be open to those
women within the community who became mothers early in life. Young
mothers frequently were devalued outside the community and, in some
respects, within the subculture as well. It would be interesting to determine if the availability of contraceptives today has affected the sexual behavior of Afro-American women and has allowed them to become sexually active without being perceived as promiscuous.

These women's responses provided rich insights into their sexual
behavior and their attitudes about factors influencing sexual expression. Though there is little, if anything, in the literature reporting sexual experiences of groups of middle-income Afro-American women,
the sample is small and does not adequately reflect the broader scope
of women's opinions—particularly those with more or less control over
their lives—because of the educational and economic stability that these
women had attained. The 43 women, as a group, appeared to have
regained their rights to "sexual ownership" in that they were consciously making decisions about their sexuality. They certainly seemed
to exhibit more "sexual ownership" than Afro-American women did
50 or 100 years ago, and they were looking for ways to develop and
maintain relationships in which to express their sexuality.

Acknowledgment

The author would like to express her appreciation to Barbara A.
Bass for her assistance in editing and collating the data for this study.

References

Bell, A. *Black sexuality, fact and fancy*. Bloomington: Black American Series, Indiana
     University, 1968.
Billingsley, A. *Black families in white America*. Englewood Cliffs, N.J.: Prentice-Hall, 1968.
Bogle, D. *Toms, coons, mulattoes, mammies and bucks*. New York: Viking, 1973.
Brunswick, A. Adolescent health, sex and fertility. *American Journal of Public Health*,
     1971, *61*, 711–728.

Burgess, E. W., & Wallin, P. *Engagement and marriage.* Philadelphia: Lippincott, 1953.

Delcampo, R. L., Sporakowski, M., & Delcampo, D. Premarital sexual permissiveness and contraceptive knowledge: A biracial comparison of college students. *Journal of Sex Research,* 1976, *12,* 180–192.

Dollard, J. *Caste and class in a Southern town.* New York: Doubleday, 1957.

Fiedling, J., & Nelson, S. Health care for the economically disadvantaged adolescent. *Pediatric Clinics of North America,* 1973, *20,* 975–988.

Gebhard, P., Pomeroy, W., Martin, C., & Christenson, C. *Pregnancy, birth and abortion.* New York: Harper & Row, 1958.

Gespert, M., & Falk, R. Sexual experimentation and pregnancy in young black adolescents. *American Journal of Obstetrics,* October 1976, pp. 459–466.

Graves, W., & Bradshaw, B. Early reconception and contraceptive use among black teenage girls after an illegitimate birth. *American Journal of Public Health,* 1975, *65,* 738–740.

Gutman, H. *The black family in slavery and freedom: 1750–1925.* New York: Vintage Press, 1976.

Hernton, C. *Sex and racism in America.* New York: Grove Press, 1965.

Hill, J. *Women talking.* Secaucus, N.J.: Lyle Stuart, 1976.

Hite, S. *The Hite report.* New York: Macmillan, 1976.

Johnson, C. Adolescent pregnancy: Intervention into the poverty cycle. *Adolescence,* 1974, *9,* 391–406.

Kardiner, A., & Ovesey, L. *The mark of oppression.* Cleveland: World, 1951.

Kinsey, A. C., Pomeroy, W. B., Martin, C. E., & Gebhard, P. H. *Sexual behavior in the human female.* Philadelphia: Saunders, 1953.

Ladner, J. *Tomorrow's tomorrow.* New York: Doubleday, 1971.

Masters, W. H., & Johnson, V. E. *Human sexual response.* Boston: Little, Brown, 1966.

Masters, W. H., & Johnson, V. E. *Human sexual inadequacy.* Boston: Little, Brown, 1970.

Poussaint, A. Blacks and the sexual revolution. *Ebony,* 1971, *26,* 112.

Rainwater, L. Some aspects of lower-class sexual behavior. *Journal of Social Issues,* 1966, *22,* 96–108.

Reiss, I. Premarital sexual permissiveness among Negroes and whites. *American Sociological Review,* 1964, *29,* 688–698.

Reiss, I. *The sexual context of pre-marital sexual permissiveness.* New York: Holt, Rinehart, and Winston, 1967.

Staples, R. *The black woman in America.* Chicago: Nelson-Hall, 1973.

Teele, J. E., Robinson, D., Schmidt, W., & Rice, E. Factors related to social work services for mothers of babies born out of wedlock. *American Journal of Public Health,* 1967, *57,* 1300–1307.

Terman, L. M. *Psychological factors in marital happiness.* New York: McGraw-Hill, 1938.

Thomas, A., & Sillen, S. *Racism and psychiatry.* New York: Brunner/Mazel, 1972.

Wyatt, G., Strayer, R., & Lobitz, C. Issues in the treatment of sexually dysfunctioning couples of Afro-American descent. *Psychotherapy: Theory, Research and Practice,* 1976, *13,* 44–50.

Young, L. C. Are black women taking care of business? *Essence,* May 1974, p. 58.

Zelnick, M., & Kantner, J. Sexual experience of young unmarried women in the United States. *Family Planning Perspectives,* 1972, *4,* 9–18.

Zelnick, M., & Kantner, J. Sexuality, contraception, and pregnancy among young unwed females in the United States. *U.S. Commission of Population Growth, Demographic and Social Aspects of Population Growth,* 1972.

Further Thoughts on a Group Discussion by Black Women about Sexuality

June Dobbs Butts

Ms. Wyatt has opened a tiny window on the psyche of today's black woman and, with this simple act of *ventilation*, has done a service to us all, black and white alike. Hers is a unique sample, which represents perhaps 4% of all black women, perhaps less. They are invisible so far as the mass media are concerned; both scientific and popular types of media focus on the largely uneducated, welfare-dependent "black matriarch" and seldom depict the kind of female sexuality that Ms. Wyatt has etched out in her exploratory study. The women whom she interviewed are indeed the cutting edge of black thought, spirit, and commitment: they cast a long shadow on world events and serve as role models for millions of women in developing countries whose skins range from light to dark, but never could be called white. Hence, the pioneering effort that Ms. Wyatt has attempted is encouraging, for it yields rich descriptive material rather than dry quantitative "facts."

However, the research sample is minuscule ($n = 45$). The data were obtained in a questionable format: two groups were assembled for frank discussion using a brief open-ended questionnaire. Ms. Wyatt does not tell us whether she had pretested this instrument or whether this was a sort of pilot study (and this reviewer hopes for the latter). While the informality of the group discussions may have fostered synergy among the participants, it seems obvious that the lack of privacy for individual thought while responding to the questionnaire facilitated

June Dobbs Butts, Ed.D. ● Assistant Professor, Department of Psychiatry, Howard University College of Medicine, Washington, D.C. 20059.

peer influence (pressure?) to an inordinate degree. Often the groups seemed defensive and accusative. In fact, the very nature of most of the questions about female sexuality was highly charged with competitiveness and bids for heightened self-esteem. Given this format, such a reaction would predictably occur in any women's consciousness-raising group. The fact that *this* one happens to be black and to feel beautiful gives this study a certain psychological élan. A final negative criticism is in order, and then we may turn to implications that go far beyond the parameters of this small study.

Ms. Wyatt has some glaring inaccuracies in her reported search of the literature of sex research that either included or excluded blacks, and of Kinsey's monumental work, which included blacks but only recently reported on their sexuality. Most white researchers express surprise when hearing of this omission, so perhaps Ms. Wyatt should not be chided for misinterpretations that even her mentors were unaware of. But the plain facts are that Alfred C. Kinsey included blacks in his late 1940s research but omitted these data from his published work on white males in the late 1940s (Kinsey, Pomeroy, & Martin, 1948) and on white women in the early 1950s (Kinsey, Pomeroy, Martin, & Gebhard, 1953). Not until 1979 did they release some of this insightful data on black subjects (Gebhard & Johnson, 1979). An update of Kinsey's work was undertaken by Morton Hunt (1974), commissioned by the Playboy Research Foundation. He found that there were no significant differences between the sexual life-styles of blacks and whites, of rural and urban people, or—interestingly enough—among married people and unmarrieds. But he did find real differences when comparing people under age 30 with those over 30.

Masters and Johnson (1966), whose pioneer observations of sexual function and dysfunction did include blacks, reported this in their publications. In fact, although their sample was relatively small, blacks appeared in every phase and cell of their research population.

But let us move on: serious consideration of black female sexuality must reflect what real people *think*, and *do*, and *feel*, not just what research scholars choose to investigate because it is topical, politically "safe," or conveniently funded by government or private backers. Black and white researchers would have to come to grips with the fantasies, myths, and misconceptions generated by those twin evils racism and sexism as they pertain to just such a sample as the one that Ms. Wyatt has studied. We all would have to reassess what women think about themselves, as well as what men think about women. And yet another oblique view of female sexuality may shed valuable light: those males whose gender identity has caused them to feel that they have a woman's mind in a man's body and thus seek surgical intervention for sex reassignment may give us insight into what *they* think is valuable about being a woman. Such aspects of the whole truth will surely lead us to view womankind as a multifaceted part of *human* sexuality, and not just the Hollywood version of commercialized sex goddesses who are "five feet two with eyes of blue." Reflecting that in my youth I was stunned by what was believed to have been the suicide of Jean Harlow and later as an adult by the apparent suicide of Marilyn Monroe, not only beautiful actresses but unabashed "sex objects" of their respective eras, I have come to support a new view of femininity. Sponsored by the as yet unintegrated women's movement, this view holds that it is the woman herself who must define her own femininity. Strengthened by such conviction, I salute Ms. Wyatt for her research, which not only tells *me* something of value about my peer group but holds something of value for my white counterparts.

REFERENCES

Gebhard, P. H., & Johnson, A. B. *The Kinsey data: Marginal tabulations of the 1938–1963 interviews conducted by the Institute for Sex Research.* Philadelphia: Saunders, 1979.

Hunt, M. M. *Sexual behavior in the 1970's.* Chicago: Playboy Press, 1974.

Kinsey, A. C., Pomeroy, W. B., & Martin, C. E. *Sexual behavior in the human male.* Philadelphia: Saunders, 1948.

Kinsey, A. C., Pomeroy, W. B., Martin, C. E., & Gebhard, P. H. *Sexual behavior in the human female.* Philadelphia: Saunders, 1953.

Masters, W. H., & Johnson, V. E. *Human sexual response.* Boston: Little, Brown, 1966.

Chapter 3

Sexual Consequences of Acculturation of American Indian Women

Marlene Echohawk

If we look at the study of human sexuality today, we find considerable attention being given to the changes taking place in female sexuality. Interest is focused on future change and the effect it will have on female sexuality. The influence of acculturation on the sexuality of American Indian women is, therefore, considered a fitting and timely topic.

Various systems of acculturation imposed on American Indian people are presented here. The interrelationship of marriage patterns of Indian women and acculturation is discussed at some length.

Much of what follows may also be applicable to American Indian men, especially regarding the systems of acculturation, but the overall emphasis is on American Indian women.

Systems of Acculturation of American Indians

Education. While it must be acknowledged that education is not exclusive to the Anglo society, the term *education*, as used here, refers to the educational system devised by Anglo people and in usage since their arrival on the North American continent.

The main goal of formal education for Indian people has been the assimilation of Indian people into Anglo society. Schools established

Marlene Echohawk, Ph.D. ● Assistant Clinical Professor, Pediatric Psychology, Department of Psychiatry and Behavioral Sciences, University of Oklahoma Health Sciences Center, Oklahoma City, Oklahoma 73126.

45

for Indian children discouraged the use of American Indian languages, customs of dress, traditional religious practices, etc. Anything native to the American Indian people, or thought of as native to American Indians, was to be suppressed; therefore, what have been taught to Indian children are the English language and Anglo values, habits, and manner of dress. There has been a total commitment on the part of educators of Indian children to the doctrine of assimilation.

The coercive methods used to establish formal education for American Indian children, in addition to the devaluation of Indian identity, may account for the fact that 400 years later, American Indians, in general, remain far from assimilated into the Anglo society. American Indian children drop out of school at a rate that is substantially higher than the dropout rate for non-Indians (U.S. Department of the Interior, 1975).

While assimilation is far from complete, certainly the educational process has exerted a profound effect on the traditional life-styles of American Indian tribes. Perhaps the most notable effect is the almost universal knowledge of the English language by Indian people. Many Indian women know and use only English, others are bilingual, and few use only their native language. Exact figures are not available regarding the language patterns of American Indian women.

RELIGION. A universal custom of all cultures is the incorporation of religious beliefs and practices into their traditions. American Indians are no exception to this custom.

In cultures as ancient as the American Indian one, it is not surprising to learn that many traditional religious beliefs still exist today. However, given the emphasis here on systems of acculturation, it is important to mention that Christianity did exert an influence on the life-styles and patterns of marriage of Indian women.

Among the earliest contacts that Indian tribes had with Anglos was the missionary work of Christian church groups (Layman, 1942). The main goal of the early missionaries was to convert Indian people to Christianity, but the education of Indians was also a major undertaking of the churches. Therefore, when referring to missionaries and their work among American Indian tribes, it is almost impossible to separate the Christianizing aspect from the educational process.

Certain Christian sects practice the removal of young Indian children from their homes and families, while other groups make an effort to maintain and strengthen family ties (Swenson, 1977). The purpose of mentioning these two different approaches is not to take a value position, but to inform the reader that various approaches to converting American Indian people to Christianity exist. Christianity has been, and perhaps still is, influential in the acculturation process of American Indian women.

The original goal of Catholic and Protestant churches was to discourage the traditional religions of American Indian tribes. Nevertheless, at the present time, religious practices among American Indians range from traditional religion, to a modification of traditional religion (intermingled with elements of Christianity), to complete acceptance of and membership in Christian churches.

SOCIAL SERVICES. Another major influence in the acculturation of American Indian women has been in the quality and the availability of social services.

Individual Indian tribes have negotiated treaties with the federal government and, in some instances, with states. Treaties recognizing tribal sovereignty have not always been honored, and the result has been jurisdictional dilemmas for the American Indian population (Echohawk, 1977). Ultimately, their dilemmas have had a significant effect on the lives of Indian women and their children.

While treaty rights have not been abrogated and technically tribal sovereignty still exists, in reality certain states have enacted legislation that undermines tribal sovereignty. The net result of such legislation is that many tribes are obliged to deal with the states in the delivery of social services. Therefore, state social-service employees working with Indian tribes are obligated to apply non-Indian state standards to a reservation setting or to an Indian community, such as that of Oklahoma, which has no reservations in the legal sense of the term. As a result, many Indian children are removed from their parents and placed in non-Indian, Anglo homes as Indians are made to comply with state standards. Many young Indians have grown up in a non-Indian environment and have lost their sense of identity with Indian people. Of course, such practices have an effect on Indian women. An Indian woman's choice of a marriage partner is influenced by the culture of her childhood.

DEVELOPMENTAL ISSUES IN AMERICAN FEMALE SEXUALITY

It is difficult to make a meaningful contribution to the topic of developmental issues in American Indian female sexuality based only on a reconstruction, derived from the contemporary Indian life-style, of traditional American Indian culture. The lack of empirical findings makes this task even more difficult.

The last 200 years have seen various forces—educational, religious, and legislative—exert their influence on traditional American

Indian life-styles. The present-day picture is considerably blurred by those outside forces. Nevertheless, it is still considered worthwhile to present information for discussion, derived from personal and professional observations, focusing on developmental issues regarding sexual identity, role, and behavior as they are believed to exist today among American Indian women.

The extended-family concept is still quite strong within American Indian cultures, so that most Indian children grow up in a group type of household. Because of the close physical quarters, Indian children view the primal scene at a very early age. What this experience means for the Indian child psychologically is not exactly known; however, assumptions about the influence on sex differences, sexual behavior, and attitudes toward sex can be made.

Learning quite early in life the function of the sex act minimizes the necessity of lengthy explanations about sexual intercourse for Indian children. Also, male and female anatomical and sex differences are learned very early, so that sex education as such becomes superfluous. However, some tribes still recognize the female's entry into "womanhood" by a ceremony held on the occasion of her first menses.

The physical exploration of one's own body is accepted as a normal stage of development in the young child, and masturbation is considered nothing more than childhood curiosity about the nature of one's own body. It is doubtful that American Indians place the same stigma on masturbation that the Anglos do. There is the expectation that the physical exploration phase will eventually be replaced by the usual male–female attraction and physical relationship. As far as is known, that is what occurs.

The close physical arrangements of most Indian households can place some restrictions on "creative" sexual styles. The opportunities for variety in sexual styles, for prolonged sex play, and for the use of sexual words are limited by the knowledge that there is very likely to be an audience, even if that audience is made up of infants or small children. The group life-style may lead to a constriction of sexual feelings, which in turn leads to a higher tolerance of sexual tension. The release of anxious feelings resulting from sexual tension is seen in the teasing in which Indians engage regarding their sexual needs. This teasing carries with it the implication that anyone who cannot handle his or her own sexual impulses is immature. There is still the strong notion among American Indians that the function of sex is primarily to have children. The lighthearted teasing about sex for pleasure recognizes this need, but minimizes its importance.

American Indians' view of the function of sexual intercourse as mainly for the purpose of having children maximizes the importance of the pregnant female and pregnancy. The importance of the female role (to bear children) may be reflected in the extremely low incidence of homosexuality among American Indian women. While there are no exact figures available regarding the incidence of homosexuality, the author has obtained a consensus of opinion from a variety of American Indian professionals who report nonexistence to extremely low incidence.

Another indication of the importance of bearing children to American Indian women is the negative attitude toward contraceptives. There is great value placed on self-control as a means of contraception. Traditionally abstinence from sexual intercourse was practiced after a woman became pregnant until the infant was several months old. This practice stressed the importance of children already born and the protection of the mother's health by spacing pregnancies.

Indians have a negative attitude toward abortion; abortion is the equivalent of genocide in the minds of most American Indian people.

The importance of the male to the physical survival of American Indian tribal groups increased the desirability of having sons as opposed to daughters. Even though living conditions have changed significantly over the past 200 years, the importance of male children to Indian people still persists.

The social forces of prejudice and discrimination have been more vigorous against Indian men than against Indian women and have taken their toll on the economic advancement and self-esteem of American Indian men. Consequently, American Indian women have worked to help support their families. Many American Indian women considered themselves liberated, sexually and economically, long before the present-day emphasis on the women's movement.

To summarize, it would seem that the physical living arrangements of American Indian households have influenced the sexual attitudes and behavior of American Indian women. Additionally, social forces have imposed a liberated life-style on American Indian women.

Acculturation Effects on Marriage Styles of American Indian Women

Interracial Marriages. Indian women have married men of various ethnic groups, but the term *interracial marriage* here refers to marriages between Indian women and Anglo men.

It must be admitted that there are no methods currently available to measure the exact level of acculturation, but it is fair to state that the use of and the preference for the English language is a good indicator of acculturation. Working and living in an urban area are other visible signs of acculturation. An even more obvious effect of acculturation is a marriage between an Indian woman and an Anglo man.

The fact that an Indian woman chooses to marry an Anglo man is, in itself, a change in the traditional Indian practice of marriages arranged by parents.

There are no statistics available regarding interracial marriages; consequently, the following statement can be challenged. Interracial marriages seem more prevalent among the coastal tribes (East and West Coasts), the Northern Plains tribes, the Oklahoma tribes, and the Southwest tribes, in that order.

Logically, if there is a correlation between acculturation and interracial marriage, then we might expect to find that the Indian women who marry Anglo men have more formal education, accept Christianity rather than traditional religions, and identify more with the Anglo culture, especially if they have been raised in a non-Indian environment. There are no studies on a national scale to support or refute the hypotheses above. One study (White & Chadwick, 1972, pp. 239–249) of Indians in Spokane, Washington, reported results that tend to support the hypotheses, but the sample was not exclusively of Indian women.

In interracial marriages, there usually seems to be a decision, spoken or unspoken, regarding which culture predominates in the marriage. If the Indian culture predominates, then the couple participates in most of the social events of Indian people. The Indian wife's family and friends are significant people in the lives of the couple. On the other hand, if there is a preference for the Anglo culture, the wife's immediate family may be the couple's only contact with Indian people.

The interracial marriages that survive seem to be those in which there is a clear-cut dominance as to cultural ties. The failure of interracial marriages may be a result of a cultural clash, in which cultural factors outweigh the physical attraction that prompted the marriage in the first place.

It seems paradoxical that many Indian women who marry Anglo men and have children by them, whether the marriage survives or not, become very strong advocates of Indian people as an oppressed minority group. Perhaps they are sensitized by the cultural conflict that their own children are experiencing. Their militancy seems to far surpass that of Indian women who have married Indian men and have full-blooded Indian children. Other possible reasons could be their ability to articulate their thoughts better in English or more confidence in expressing their beliefs. For whatever reason, their aggression belies a passive feminine role.

Consequences for Children. The lives of the biologically mixed Indian-Anglo children are apt to include an identity problem. The children are considered Anglos by Indian people and are considered Indians by the Anglos and are likely to feel a sense of rejection by both of their own ethnic groups.

If the Indian mother has maintained her ties to the Indian community or has continued to live in an Indian community, it is not surprising to find that often her offspring prefer to keep their Indian identity.

The biologically mixed Indian-Anglo females show physical differences. As a consequence of their modified hair color, eye color, and skin pigmentation, it is much easier for those females to identify with, and eventually marry into, the Anglo society. However, observation indicates that those with mixed blood tend to find and marry others with mixed blood. In many instances, there is a reluctance to deny or to move away from an Indian identity. This tendency seems to have increased over the last 20 years. The activism of the 1960s may have added an impetus to this current tendency. There seems to be a pride in one's "Indianness."

Consequences for the Mothers. The Indian mother married to an Anglo usually has little in common with her in-laws from a cultural standpoint. This does not necessarily mean that she is incompatible with her in-laws. There would very likely be some pressure on the mother regarding which culture is to dominate in the lives of her children.

The mother does not have the same help from the extended family that exists in an Indian–Indian marriage. While the Indian woman herself may be comfortable in another culture, members of her family may not be. Therefore, members of her family may remain aloof from or inaccessible to the mother. In that case, the mother may become more independent in raising her own family.

Since most mothers appreciate some form of support in the rearing of children, the Indian mother might be expected to have a similar appreciation of a support system. If she is denied the support of an extended family, or comes from a small family, she is more likely to join community resources such as a church group or the PTA. If she extends herself to the community, she is well on the way to being labeled as acculturated, or at least as becoming acculturated.

In the case of an Indian mother who is unwilling to separate herself from her family and tribe, there is the possibility of serious marital discord, sometimes leading to divorce.

An Indian mother must inevitably choose which culture will predominate in the lives of her racially mixed children. If the children identify with the Anglo culture but are reacted to as Indians by society, or vice versa, they may be subjected to the pain of an identity crisis. The usual stress in the transition from adolescence to adulthood is intensified.

INTERTRIBAL MARRIAGES. The situation of American Indian women who choose to marry Indian men from a different tribe may be similar to that of the Indian women who marry Anglo men. They must be able to use a language that their future husbands understand in order to communicate. Invariably, the language they have in common is English.

The educational system has made it possible for Indians from various tribes to become acquainted and eventually to marry. While the language barrier may have been overcome, there may be other differences that have to be resolved, such as specific tribal customs.

It seems that Indian women marrying intertribally still retain much of their connection to their own ethnic group, as well as to their own tribes. They generally use English more than their own tribal language, and they may not even be fluent in their native language. They participate more in traditional Indian social life, of their own tribes and of their husbands', than in Anglo social life.

Since about one-half the Indian population is currently living in an urban setting, there may be little opportunity, time, and money for an intertribally married couple to return to their tribal areas often. The practice in most cities that have an Indian population of any size is to establish an Indian center where Indian dances and other social activities may be held. The knowledge and use of a common language, English, provides an opportunity for further interaction between the members of many tribes. Indian women who want to marry Indian men, not necessarily from their own tribe, have more opportunity through the knowledge and use of English.

Role of the Extended Family. The intertribal marriages of Indian women have more support than interracial marriages from paternal and maternal relatives. This network support for the mothers can be positive in times of stress. For instance, when baby-sitters are needed and the budget will not allow for a paid baby-sitter, family members are usually available. Also, having an extended-family relationship allows for more social interaction, as well as having someone to talk to when advice is needed.

The same extended-family relationship can also be the cause of added stress rather than relief from stress. Members from either side of the family feel free to go into the couple's home unannounced, for just a short visit or for a prolonged stay. In the latter case, the stress placed on the wife may be considerable, especially if she has a job and must do extra work at home for her "company." It is a difficult conflict situation because she knows that if she confronts anyone concerning the situation, her marriage could be in serious trouble. However, many Indian women reconcile themselves to their relationships.

WITHIN-TRIBE MARRIAGE. As mentioned earlier, there are no data available on the frequency of each type of marriage. Many tribes are small and previous generations have intermarried, which means that many Indian women are related to most of the young men within the tribe. Therefore, if data were available, we might find that there are fewer within-tribe marriages than intertribal marriages.

Within-tribe marriages seem to survive better than other kinds of Indian marriages. This statement is not an attempt to convey the notion that this type of marriage is of the "made-in-heaven" variety. It's not at all uncommon for a woman married within her own tribe to separate from her husband during times of marital conflict. However, the wife usually reconciles with the husband and the marriage remains intact. Several factors may contribute to the longevity of within-tribe marriages.

One obvious factor is the couple's having more in common as far as status, philosophy, and religious beliefs are concerned. Thus, conflicts regarding tribal customs and traditions are minimized.

Another may be the common economic land base of both marriage partners, or of their families in the same community. The couple's long-range goals would most likely be involved with the same community.

Within-tribe marriages are the basis of an Indian tribe, and in turn, the support of the tribal community no doubt helps to maintain the couple's marriage. The extended family includes the entire tribe in traditional Indian relationships.

Identity Crisis Diminished. It is easy to understand how the identity crisis would be less for an Indian woman marrying within her own tribe than for an Indian woman marrying outside her tribe or her ethnic group.

The full-blooded Indian woman's physical features are clearly identifiable with her ethnic background. Several thousand years of tribal culture provide her with customs and traditions. She may still understand and speak her own tribal language, as well as English.

The problem most often encountered by the full-blooded Indian woman is cultural conflict, rather than identity crisis. The security in her own identity makes overcoming the cultural conflict less of a trauma. However, if she was separated from her family during a critical stage in her development, such as when attending an Indian boarding school or while living in a non-Indian foster home, she may truly experience an identity crisis.

Much more could be written regarding the early removal of Indian children from their families, but that would take us beyond the scope of the present topic.

VIEWS OF PROMISCUITY

What constitutes promiscuity in one culture may not in another culture. The term *promiscuity* as used here refers to many casual and short-term "living-together" relationships.

First of all, it must be pointed out that prior to Indian–Anglo contact there were no written records of tribal marriages. With the advent of recorded marriages, many Indian women have been married according to state law. However, given the economic situation of Indian people, it is not unusual to find Indian women living in common-law marriages. In some instances, the money for a marriage license and the state-required blood test may not be readily available. In general, common-law marriages are recognized as valid. Therefore, Indian women living in such an arrangement are not considered promiscuous by their tribes or by the Indian communities in which they live. Many Indian people teasingly refer to a common-law marriage as being "married Indian style."

A great number of Indian women no longer live in tribal settings; therefore, the custom of making a public marriage announcement to the entire tribe at once is difficult to uphold. However, most American Indian tribes are numerically small, and marriages become known in a relatively short time.

Considering the prevalence of common-law marriages, Indian women may be viewed by Anglo society as being promiscuous in their relationships. Nonetheless, to Indian women common-law marriages are legitimate, and the same commitment is expected in those relationships as in marriages by civil law. Such marriages have been known to last for years, or until the death of one of the partners.

Promiscuous behavior, for an Indian woman, is living with someone else's husband, or living with another man while she's still married (adultery). She will most likely not try to hide the way she is living. Indian people react to her misbehavior by never questioning her about her actions. The "punishment" for her is that she is never given the opportunity to defend her behavior. She is left alone to face, or not to face, her own guilt. Doing combat with one's own conscience is never easy. To non-Indians, an Indian woman's irregular relationship may appear to be condoned, because there is generally less of a public issue made of her behavior.

Another form of behavior considered promiscuous by Indians is many short-term living-together relationships, with or without the use of alcohol. An Indian woman living such an existence is looked on as a person more to be pitied than to be scorned. She usually lives in an urban area to be near the drinking crowd. Such a woman, while not given high respect in the Indian social structure, is never publicly ignored when she is sober. If tribal acquaintances or relatives happen to meet her on the street, for instance, they will not ignore, ridicule, or preach to her. However, they will avoid her if she is drinking.

Non-Indians, unfamiliar with the Indian social structure, may interpret the acceptance of the way an Indian woman chooses to live her life as condoning promiscuity. One would have to be thoroughly familiar with tribal culture to recognize the difference between acceptance of the way she chooses to live her life and acceptance of her as an integral part of the tribal community.

Conclusion

We have seen how the various systems of acculturation, education, religion, and state social services have worked toward the goal of assimilating American Indian tribes into the current American culture. Although the complete assimilation of American Indians has never been accomplished, acculturation has influenced the marriage styles of Indian women. The sexuality of American Indian women appears to vary as a function of the level of acculturation, as noted through observation and not through the actual accumulation of data.

Acknowledgments

The author wishes to thank Mr. Emanuel Moran, Ms. Gayla Twiss, and Ms. Martha Primeaux for their valuable help in critiquing this paper.

References

Echohawk, M. *Native American jurisdictional and delivery of services issues related to child abuse and neglect.* Paper prepared for the National Institute for Advanced Studies, Washington, D.C., September 1977.

Layman, M. E. *A history of Indian education in the United States.* Unpublished doctoral dissertation, University of Minnesota, 1942.

Swenson, J. P. *Supportive care, custody, placement and adoption of American Indian children.* Proceedings of a national conference sponsored by the American Academy of Child Psychiatry, Warm Springs, Oregon, April 1977.

U.S. Department of the Interior, Bureau of Indian Affairs. *Facts about American Indians and Alaska natives.* Washington, D.C.: Author, 1975.

White, L. C., & Chadwick, B. A. Urban residence, assimilation and identity of the Spokane Indian. In H. M. Bahr, B. A. Chadwick, & R. C. Day (Eds.), *Native American today: Sociological perspectives.* New York: Harper & Row, 1972.

Myths in the Midst of Missing Data

Joan Crofut Weibel

In view of the almost nonexistent ethnographic or psychological literature and/or research on the sexuality of American Indian women, Dr. Echohawk's paper must be thought of as a highly speculative and thought-provoking set of hypotheses yet to be tested. She does present several fascinating suggestions of possible change agents. However, it is unclear what changes these influences have effected on the sexual behavior of American Indian women or the direction in which these changes have occurred.

The meaning of the statement, "The coercive methods used to establish formal education for American Indian children, in addition to the devaluation of Indian identity, may account for the fact that 400 years later, American Indians, in general, remain far from assimilated into the Anglo society" is unclear. Is she saying that because the acculturative measures taken by missionaries, boarding-school personnel, etc., were so severe and repressive, the American Indians subjected to these repressive measures rebelled and rejected the imposed influences? If so, how does that fact affect changes in sexual attitudes and behaviors among Native American women? Have sexual attitudes also not changed or have they been synthesized *because* of the repressive nature of the acculturation process? This hypothesis is not supported by documentation.

I wish Dr. Echohawk had demonstrated the association between the predominant use of English and its effects on American Indian women's sexuality or, for that matter, the association of the introduc-

Joan Crofut Weibel, Ph.D. ● The Alcohol Research Center, Neuropsychiatric Institute, University of California at Los Angeles, Los Angeles, California 90024; Assistant Professor, Anthropology Department, University of Southern California, Los Angeles, California 90006.

tion of Christianity and its profound influence on indigenous sexual mores. Future research into the writings of early missionaries might give evidence of the consternation with which the pioneering missionaries viewed premarital sex, seminudity, and polygamy in the Native American societies in which they proselytized and the steps by which the early missionaries inculcated the concepts of modesty, guilt, and original sin among their newly baptized Indian flocks. These attitudes must have influenced the way Indian women thought about sex and their own bodies; we need further exploration and expansion of these influences.

We are told that jurisdictional dilemmas over treaty rights have affected the lives of American Indian women and children. We need expansion and explanation of how these problems have affected the American Indian woman's sexual behavior. How do the removal of Indian children from their biological homes and the "state standards" with which the Indian family has had to comply affect the development of sexuality? Dr. Echohawk offers these as provocative independent variables with which no satisfactory outcome variable is associated.

Obvious governmental impositions such as the insistence by state and county governments on legal marriage contracts and the labeling of children of unwed mothers as illegitimate must have had an influence on American Indian women and their sexual behavior. And the influences that the introduction of medically induced legal abortions, contraceptive devices, instruction in family planning, and the welfare system, which rewards unwed motherhood, have had on American Indian family life and sexuality are other areas that could be explored more fully.

The statement that masturbation is practiced with relatively high toleration among Indians would have more credibility with a literature citation or two, though none may be available. The discussion of verbal sex play as a tension releaser for thwarted sexual activity in constricted households is fascinating. The statement that there is extremely low incidence of homosexuality among American Indians, even though there are no exact figures, is provocative. It obviously requires further investigation and verification, since the cultural roles of *berdache* and *contraire* [1] are well documented as means by which sex-role

---

[1]Cheyenne men who did not wish to accept the normative adult male roles of warrior and hunter had two alternative institutionalized roles available to them. Some men dressed in women's clothing, did tasks customarily assigned to women, and were called *berdaches*. Others chose to exhibit behavior that mirror-imaged normative Cheyenne activities. They laughed when it was appropriate to cry, rode their horses backwards, and said east when they meant west. For obvious reasons, those men who chose to live lives of contradiction were called *contraires* (Hoebel, 1969).

deviancy was institutionalized in nineteenth-century Indian societies.

While the importance of women as procreators of their people is consistent with the attitudes of women with whom I worked at an urban Indian free clinic, I found that, increasingly, urban Indian women are accepting the idea of planned parenthood and the use of prescribed contraceptive devices as ways of coping with the economic constraints of urban life and, indeed, nineteenth-century Indian pharmacopoeias included herb and root drinks to be used specifically for contraceptive purposes (Foreman, 1857).

The argument that sons were (and are) preferable to daughters overlooks the importance of women as clan mothers in matrilineal societies. Again, generalizing about Indians allows for this oversight—a major one—since male–female interactional styles are greatly influenced by patterns of matrilineality or patrilineality. And eons ago, matrilineality had as much to do with American Indian women's sexual and economic liberation as has their more recent inclusion in the country's labor force.

The discussion of culturally defined differences in the use of the term *promiscuity* and the social consequences of promiscuous behavior is valuable information. From my experience in contemporary Indian communities, I would agree that there is a high tolerance of early, premarital sex. And the social and familial stigma of teenage and single-mother pregnancies is minimal in contemporary American Indian society.

Echohawk states that "In interracial marriages, there usually seems to be a decision, spoken or unspoken, regarding which culture predominates in the marriage" and "The interracial marriages that survive seem to be those in which there is a clear-cut dominance as to cultural ties." These hypotheses are, as yet, untested but are other areas in which research could be directed. Echohawk's concluding statement, "The sexuality of American Indian women appears to vary as a function of the level of acculturation, as noted through observation and not through the actual accumulation of data," seems little supported by the generalizations from informal observations provided.

I suspect the influence that the mass media exert on all our sexual mores has had as significant an acculturational effect on American Indian women's sexual behavior as any other contributing factor. Films, television, radio, bill board advertisements, literature, and pop magazines all shape our conceptions of ourselves as women, mothers, and sexual beings from the time we pick up our first copy of *Seventeen* to the time we identify with Maggie Kuhn and/or Mae West. Mass media presentations are no less accessible to maturing American Indian women than they are to the general population. One suspects that shifts in American Indian women's sexual mores would be as much affected by the visual and verbal onslaughts of mass media "ideal feminine types" as they are by the acquisition of English, the prohibitions of Christianity, or interracial marriages.

As a general comment on the assumptions and hypotheses stated in this paper I want to caution the reader that it is always dangerous to talk about Indians as a cultural totality. The widely divergent tribal groups are as culturally distinct as are England and Uganda or Sri Lanka and Paraguay. General statements about all Indians made from an unknown number of "personal and professional observations" can, at best, be only highly speculative.

No rigorous body of research supports Dr. Echohawk's informal observations and speculations. I suggest that the effectiveness of this chapter is that it clearly illustrates serious gaps in our knowledge of contemporary American Indian family life and sexual mores and the need for well-thought-out and well-executed research in this area.

REFERENCES

Foreman, R. *Indian guide to health: The Cherokee physician.* Norman, Okla.: Hooper Printing Co., 1857.

Hoebel, E. A. *The Cheyennes: Indians of the Great Plains.* New York: Holt, Rinehart and Winston, 1960.

Chapter 4

Sex and Sexuality

Women at Midlife

LILLIAN B. RUBIN

> Sex? It's gotten better and better. For the first years of our marriage—maybe
> nine or ten—it was a very big problem. But it's changed and improved in
> lots of ways. Right now, I'm enjoying sex more than I ever did in my life
> before—maybe even more than I ever thought I could.

"It's gotten better and better." That's what most women say. Better than what? Where did they start from, these midlife women? Where
have they gone?

To answer those and other questions, I conducted intensive, in-
depth interviews with 160 women whose average age was 46.5 years.
They were all women who were or had been married, who had borne
and raised children, who (except for 10) had none under 13 years old
left in the house, and whose class backgrounds ranged from working
class to professional upper-middle class.[1]

It is simple enough to cite statistics on the sexual behavior of the
women I met. Over half of those who were married had sexual intercourse once or twice a week; another 20% did so three or four times a

Chapter 4, "Sex? It's Gotten Better and Better" (pp. 74–103) in *Women of a Certain Age: The Midlife Search for Self* by Lillian B. Rubin. Copyright © 1979 by Lillian B. Rubin. Reprinted by permission of Harper & Row, Publishers, Inc.

[1]The women were drawn into the study by the snowball method of sampling. Each
respondent was asked for referrals. Subsequent interviewees were chosen on the basis
of having the most distant connection—both geographically and emotionally—from the
person making the referral. Such precautions assured that the study would not be biased
by being composed of friendship networks.

LILLIAN B. RUBIN, PH.D., M.F.C. ● Research Sociologist, Institute for Scientific Analysis, San Francisco, California 94123. Research supported by the Behavioral Sciences Research Division, National Institute of Mental Health, Grant No. MH 28167.

week.[2] Close to 90% were currently capable of achieving orgasm, well over half doing so more than half the time. About two-thirds engaged in oral–genital sex, almost half of them often enough to consider it a standard part of their sexual repertoire.[3]

But having said those things, what do we really know about the *quality* of their sexual interaction, about its *meaning* in their lives, about its *history*? Ask midlife women about their sexual histories, and the stories come tumbling out—stories of their early sexual repression:

> During the dating years, I was constantly putting on the brakes, and I just couldn't reverse on command. It took years of feeling inadequate and of hating myself, which didn't help me *or* our sex life,

stories of their painful struggle to bring to life that repressed part of the self:

> Sex was a constant source of difficulty for me as an individual and created nothing but conflict in my marriage. I was so closed off sexually, I really thought of myself as an asexual person. Getting through all that took lots of years and meant some terrible suffering for both of us—my husband *and* me. [*A look of angry distaste on her face.*] God, what a waste; what an unnecessary waste.

With only a few exceptions, the memories of marital sex in the early years brought with them an outpouring of deep feelings:

> What words can I use? They were *hard* times, *plain hard times*. It was the key issue in our marriage for years. It was the one that nearly wrecked us. [*A combination of anger and bewilderment in her voice.*] And it wasn't anybody's fault. We were both incredibly ignorant. Both of us were only doing whatever was expected; you know, what we learned God knows when—maybe with our mother's milk. All I know is that for me, sex was all one big "NO."

Over and over those memories called up these women's anger about the bind they found themselves in—a bind born of the mandate of virginity and the expectation that they would turn into sexual sirens at the pronouncement of the marriage vows[4]:

---

[2]Although just under 22% of the women in this study were divorced, since the sexual issues they face generally are quite different from the issues facing those who remain married, this paper deals only with women who were married or in a stable, marriagelike relationship. At the developmental level, there are, of course, no differences. But at the behavioral level, sexual issues for divorced women at midlife are likely to be felt most keenly in the unavailability of what they would consider appropriate partners.

[3]For more detailed data on sexual behavior among women of this generation, see Hunt (1974) and Kinsey, Pomerantz, Martin, & Gebhard (1953).

[4]Over 60% of the women I met were virgins when married—a figure that corresponds roughly to the Kinsey *et al*. (1953) data.

> It was terrible at first, just terrible. He wanted me to be a virgin—that was very important to him before we were married—and he also wanted me to be skilled in bed right from the start. Imagine! It wasn't just awful, it was *impossible*. When I think of it now, I feel outraged because it wasn't even our fault. We were both just playing our parts, like puppets on a string.

What "parts" were they playing? Who was pulling the "string"? The parts, of course, were those assigned by the culture—the stereotypical versions of sexuality with which girls and boys of that generation grew up. These were women and men who came to adulthood in the 1940s and 1950s. The wave of sexual liberation of the 1920s that had brought the Victorian era to a screeching halt was past. The reaction had set in. Two decades later, it was clear that the Victorian heritage was not gone, that the double standard of sexual behavior had not been wiped out by the revolution of the 1920s. It had simply changed its form. By the 1940s, it was granted that women were capable, even desirous, of sexual pleasure. But the time, place, and manner were carefully circumscribed—limited to only one man, only in marriage.

Thus, almost without exception, the women who came to the marriage bed were naive, repressed, and inexperienced. Even among those who had had premarital intercourse, it was the rare woman who found the experience enjoyable, rarer still the woman who had orgasms in that period of her life. Indeed, most described those experiments in illicit sex as unsatisfactory and guilt-ridden, usually acts so hasty and rudimentary that they barely qualify as full-fledged sexual intercourse. But about that, there were no complaints. They were, after all, engaged in forbidden behaviors. Most women didn't expect to enjoy them.

After marriage, though, after sex became licit, then, it was a different story. Then, all of them—technical virgins or not—expected something more, something special, something magical to happen. They were filled with romantic fantasies that their own special prince would unlock the secrets of their bodies, their souls. They dreamed that "bells would ring," that "the earth would move," that "waves would be crashing on the shore" as they were swept away by his magical touch. And, of course, they were bitterly disappointed:

> The first time I had intercourse, I thought: Is this what I've been saving myself for? [*Her expression registering the surprise she felt so long ago.*] *I couldn't believe it: it was such a big nothing.* I had read all those romantic novels about violins playing and bells ringing, and I absolutely believed some fantastic things would happen. My god, what a disappointment it was.

This was the "gift" of the liberated sexuality of that era—incredible fantasies and magical expectations that were bound to fail:

> I had tremendous hopes that I would flower as a sexual being after we were
> married. I looked to my husband to give me all the sexual pleasure I was
> afraid of before marriage. And when he couldn't, I was bitterly disap-
> pointed and resentful.

But the disappointment and resentment were not the women's alone, for the men shared this package of impossible expectations. Both wife and husband believed that it was *his* responsibility to open up the mysteries of sexual pleasure for her; both believed that *he* held the secret key.[5] For both, it was a distressing surprise to find that a life-time of sexual repression exacted a price, that a woman couldn't spring into sexual responsiveness on cue. When the fantasies didn't come true, both husband and wife were caught in a bind, where each oscillated between angry blaming of the other and a deeply felt sense of personal inadequacy—often creating a vicious circle where the more the inadequacy was experienced, the more it was externalized as anger against the other:

> We came to the marriage with such high hopes. But our sexual maladjust-
> ment turned it into a nightmare of self-consciousness and resentment. It
> seemed as if there was no peace. I was either angry at myself or angry at
> him. And I think he felt pretty much the same way.

But, one might ask, were there no women who were sexually responsive right from the beginning of marriage? The answer: very few. It's true that some speak of sexual pleasure in the early years. But very rarely did that pleasure include orgasms. What was it they enjoyed then?

Some valued the sexual experience because it was the major means of communication in the new marriage—not exactly the life they had dreamed of, but better than nothing:

> I never even knew what an orgasm was then. I enjoyed sex because it was
> a coming together in an intimate-type way. It was the most intimate thing
> we ever did in those days because we didn't do much talking.

For others, there was something else as well—the satisfaction that comes mostly from giving pleasure, a quality of caring and nurturing for which women are well schooled:

> Long before I ever had an orgasm myself, I used to have a feeling of joy
> out of giving him joy. It didn't make a big difference if it wasn't such a
> great thing for me. Having someone in my arms whom I loved and to
> whom I was giving satisfaction was very important and gave me real plea-
> sure.

[5]The popular marriage manuals of the day are quite explicit on the issue of male re-sponsibility for female orgasm. See, for example, Chesser (1947), Van de Velde (1930), and also Gordon and Shankweiler (1974) for a review of recent marriage manuals.

An interesting and provocative issue this: women who take such satisfaction in giving pleasure that their own unfulfilled sexual longings become relatively unimportant. In this age, when the emphasis is so much on *taking* pleasure, we might be tempted to label such women with pejoratives—to speak of their socialization to passivity, to bemoan their tendencies toward masochism and self-denial. But that's too easy. And it leads too often to a call to arms, to a shrill and insistent demand for change, that leaves many women feeling confused and angry, inadequate or misunderstood. Worst of all, it leaves them feeling as if some prized part of themselves were being denied and invalidated—the part that's tender, giving, nurturing; the part that gets "joy out of giving him joy."

But what does this say? What of the often tragic consequences of traditional socialization practices that encourage passivity, masochism, and self-denial in women? No denying those; no denying either that the behavior I speak of here may be related to those tendencies. But let's not deny the reality and complexity of their experience when women speak of the importance of being able to give pleasure to a loved one. Let's not wipe out such giving with words of disparagement. Indeed, to do so invalidates any possibility of an authentic altruism—that kind of behavior that was glorified in the pre-Freudian age, that once was lauded as the height of virtue. It's true that the post-Freudian view that directs us to the potential pathology in such altruistic behavior is an important corrective to our earlier romantic notions about saintliness and self-abnegation. But it has been carried too far if in this era of human history we can no longer distinguish at all between the authentic desire to give and its pathological distortion: masochism.

When it comes to sex, it is this very quality of giving that is necessary to turn the sex act into a relationship. Only when two people wish to give at least as much as they wish to take does sex become a nourishing and enriching experience. Only then is the uniquely human separated from the animal.

Of course, it takes two. And until now, there too often has been only one—the woman—to do this kind of giving. The task now is *not* to exhort women to change or to thwart that capacity in themselves, but to encourage men to develop it more fully. No easy task, to be sure, but a necessary one if sexual relations between women and men are to fulfill their promise.

Unfortunately, in this culture, facile answers too often take the place of real struggle. Thus, we now have a whole new vocabulary of assertiveness for women and a profitable industry to match. Yet much of the rhetoric mistakes "assertiveness" for selfishness and seeks to teach women to abandon those giving parts of themselves. In fact, *real* assertiveness would mean that women would respect those gentle, tender, giving qualities enough to assert their value. *Real* assertiveness would mean that they would continue to give such care and concern in their relationships *and* would insist on getting it from their men as well. Difficult demands for women to make—made especially difficult in a culture where such values and ways of being have been consistently devalued with the label *feminine*.

These reflections aside, there was pain in the early years of marriage. And there was conflict. But most women eventually win a victory in the struggle with their repressed sexuality—a victory of nature over culture, the triumph of female sexuality over the forces that for so long have conspired to obliterate it.

As long ago as 1953, Kinsey showed that the proportion of women experiencing orgasm in marriage rises steadily through the years.[6] So it is with the women I met. "I'm enjoying sex more than I ever did in my life before, maybe even more than I ever thought I could"—common sentiments, spoken repeatedly. But it took time. For some, it was a year or two before they experienced their first orgasm; for those less fortunate, it didn't happen for a decade or more. Others commented on the dramatic change after the birth of the first child, telling not only of having their first orgasm but of experiencing spontaneous sexual feelings for the first time in their lives[7]:

> All of a sudden, I knew what it was like to feel sexual. I mean, I would get sexual feelings before that when I was stimulated, but they didn't just come by themselves. I used to wonder what people meant when they talked about being horny, but I never knew until after Lisa was born.

Unfortunately, for women who are new mothers and who must bear the burden of child care alone, increasing sexual responsiveness is not an unmitigated blessing. For it's one of life's hapless paradoxes that the physiological development of this stage of the life cycle is so poorly matched with its demands. Certainly there's joy in those early months of motherhood, but there's also exhaustion. Of course there's the wonder of a new life and a new love, but there's also anxiety. Am I a good enough mother? Will I spoil my baby by holding her now?

[6]Kinsey *et al.* (1953) showed that by the 15th year of marriage, only 10% of his sample never reached orgasm in marital coitus, and that by the end of 20 years of continuous marriage, 47% were having orgasm all or most of the time. These figures comport with the findings of the present study, where close to 90% of the women were orgasmic, over 50% more than half the time.

[7]For a compelling argument about the physiological reasons for the increase in orgasmic potential after childbirth, see Sherfey (1973).

Or will I damage him forever if I don't? Is there something wrong with me that I sometimes feel restless and discontented? How could I have been so angry yesterday—she's only an innocent child? Question upon question, born of the myths and the mandates that attach to motherhood in our society—the myth of the all-loving, all-nurturing madonna-mother; the mandates that remind her repeatedly that she alone is responsible for the healthy development of her child.[8] Preoccupied with such fears, anxious about her adequacy in this new and demanding role, the young mother finds it hard to care much about sex. In fact, for most women in this study—including those who by then were enjoying good sexual relationships—the arrival of the first child marked a significant drop in both sexual activity and sexual pleasure.

Even among those who experienced orgasm for the first time after giving birth, it usually wasn't met with pure pleasure. Rather, it was pleasure mixed with relief at finally having achieved that long-sought goal. And there was frustration and anger as well.

> It was a damned irony. Just when I couldn't have cared less, it happened. And then for years, I was too tired and too preoccupied to want it much. God, what an aggravating time that was.

In fact, from the time they're born until they leave home, the presence of children generally inhibits a woman's sexual responsiveness—a fact that is a constant source of conflict between many wives and husbands.[9] At first, the strain of a newborn infant leaves her tired and edgy much of the time. Later, other concerns about the care and welfare of children dominate her attention:

> He could be ready at any time of the day or night, no matter what was happening; and it made me very uncomfortable. You know, a child could be banging at the door, and he wouldn't be interrupted for anything. Or you could hear a kid screaming down the hall, and it wouldn't faze him at all. Well, I couldn't very well get into it under those circumstances.

These are trying times in a marriage. Whether at the breakfast table or dinner, in bed or out, young children are difficult, demanding, and often irritating companions. Even when they're at their an-

---

[8]Several recent accounts of motherhood, written by women who are also mothers, speak to the joys and pains of what Adrienne Rich (1976) calls the "institution of motherhood." All make clear that many of the problems experienced by mothers in relation to their children are related to the cultural myths around motherhood and the guilt women experience from the internalization of that package of impossible expectations (Hammer, 1975; Lazarre, 1976; McBride, 1973; Rich, 1976).

[9]See Hobbs and Cole (1976) for a replication of their 1963 study, which shows that decreased sexual responsiveness in women continues to be a major problem in the transition to parenthood.

gelic best, spontaneous interaction and communication between adults is limited just by their presence.[10] That means there's often some distance between wife and husband—distance born of the fact that their daily lives are separate while their evenings are too short, and altogether too full of distractions, to allow them to reestablish a connection quickly.[11] For most women, that spells difficulty in the sexual relationship—a consequence of the fact that for women, more than for men, sex is *part* of the total relationship, not something that stands *a*part from it.[12] Over and over, they speak of not being able "to turn on the minute the kids go to bed," of needing "some time together before jumping into bed," of not feeling "very close or sexual after we've barely talked to each other for a few days." And over and over, they also tell of the conflict these differences with their husbands create.

When children get older, they need less and demand less. But then the irritation of their seemingly unceasing demands, the constriction of their constant presence, and the worries about their physical and psychological well-being are replaced by embarrassed concern about what they might think their parents are doing behind the closed door, or what they might hear in the night:

> Just knowing that the bed could squeak or they could hear some noise makes it hard to get into sex sometimes. I feel nervous that they could walk in any time, too. We've thought about putting a lock on the door, but after 20 years of not having a lock on the bedroom door, I feel embarrassed to suddenly have one show up. What would I tell the kids? Even if they didn't ask any questions, I know what they'd be thinking, and I feel like I'd have to explain. But what would I say?

The fear of pregnancy is another important inhibitor of sexual desire and activity in women. Despite almost universal use of birth control measures, that concern remains alive for most women in their childbearing years. For some, usually those who have had the experience of an unwanted pregnancy—a child born of a birth control device that failed—concern turns to fear.

To deal with this fear, just over 15% of the men have had vasec-

---

[10]See Miller (1976) for a recent study showing that children tend to decrease the frequency of marital companionship; therefore, their presence generally means also a decrease in marital satisfaction.

[11]Hobbs and Cole (1976) show that among the top seven problems that men and women experience in the transition to parenthood is "feeling more distant from spouse."

[12]Gagnon and Simon (1973) argued that this split between sex and love, this separation of sex from the total relationship, is the hallmark of male sexuality in the American culture.

tomies.[13] Without exception, the result has been more relaxed and frequent sexual activity between wife and husband—the woman sometimes becoming orgasmic for the first time. When this happens, a woman credits her newfound sexual responsiveness to the freedom from fears of pregnancy:

> It made all the difference in the world not to lie there scared to death that I'd pay for this for the rest of my life. The last thing I wanted was another baby, and I never felt secure with either condoms or a diaphragm. After he had the vasectomy, I could begin enjoying sex for the first time in my whole life.

"The last thing I wanted was another baby"—no reason to doubt her words. But there's still another issue, perhaps equally important, in this complex drama between wives and husbands. Very often, a woman sees her husband's willingness to undergo vasectomy as a statement of his caring and concern for her, a statement of his commitment to something besides his own gratification and pleasure. Both together—the release from the pregnancy fears *and* the reassurance about his love and commitment that the vasectomy seems to her to imply—become powerful forces in freeing a woman to more sexual responsiveness.

In several families, there was conflict about whether or not a man would take this step. And always, for the wife, that conflict centered on both these issues, as these comments from a woman in a deteriorating marriage show:

> I can honestly say to you that from the second year of our marriage to the fifteenth, I enjoyed sex as much as he did. But no more. Not one of my children was planned. No matter what kind of birth control we used, something always happened. Five years ago, I got pregnant again for the fifth time. Fortunately, I had a miscarriage, so I didn't have to have the baby. But it turned me off sex, and ever since we have big rows over it for the first time in our lives. [*Tears streaming down her face.*] But dammit, he can do something about it instead of just bitching at me. He could have a vasectomy and take care of me in that way—finally. Until now, it's always been my job. Well, since it didn't work for me, it's his turn. If he cares enough about something besides himself, he'll do it. But I just don't think he does.

It should be clear by now that both life cycle and culture influence women's sexual responsiveness. At the beginning, it's youth, inexpe-

---

[13]Westoff and Jones (1977) showed striking increases in the use of vasectomy as a means of sterilization in the years between 1965 and 1975. Among white couples continuously married for 15–19 years, the proportion of vasectomies jumped from 4.4% in 1965 to 19.5% in 1975. Among those married 20–24 years, the corresponding proportions were from 5.9% to 19.5%.

rience, and the prohibitions against female sexuality that have to be overcome. Later it's children—small ones or teenagers—and the fear of another pregnancy that impose constraints. Through all this, however, most women move steadily toward a more expansive and open sexuality—partly because some life-cycle issues are resolved, and partly in response to the changing cultural context.

Between the time these midlife women grew to sexual maturity and the time they were raising their own daughters to womanhood, profound changes in the boundaries of acceptable sexual behavior had taken place. Whether in marriage or outside of it, what for the mothers had been inconceivable for their daughters has become commonplace.[14] While a few of the most daring of the mothers had premarital sexual relations furtively, now most of their daughters are doing so openly—many living in arrangements their mothers once would have considered sinful. While most of the mothers speak with pride—albeit tinged with some sadness—about their premarital sexual naiveté, their daughters would be embarrassed to make such an admission.

I have written elsewhere about the costs to young people of this revolution in sexual behavior, of the difficulties they suffer as they struggle to cast off their parents' teachings and to change their old consciousness to match the new behavior.[15] Imagine the impact on the parental generation. Suddenly, they find themselves living in a culture that not only gives license to formerly forbidden behaviors but exalts them. Suddenly, their unmarried children become sexually active, shocking their mothers, but reminding them also of their own repressed girlhood and young womanhood, of the moments now when they dare to wonder—quietly and to themselves, to be sure—whether those old ways were indeed the best ways:

> When my daughters got old enough to have sexual relations with boys, I had to ask myself some very hard questions. Was it better the way I was? Did I want them to spend the first ten or twelve years of their marriage getting through the sexual hang-ups my husband and I had? I guess I was somewhat jealous of the opportunities they had even though I was upset about what they were doing and afraid for them.

Sexually, it seemed as if the culture were exploding. Wherever they turned—on film, on stage, in print, or in life—they were bombarded with what seemed like a newly liberated sexual energy, reminded of what they might be missing, told these joys could also be

[14]Hunt (1974) compared sexual behavior in the 1970s with the data from the Kinsey studies of the early 1950s to document the sweeping changes in sexual behavior across the generations. See also Rubin (1976) for data and analysis of the *meaning* of such large cultural changes in the lives of the people who are trying to live with them.
[15]Rubin (1976); Chapter 8 "The Marriage Bed," pp. 134–154.

theirs. Simultaneously, for the first time, relatively large numbers of women were speaking and writing about female sexuality, launching a concerted attack on established myths and stereotypes. For the first time, women were speaking to and for women, insisting on defining their own experience and challenging existing interpretations of female sexuality—from the general conception of sexual inertia in women to the more specific myth of the vaginal orgasm.

But these messages of liberation bring with them also a new set of constraints, new rules for acceptable sexual behavior. Thus, despite some changes wrought by the public discussion of female sexuality by feminist writers, women still tend to see their sexual behavior in highly individualistic and personalized terms, suffering from guilt, feelings of inadequacy, and sometimes desperation, when they are not meeting whatever may be the current standards for sexual behavior. This is the paradox of the new sexual freedoms: they are not simply "freedoms" but very often new coercions—new mandates for behavior that evoke guilt and discomfort in much the same way as did the old restrictions. Indeed, in our highly conformist and goal-oriented society, these new directives for sexual behavior can be more oppressive than the old ones since, when oppression comes in the name of *freedom*, it's more mystifying, hence harder to grasp and overcome.

Thus, if some women are found to be capable of multiple orgasms, it's not just a matter of pleasure for those who can or wish to, it becomes a requirement of adequate sexual performance—the goal toward which sexual activity is directed. The pleasure a couple may have experienced before the new "discovery" too often gets lost in the determined, sometimes tortured, march toward the new goal. If she doesn't have multiple orgasms, *she* feels terrible; if he can't "make her," *he* suffers as well. From blaming themselves, they shift to blaming each other, and back again. Wherever they come to rest at any given moment, their sexual relationship suffers—all in the service of the quest for something more, something "better." Nothing wrong with the search, of course; only in the way it's conducted, only in the fact that it's alienated from internal needs and longings, dominated by the latest sexual fad. This year it's multiple orgasm, last year it was vaginal—a quest that brought needless pain and suffering to millions:

> We kept trying and trying to get me to have a vaginal orgasm. That was the Big "A"—"A" for being female, "A" for validating your husband. It was the focus of all our sex. We were no longer human beings, but guinea pigs in our own experiment.

But it wasn't, in fact, their own experiment. They were responding not to some inner mandates but to external, social ones. To some, it must seem like the ultimate paradox that, while using the language of pleasure, the recent sexual revolution has managed to do to sex what even the Puritans couldn't quite achieve: to turn it into hard work.[16] Our concern about performance and technique leaves little or no room for a playful, pleasurable, sensuous sexuality—the kind of sexual play that would lead quite naturally to a woman's orgasm. Instead, we speak with a kind of grim resolve about the techniques for "getting her ready," both women and men missing the pleasures and delights to be found in the process. The word we use to describe this part of the sexual interaction tells the story: *fore*play, the part that comes before the real thing. If we understand the social context in which language, culture, and behavior interact, this comes not as a surprise, but as another demonstration of the many contradictions in the American culture—in this case, the tension between work and pleasure that dominates public policy as well as individual life, a tension built deep into the American consciousness, part of our Puritan heritage.[17]

In this context, let's look anew at the issue of faking orgasm and its meaning to women who do it. A very small proportion of the women I met fake orgasm all or most of the time. But most have done it at some time in their married lives, and almost half still do it at least once in a while.

That's no big news. The issue claimed my attention only because most of the women who fake orgasm, even those who do it only occasionally, speak intensely about the guilt and discomfort they feel now that the phrase *faking orgasm* has become practically an epithet. They tell of reawakened fears about their sexual adequacy; they talk about feeling judged. Most of all, they plead to be understood, wanting the meaning of what they do in bed to be known before the judgments are rendered.

But who's judging? Surely not the feminist writers who have spoken out so passionately about contorted social definitions of female sexuality. Surely not those same women who have written with such compassion about the sexual conflicts women face as a consequence of those distortions. Ask the women, and they'll say they don't know who, only that they feel they're being judged and found wanting, that

---

[16]See Slater (1976), who also argues that our preoccupation with orgasm and the techniques for achieving it is a natural extension of the Protestant work ethic, in which nothing is to be enjoyed for its own sake except striving.

[17]One can see this tension between work and pleasure played out in the public policy debates about unwed mothers, where the discussion repeatedly focuses on their alleged "licentious" and "pleasure-seeking" behavior. In reading or listening to these discussions, it is difficult to escape the conclusion that our national rage is directed not simply at their sexual behavior but at the pleasure we fantasy they take in it.

they feel misunderstood because there's not enough talk about what it means to them to fake orgasm, why they do it:

> It's every place you turn these days. And it makes me uncomfortable because I don't think those women who shout about how terrible it is to fake it understand what it's like and why a woman would do it.
>
> *And why do you do it?*
>
> It's just easier sometimes, that's all. I never tell a lie about it; it just happens. [*Squirming uncomfortably in her chair.*] Joe doesn't ask me, right? He doesn't say, "Did you or didn't you," right? So what if I just let him think I did? He needs to believe it's that way. So what if I just give him that impression?

The "so what" is that she—and others like her for whom these comments are typical—is asking those questions of herself, not of me, suggesting that she's not so sure anymore that it's really all right:

> *You sound as if you're asking yourself that question, not me.*
>
> Yeah, I never did before, though. I never thought it was a problem. I've never talked about my sex life to anyone, *never*. But there's so much talk about things like that now, you can't help hearing and reading things. And lately, people are talking about women faking it, so I worry about it. I guess now I ask myself if it's honest or not. [*Hesitantly.*] And you know, I begin to think maybe there's something wrong with me that I don't have an orgasm every time.

How does it happen that way? How does it happen that she's angry at "those women who shout about how terrible it is to fake it"? How does it happen that she worries that "there's something wrong with me that I don't have an orgasm every time"? Certainly, the feminist discussion about faking orgasm has dealt with the *why*; certainly it has tried to place the behavior in the context of social expectations, not personal responsibility. Then, how does it happen that this woman, and so many like her, haven't been able to hear that message?

Perhaps women fail to hear the reassurances because their own internal anxiety about what they do is so great that it must be disowned—projected outward onto anyone who calls attention to it. Perhaps they have trouble listening because the emphasis on the social sources of their sexual behavior indeed misses something in their own experience that makes those explanations seem alien. Perhaps they don't integrate the message because there's so much noise in the social world about sexual issues that it's hard to know who's talking, hard to know what's being said—perhaps also because they have had quite enough of the changing and often contradictory cultural expectations that influence and shape their sexuality.

I came to the issue of faking orgasm with my own biases, believing that the only reason a woman fakes it is to please her partner and that, no matter what, no woman ought to deny her own experience and sexual needs in this way. But the women I met taught me anew that human behavior is never so simple, and that changing it requires understanding, not injunctions—understanding, not just of individuals, but of the social system in which they live.

It's true, of course, that one reason women fake orgasm is to please their partner. But rather than viewing that in its negative sense, let's turn the prism a bit. Then we see that the behavior is born of their caring concern for him—a gift that's born of love and the ability to give of which I spoke earlier:

> It isn't as if he's not a good lover, because he is. He doesn't rush and he's not abrupt. I need a lot of attention and loving, and he gives it. So why should I make him feel like he's fallen short or he's a failure just because I don't have an orgasm every time?

But there's another reason that women fake orgasm—one that speaks more to their own needs than to their husbands'. Women's orgasms are now big business—books, films, therapies, and the like, all part of a highly profitable industry devoted to telling us how to make it happen, all selling the notion that good sex must end in orgasm. Anything else is portrayed as not quite good enough, not quite the real thing. That means that women are now under the same performance pressures that men have experienced for so long—pressures that sometimes feel incompatible with internal needs, since many women insist that it's not necessary for them to have an orgasm every time they have sexual intercourse, that sometimes they can be quite content with a loving, tender sexual experience that does not culminate in orgasm.

Whether in men or in women, such pressures ultimately generate a response. Men may become impotent. But there's no such out for women, no physiological response that makes them absolutely unable to participate in sexual intercourse. For them, faking orgasm is one way to make *in*congruent demands feel more congruent—a reasonable response to an unreasonable situation, perhaps the only way to take some of the pressure off:

> I never thought it was a big thing until now. After all, I don't have to have an orgasm every time. Sometimes I just don't need or want one, but it's important to him, so I just let him think I have it.

For some women, then, faking orgasm may be the most effective protective device available—a way of dealing with sexual mandates from a culture and a husband that are experienced, if not always consciously understood, as alien and alienating; perhaps the only way a woman has at any given moment of pleasing her man, who may be trying so hard, yet unsuccessfully, to please her.

Still, the act of faking is alienating in itself, one might argue, and ought to be dealt with in that context. Indeed, that's an important and complex issue for both women and men—one major reason that they must learn to be more open with each other about this and other sexual issues. But that alienation doesn't start with faking orgasm. Faking it is only a symptom of alienated sexuality that begins early in childhood when girls begin the process of internalizing social definitions of female sexuality that distort their experience and alienate them from the messages of their own bodies. From the beginning, it's those external cultural definitions of sexuality that dominate our consciousness, circumscribe our behavior, and define our relationship to the sexual side of our personal identity. And it's those cultural definitions and the way they are responded to that deserve our closest attention. For to allow the discussion of faking orgasm to take place outside that deeper cultural context is to burden women and men with yet more reasons for guilt and more feelings of personal inadequacy.

With all the constraints, with all the problems, there's also a liberating side to the public discussion of sex and sexuality. Whether young, middle-aged, or old, women have been listening intently, hearing the new words, daring finally to believe their own experience, to give legitimacy to the messages of their own bodies:

> God, it was like a heavy load lifted from me—from both of us—to find we were okay. But it didn't come easy. It took years of reading all this stuff that's been coming out about women's orgasms, as well as some therapy, before we began to be able to accept that whichever way I get it, it's okay.

It's true that some few still speak sadly about being unable to take advantage of a cultural climate that offers permission for more sexual freedom than they ever before dreamed of:

> I wish I could be free sexually like the kids, but I can't. It just doesn't work for me. Too many years of repression, I guess, and too many lessons that I learned too well.

But for most of the midlife women I met, life cycle changes and a culture that encourages more sexual experimentation have come together to permit the opportunity for more gratifying sexual relationships even in long-term marriages. The years of sharing the same bed means they know each other better, are more likely to know what will bring sexual pleasure, are more trusting, and, therefore, are more able to be interdependent. With the children grown, there's more privacy, more opportunity for relaxed time alone:

> We're a lot freer sexually now than we ever were before. And now that it's just the two of us in the house, you can do it when you feel like it, and you can take your time—you know, just lie there together for an hour or

> two, or even more. It makes all the difference when you don't have to
> worry who's listening in one of the upstairs bedrooms.

Such changes in personal sexual behavior do not come easily, nor
do they come all at once. For some, one small change has led to larger
ones; for others, one has been quite enough. And most of the time,
they are changes that, by current standards of sexual practice, are small
indeed. But that they have come at all is testimony to women's will to
struggle toward change, testimony to their capacity for growth and
development in the face of repressive early training that presents for-
midable obstacles.

But this expanding sexuality in women is not without its paradoxical effects, not without its positive and its negative sides. For just as
there is a distinct and different pattern in the work careers of women
and men, so there are differences in their sexual careers and development as well.

We know that for men the passage of years means a diminution
of the sexual imperative. That lessening of sexual capacity has been
discussed at length, usually with expressions of regret and sadness for
the lost virility of youth. But rarely do we hear about the positive
impact of that fact on midlife marriage:

> It's not as frequent as when we were younger (it just seemed like all the
> time then), but it's more meaningful and it's more enjoyable. I don't ever
> feel pushed into it anymore, and that's good for both of us. We don't start
> out with all that stuff between us—you know, his wanting it and me re-
> sisting it. Now I want it as much as he does—sometimes even more. So
> sex now is really very good and much more varied than it ever was. [Laugh-
> ing.] I guess this is one time when less is more. I mean, there's less quantity
> but more quality—a lot more.

Indeed, for many women, the waning of the intensity and frequency of their husband's sexual need brings an important new dimension to their own sexual experience. Until this happens, many
women never have the chance to feel the full force of their own sexual
rhythm, never get to experience the frequency or potency of their
own sexual desires. For until this time, that rhythm, that force, was
coopted by the urgency of their husband's sexual demands. For the
first time, many women discover that their sexual responsiveness is
cyclical, the waxing and waning of its intensity related to the menstrual cycle:

> I'd heard talk that women were supposed to be sexier around their period,
> but I have to tell you that I didn't know anything about it firsthand until
> recently. I always just thought I wasn't very sexy and that I didn't have
> any peaks and valleys [with a self-mocking laugh], just valleys, you know. It
> was kind of a wonder to me to find out about the peaks, which happened
> after my husband kind of slowed down.

It's not that this woman, and others like her, didn't often enjoy the sexual encounter in the earlier years. The point is simply that the initiative then usually came from the men and was related to *their* wishes, needs, and sexual rhythm, not to the women's. When that changes, when the men's sexual need is no longer so clamorous, women often learn for the first time about their bodies' capacity for sexual response:

> I didn't even know it then, but I never knew what it was like to feel horny. He was always there waiting and ready, and most of the time I felt as if I had to say "yes" even if I didn't feel like it. Now I *love* feeling that I'm a sexual person for the first time in my life. It's sometimes hard to believe the change.

And now the paradox. For this very shift in the urgency of male sexual response that makes life easier in so many ways also means that women again are stuck with having to quiet their own rising sexual needs. For men, there seems to be no anxiety worse than the fear that their sexual powers are waning. Thus, at the first sign of diminished sexual capacity, a woman is likely to act as if on automatic pilot to protect her man from having to confront that reality. That means she doesn't initiate a sexual encounter even at the cost of muting her own heightened sexual imperative. For her, that's not so hard. She has, after all, been trained almost from birth to repress such feelings, to deny their existence:

> There's nothing worse than to push him and have him unable to perform. If he fails, it causes more problems than it's worth. It's a shame because I feel deprived now when I never would have before. But I worry more about him than I do about myself. So I just wait for him to ask me. That's easier all around.

Perhaps she's angrier about it now than she might have been in another era and at another time in her life—angrier because now the repression is more difficult to achieve, the deprivation experienced more keenly, and the culture somewhat more permissive of her acknowledging and expressing those feelings:

> I know now that this is denying oneself, that it's an enormous part of life that I've denied for a long time. It's denying feelings of self-affirmation that you need more as you get older. I can't deny those feelings so easily anymore, and sometimes I get mad that I still have to because now he can't have sex so easily anymore.

Generally, however, most women don't speak that anger very readily—and surely not to their men. In fact, a woman who experiences this sexual turnabout in a marriage is likely to tread very gingerly. She's frightened for her husband—frightened that his fear of losing his sexual potency will, in fact, become a self-fulfilling prophecy. And she's frightened for herself—frightened because she knows his sense of manhood rests on his sexual performance; frightened because she understands how dangerous to him, to her, and to their marriage is any threat to that sexual capacity:

> It's a shame men are so sensitive about their virility. But it's true. When impotence hits a man, it's a real trauma. I don't want to put him in a position of having a failure and feeling so terrible that he won't be able to make it next time. Sure, I like sex; I enjoy it. But I'm not going to die without it for a while. So I just wait.

It's true, she won't "die without it," but she will temper her sexual desire because of her concern for her husband's sense of manhood, moderate her own yearning because of his need to believe in his sexual competency. And although almost always she'll speak words of understanding, she's usually ambivalent, if not downright angry, about the situation:

> [Bursting out spontaneously.] It makes me furious that just when I become a real sexual being, he cops out. [Then immediately wanting to modify the anger.] Oh, that's not fair, is it? It's not *his* fault. Sex has always been so important to him, and I know how hard it must be not to be able to do it all the time. I guess he was what you'd call a sexual athlete until a few years ago, when that all changed. I feel very badly for him, I really do. But I guess I can't help feeling bad for myself, too. It just seems like one of life's rotten tricks.

Half a lifetime of struggling with her repressed sexuality and a woman awakens to find her husband getting ready for sleep. Indeed, one of life's ironies, "one of life's rotten tricks"—especially galling because for so many years the situation was reversed, especially so because for so long her active sexual interest was what he pleaded for, argued for. Finally, she's the one who would like to initiate sexual activity. And she can't—restrained by the fear that he'll experience it as pressure, that he won't be able to complete the act.

How often does this happen? Often enough to engage the attention and concern of about half the women I spoke with. To whom does it happen? It's hard to discern a clear pattern. But age makes a difference. The women in this study between 45 and 55—all married to men from 2 to 10 years older than they are—spoke about the waning of their husbands' sexual capacity more often than those who were younger. But even among the 40-year-olds, it was already being felt, already a subject of concern.

It's tempting to speak only of physiological differences—of the divergent developmental paths that put the peak of male sexuality a decade or more before the female sexual peak—to explain the diminution of sexual interaction in midlife families. But there's more than biology here, more than a regrettable physiological process at work. Indeed, that's too easy an answer, too static a notion—one that fails to take into account that sexual behavior takes place in the context of a relationship, that it is an *interaction* between two people, that much of the complexity of the total relationship is expressed in the sexual interaction. Ask yourself: If it were *just* biology, how could we explain the man whose impotence or waning sexual interest is replaced by a clamoring sexuality immediately after a divorce?

In fact, where serious incompatibility of sexual desire exists, it's often related at least as much to power struggles in the marriage as to distinctly physiological issues—power struggles that, as anyone who has lived in a marriage knows, tend to get played out in bed.[18] Certainly, it was true in over one-fourth of the families I met where those power struggles were alive, dominating the sexual interaction, determining its context and frequency. In some families, they were very old; in others, they were much newer—the product of a wife's emergence as a force to be reckoned with in this era when so many women are beginning to make their presence felt in new ways.

Where the struggle has a long history, it is played out in the sexual interaction in one of two ways. Either the husband is relatively indifferent to his wife's needs, taking what he wants sexually while she simply submits, or the wife withholds—sometimes physically, by refusing to participate, more often emotionally, by becoming inorgasmic. Where the struggle is more recent, it's usually manifest by a husband's failing sexual interest at exactly the time when a wife's increasing independence outside the home begins to make itself felt inside the home as well—whether in the kitchen, in the living room, or in the bedroom. She may be trying her wings on a job or at school at the same time that she's beginning to experience and assert her sexual needs and desires. After years of hearing his complaints because she doesn't initiate sexual activity, she finally does. And he turns off:

> He always wanted me to take the first step, but when I began to do it, he was always too tired or [*mimicking his posture and voice*] he just didn't feel like it.
>
> *How did you feel about that?*
>
> I didn't like it, but what can you do? With a man, you can't make him, can you? You just have to wait it out.
>
> *What do you think was going on for him?*
>
> I don't *think*, I know. I had just gotten my first job and was very excited with my life. Things were changing around here and he didn't like it.

[18]See Rubin (1976) for an extended discussion of the ways in which power struggles are played out in a marriage at any age and at any stage of the life cycle.

"Things were changing around here and he didn't like it"—a common story in families, especially common as women begin to assert their needs and expect some cooperation from their husbands in getting them met. In all families, such changes in long-standing interaction patterns are difficult. In some, they are met with resistance that expresses itself in a number of overt and covert ways—not least of them in the sexual dynamic:

> When we do have sex, it's good, and I always experience orgasm now, although it's a new feeling for me to feel as if it's not often enough. There's nothing much I can do about it right now because he doesn't want me to be the aggressor. [*Her eyes bright, voice tinged with a mocking anger.*] Oh, he doesn't say that; he has said exactly the opposite for years, in fact. But he doesn't have to say it; there are other ways to get the message across.
>
> *What do you mean? What other ways?*
>
> I went through a period of time a year or so ago when I took him at his word. I mean, I got fairly aggressive and let him know when *I* wanted sex. It didn't take long to see how uncomfortable that made him.
>
> *If he didn't say that, how did you know he was uncomfortable?*
>
> It was easy; he just wouldn't be interested. After the first couple of times, he'd just be too tired or too something. Whatever he was, he wasn't interested. In fact, he hasn't been terribly aggressive himself for the last few years.

"The last few years"—precisely the period when she was appointed to a municipal commission in her city of residence and enrolled in college to begin study for a bachelor's degree. When these activities come together with a new assertiveness at home, as eventually they must, the change can be overwhelming indeed, seeming to both wife and husband to threaten the stability of the marriage.

One unconscious mechanism for coping with the anxieties stirred by such a threat is to seek to reestablish the former equilibrium—which means trying to restore the relationship to the way it was. Even when that "way" is recognized by both partners as far from ideal, they generally collude in the struggle to return to the past, since it is, at least, known. And psychologically, the *un*known can be more terrifying than the known, however bad that may be.

The sexual sphere, laden as it is with so many repressed emotional and cultural burdens—guilt, shame, rigidly sex-stereotyped notions of appropriate behavior—probably is the most readily manipulable, the most easily restored to the old balance. Thus, she stops being "aggressive," and he regains the sexual initiative—not a perfect solution but a tolerable one, one that allows both to retain something: she, her outside activities; he, the feeling that he remains in control.

The issue, then, is not just sex but also power—the struggle for one affecting the other in a continuing dynamic interaction. It's true, however, that the fact that these struggles are acted out in this particular way in the sexual arena is likely to be age-related. Male impotence or sexual withholding is a more probable weapon—one not so hard on the person wielding it—at 50 than at 25.

There we have it: a complex picture of a delicate and complex part of life: sex and sexuality. For women, there seems to be a disturbing disjunction between sexual development and sexual behavior. At the developmental level, women's sexuality breaks the bonds of the early repressions and gathers force and power as they move into midlife. But at the behavioral level, something else happens. There, we see that despite the development and recognition of their own internal needs and sexual rhythm, despite all the talk about the liberation of sexuality for both women and men, we still can't discuss the sexual behavior of women in marriage outside the context of their relationships with their husbands [19]—at least, not when looking at the present generation of midlife women. No matter how we turn the prism, no matter what facet of the sexual interaction we examine, women still are largely reflectors of their men's needs and wishes—responding to male initiatives and imperatives, subduing their own.

It's true that, like all peoples in subordinate positions, women have ways of striking back—covert ways that even they don't fully understand. Thus, women who are constrained from acting directly and forcefully by a lifetime of training to appropriately "feminine" behavior may become nonorgasmic or unresponsive in an unconscious attempt to assert themselves and claim autonomy. Or they may fake orgasm to protect themselves from unwelcome demands. But the price for such behavior is high indeed, since it hurts the woman who does it at least as much as it deprives the man who is the object of it.

Whether their daughters' generation will effect some fundamental change is as yet unknown. For that answer, we must wait another 20 years. They may, indeed, be successful finally in rising "up from the pedestal," [20] in developing a surer sense of their own sexuality, in gaining the ability to assert it, and in helping their men to develop those capacities of caring, concern, the nurturance that until now have been the almost exclusive province of women. We can only hope so and wish them well. But today, the needs and desires, the frustrations and discontents, that men bring to the relationship still dictate the behavior of most midlife women, if not their desires.

[19]While not wishing to deny other forms of the family—in particular, the homosexual family—I am speaking here of heterosexual familes only.
[20]This felicitous phrase is borrowed from the title of Kraditor's (1968) volume of feminist writings.

Still, there's something left to be said. With all the complexity, with all the difficulties, most midlife women will say, "Sex? It's gotten better and better." A remarkable experience this, given the level of sexual repression with which they have lived for so long. A remarkable experience, given the number and magnitude of issues that beset the sexual interaction in marriage. And a remarkable expression of the strength, the tenacity, the force, of female sexuality. Despite all attempts to sublimate it, repress it, and deny its existence, it forces its way into life and consciousness—there to be given a warm welcome by women who have spent a lifetime struggling to claim their sexuality, to define themselves as sexual beings.

REFERENCES

Chesser, E. *Love without fear*. New York: Roy Publishers, 1947.

Gagnon, J., & Simon, W. *Sexual conduct: The social sources of human sexuality*. Chicago: Aldine, 1973.

Gordon, M., & Shankweiler, P. Different equals less: Female sexuality in recent marriage manuals. In A. Skolnick & J. Skolnick (Eds.), *Intimacy, family, and society*. Boston: Little, Brown, 1974.

Hammer, S. *Daughters and mothers: Mothers and daughters*. New York: Signet, 1975.

Hobbs, D. F., Jr., & Cole, S. P. Transition to parenthood: A decade replication. *Journal of Marriage and the Family*, 1976, *38*, 723–731.

Hunt, M. *Sexual behavior in the 1970's*. Chicago: Playboy Press, 1974.

Kinsey, A. C., Pomeroy, W. B., Martin, C. E., & Gebhard, P. H. *Sexual behavior in the human female*. Philadelphia: Saunders, 1953.

Kraditor, A. S. *Up from the pedestal*. Chicago: Quadrangle, 1968.

Lazarre, J. *The mother knot*. New York: Dell, 1976.

McBride, A. B. *The growth and development of mothers*. New York: Harper & Row, 1973.

Miller, B. C. A multivariate developmental model of marital satisfaction. *Journal of Marriage and the Family*, 1976, *38*, 643–657.

Rich, A. *Of woman born: Motherhood as experience and institution*. New York: Norton, 1976.

Rubin, L. B. *Worlds of pain: Life in the working-class family*. New York: Basic Books, 1976.

Sherfey, M. J. *The nature and evolution of female sexuality*. New York: Vintage Books, 1973.

Slater, P. E. Sexual adequacy in America. In C. Gordon & G. Johnson (Eds.), *Human sexuality: Contemporary perspectives*. New York: Harper & Row, 1976.

Van de Velde, T. H. *Ideal marriage: Its physiology and technique*. New York: Random House, 1930.

Westoff, C. F., & Jones, E. F. Contraception and sterilization in the United States, 1965–1975. *Family Planning Perspectives*, 1977, *9*, 153–157.

Midlife Women

Lessons for Sex Therapy

Leslie R. Schover

As a psychologist trained in the treatment of sexual dysfunctions, I found Dr. Rubin's chapter of great practical interest. In fact, the day after I read it, I evaluated a midlife couple for sex therapy. It was like déjà vu when the wife said:

> You know, once the kids were grown up, sex was really great. I used to worry that they'd need something, you know, right in the middle, but after they were out of the house I could relax and really enjoy it . . . until my husband started having these problems, I mean.

I was eager to read further in the literature on sexual responsiveness and problems in midlife women—until I discovered that no such work existed. There were several recent articles on male sexuality in middle age and a number of publications on sex in the elderly, but Dr. Rubin's survey stands alone as a detailed study of women in this crucial life period. I say crucial, because clinically we treat far more midlife than elderly couples for sexual problems.

It is also a crucial group of women for research. One thing I did discover was that such widely read books as *The Hite Report* (1976) and Helen S. Kaplan's *The New Sex Therapy* (1974) agree with Dr. Rubin's finding that sex for midlife women has gotten "better and better." Thus, we have a group of women who have overcome their early sexual problems without professional help. Why are so many women able to become orgasmic, sexually assertive, and relaxed, while others remain inhibited and dissatisfied throughout their lives? Re-

---

Leslie R. Schover, Ph.D. ● Assistant Professor of Urology (Psychology), Department of Urology, M. D. Anderson Hospital and Tumor Institute, Houston, Texas 77030.

search is needed to compare women at midlife who seek sex therapy with a matched group who had early sexual difficulties that are now resolved. Can we separate the two groups according to such factors as childhood or adolescent sexual history, adult personality, or the quality of their marriage relationships? This kind of knowledge can help prevent sexual problems in future generations.

In addition, we might be able to improve sex therapy techniques if we knew what the learning process was like for the sexually satisfied women. Dr. Rubin's work suggests they were able to feel more sexually free as society's values changed, and that they communicated their new desires to their husbands. Sex therapists certainly teach attitude change and communication skills. We also focus on the woman's taking responsibility for her own sexual arousal, first by learning what kind of stimulation is most exciting for her, and then by sharing her new knowledge with her partner. I would guess that the midlife women who grew the most in their sexual responsiveness were the ones who were able to reject our cultural myth that men are the authorities on and providers of women's arousal and orgasm.

I agree with Dr. Rubin that altruism, in the sense of giving and caring, is a very healthy part of sex. I also believe, however, that allowing oneself to be self-centered during sex is one of the most difficult aspects of becoming orgasmic for women in our society. Joyce Walstedt (1977), a psychologist at the University of Delaware, has developed a questionnaire that measures the altruistic other-orientation in women, that is, the tendency always to put the man first. Walstedt studied a large group of women, similar in age and marital status to Dr. Rubin's sample. She found that women who were strongly other-oriented were less likely to be financially self-supporting or to have academic degrees than their less altruistic peers. I also wonder if the very other-oriented women were less likely to be orgasmic in their sexual relationships.

In our research group here at Stony Brook, Julia Heiman and Patricia Morokoff (1977) have completed a study that sheds more light on the reasons that some women have chronic sexual problems. They compared a group of women about to enter sex therapy with a group of sexually functioning women from the community. The average age in both groups was about 30. All research subjects had sexual fantasies, listened to erotic tapes, and watched sexual films in the laboratory, while their physical sexual arousal was measured. They also rated how much subjective excitement they felt. There was no difference in actual physical response between the clinical group and the "normal" women, but those who were about to start sex therapy felt *subjectively* less aroused. This finding suggests that some women are not aware of their body's state of sexual excitement, and that this lack of recognition contributes to difficulty in reaching orgasm. Heiman and Morokoff also discovered that women who said they *felt* aroused had positive emotions, such as interest and liking, toward the sexual material used in the experiment, including their own fantasies. It is easy to see, with hindsight, that Dr. Rubin's midlife women, who were taught not to have sexual feelings or to enjoy sexual situations, would have problems with arousal and orgasm.

Dr. Rubin raised the question of whether younger women are growing up in a saner sexual climate, or if our current olympic standards for sexual performance are even more destructive than Victorian prohibitions. There is evidence that college-aged men and women are more equal in their sexual responsiveness than their parents were thought to be. A number of recent studies [1] have found no differences between men and women in physical or subjective sexual arousal in response to erotic fantasies, stories, or films. Julia Heiman has even demonstrated that young women are no more apt than young men to be aroused by romantic details added to a purely sexual scenario. She also found that both men and women were most aroused by tapes that took a woman's sexual point of view, and in which the woman was the initiator of sexual activity. (It would seem that our traditional pornography is missing its market.) Since we have no reliable data on past generations, or even on those past college age in our own population, there is no way to tell if this gender equality is a product of cultural change or just the nature of the beast.

Perhaps the most striking evidence for positive change in female sexuality is the repeated finding [2] that the best predictor of a woman's success in reaching orgasm is the decade of her birth. I join with Dr. Rubin in hoping that this trend continues, and that our popular culture will work through its current fixation on multitudinous orgasms and interminable intercourse and begin to present a more emotional, sensual, and human model of sex for our daughters.

REFERENCES

Abramson, P. R., Goldberg, P. A., Mosher, D. L., Abramson, L. M., & Gottesdiener, L. Experimenter effects on responses to explicitly sexual stimuli. *Journal of Research in Personality*, 1975, *9*, 136–146.
Heiman, J. A psychophysiological exploration of sexual arousal patterns in females and males. *Psychophysiology*, 1977, *14*, 266–274.

---

[1]For more detailed accounts, see Abramson, Goldberg, Mosher, Abramson, and Gottesdiener (1975), Heiman (1977), and Mosher and Abramson (1977).
[2]See Morokoff (1978) for a review of the literature on female orgasm and its determinants.

Heiman, J., & Morokoff, P. *Female sexual arousal and experience as correlates of sexual malaise*. Paper presented at the American Psychological Association Meeting, San Francisco, Calif., 1977.

Hite, S. *The Hite report*. New York: Macmillian, 1976.

Kaplan, H. S. *The new sex therapy*. New York: Brunner/Mazel, 1974.

Morokoff, P. Determinants of female orgasm. In J. LoPiccolo & L. LoPiccolo (Eds.), *Handbook of sex therapy*. New York: Plenum Press, 1978.

Mosher, D. L., & Abramson, P. R. Subjective sexual arousal to films of masturbation. *Journal of Consulting and Clinical Psychology*, 1977, *45*, 796–807.

Walstedt, J. J. The altruistic other orientation: An exploration of female powerlessness. *Psychology of Women Quarterly*, 1977, *2*, 162–176.

Chapter 5

In Praise of Older Women

B. Genevay

What Does It Mean To Be an Older Woman?

> . . . next to not being spoken to, there is nothing worse for a woman than not being used or touched. Not in passion for that may be spent but in warmth. (Mannes, 1968)
> Do I hear whispers, "Disgusting, those old people making love"? . . . we are merely ourselves, speaking, feeling, touching, loving in our differences as human beings. (p. 58)

To be an old woman and to claim full sexual expression means one may be seen as undignified, sick, depraved—or as being a rare exception. This oppression results in our hiding one part of ourselves (our sexual self) from the rest of us, and the toll in life energy is great for many older women who repress their sexual thoughts, feelings, and behaviors. Gerontologists continue to remind us that sex and intimacy needs are of greater concern to elderly people than many of us acknowledge, and that aging women are more likely than aging men to suffer from intimacy deprivation.

How, then, are we older women to express our fullness as females at 50, 75, and 100? Since we will continue to outlive men, there are often no men to be loved by us, if we are heterosexual. We pay the price of hiddenness, or we experience the repugnance of others, if we are lesbian. And our families and friends, as well as professionals, are frequently uncomfortable when we even *talk* about our sexual identity

---

In Praise of Older Women is an erotic memoir by Stephen Vizinczey (New York: Ballantine Books, 1965). I borrow the *title only* for this chapter because "in praise of older women" expresses precisely the cultural attitude essential to viewing aging women as equal sexual beings.

B. Genevay, M. S. W. ● Consultant in Aging, Family Services of King County, Seattle, Washington 98104.

and sexual losses, past and present. In a television interview with Barbara Walters in 1976, Virginia Johnson said that there are changes in the acceptance by Americans of women's right to enjoy sex. This may be true for younger women today; it is not true for the majority of older women with whom I come in contact.

Physically, women are wonderfully equipped to love and be sexual until illness, disinclination, or death intervenes. Kinsey and his colleagues observed long ago that women tend to become less inhibited and more interested in sex as they move through their 40s, 50s, and 60s. Since women are living much longer now, we may safely add the 70s and 80s. We know also that "women are . . . not as intensely sexually oriented [as men] during youth but slowly become so and reach erotic peak in middle age, declining only slowly thereafter" (Kaplan & Sager, 1971).

Socially, we are faced with a whole new generation of older women, many of whom have been widows for 20 years or more. Increasingly, there are women in their 60s caring for their 80- and 90-year-old mothers—both generations facing sex, touching, and intimacy deprivation. We now categorize older people as young-old, middle-old, and older-old to help us conceptualize the developmental and situational differences that characterize what we once lumped together as "old age." I refuse to apply chronological ages to these three developmental stages at the end of life, for we become more and more diverse as we age. Numbers become meaningless when we see a very ill 64-year-old woman who "looks" 80, or a vigorous 79-year-old woman who functions as she did in middle age. What does it mean to be a sexually active 60-year-old woman when your 85-year-old mother, who lives with you, has not condoned sex since her menopause? How can a 70-year-old mother pursue intimacy when her 50-year-old daughter, a stroke victim, has no intimacy in her life? These kinds of sexual–personal–familial issues become more and more complex as we see an increase in three- and four-generational families, each generation and each individual espousing different sexual norms and values.

Culturally, older women are strongly affected by the American injunction that requires youth and beauty for us to be sexually eligible. Susan Sontag (1972) has ably documented this. It is an insidious norm which tells us that we are not equal in attractiveness and sexual potential to younger women, or to aging male peers. In her paper entitled "An Old Bag: The Stereotype of the Older Woman," Caroline Preston (1975) commented:

> What an evolution, what a development, what progress to move from being a "baby"—even one that's "come a long way"—to being an old bag whose only concern for either herself or her mate is their respective "regularity" or their "iron-poor tired blood." (p. 42)

Many older women decide to opt out as sexual beings when they feel they can no longer compete with firm breasts, bellies, and buttocks. The caricature of the old woman who continues to pattern her behavior after youthful sex symbols is hardly a model for the majority of aging women, who may seek some kind of societal permission for continuing to be their sexual selves. The following example illustrates what I mean.

Dody Goodman, a very attractive actress well past middle age, was interviewed by Merv Griffin on his television show on August 24, 1978. Ms. Goodman and Merv, along with other guests, colluded in a running ageist–sexist patter that focused primarily on references to intercourse, female body parts, and phallic symbols. Their conversation abounded with comments like Ms. Goodman's "the first time I've ever 'done it' on the air," and "how 'hard' it is." The actress modeled a parody of a shallow young female sex symbol. The message seemed to be: old women who "look" young and don't mind being a curiosity can still get attention by making fun of genital sex. This kind of media handling of aging femaleness is scarcely a compliment to the sexual caring, wisdom, and experience of mature older women.

It is clear that (1) the physiology of the older woman proclaims "all systems go!" sexually; (2) older women are faced with a lack of sanctioned partners with whom to express sexuality; (3) we face an increasing number of years of potential sexual void because of our longevity; and (4) family, peer-group, and cultural mores often hinder the sexual behaviors and imagination of older women. We become more complex and diverse as we age, sexually as in all other ways (if we so desire). Yet we are on a developmental frontier with few models for sexual and intimate behavior in the 60s, 70s, 80s, 90s, and 100s.

A picture of female sexuality might begin with a black-and-white line drawing representing the tenuous, irregular sexual expression of youth. By middle age, color and stronger lines may "flesh out" our sexual portraits: some splashed with the magenta and orange of sexual variety, others delicately washed with the beiges and yellows of gentle experimentation and ripening. Whenever "old age" begins, and this may vary from age 40 to never—depending on self-image, illness, compounded losses, and many other factors—the portrait becomes three-dimensional. The facets of sexuality simply multiply with aging, if we choose. The older woman is able to draw on who she was in the beginning, is now, and still has the possibility of becoming! And she may use all the sensory, sensual, nongenital, and genital thoughts, feelings, fantasies, dreams, and behaviors of her rich life history.

Intimacy is a much more meaningful word to use in describing aging female sexuality, for it touches on all the closeness and distance in human interaction that the jaundiced word *sex* cannot possibly convey in our culture today. I seldom ask an older woman about her sex life, for she may not know what it is I want to know out of all those past life experiences. If she's asked about those people she's been close to, she can select the sexual experiences she wishes to share. What does it mean sexually to be an older woman? It can mean a very broad avenue of sexual history, with a many-splendored possibility of continuing to be a sexual being until the end of life.

Sexual Options of Older Women

One of the difficult things for us as older women is to imagine enough possibilities for ourselves as we age that we can embrace those sexual options that do lie in wait for us in the world. Minimally, the continuum of sexual options is that shown in Figure 1. Just as one person cannot whistle a symphony, so must we be aware that there is more than one variation on the theme of sexual options for older women. The one requirement on the part of the aging female is that she allow herself as many possibilities as her mind, body, and emotions can encompass. As our bodies diminish in functioning, we might look to younger disabled women for their modeling of sexual options and possibilities. The example of a young spinal-cord-injured paraplegic woman speaks to the older woman who claims disability as a reason for opting out of sexual life:

> People think just because you're in a wheelchair, you can't have sex
> . . . I got a lot of questions from women when I was pregnant. They realized
> then, of course, that I had intercourse. They were really surprised. I'd tell
> them, "Of course people in wheelchairs make love." (Hale, Norman, Bogle,
> & Shaul, 1977, p.4)

Even with severe physical disability, the older woman can avail herself of at least half of the sexual options on the continuum in Figure 1. Following are examples of sexual options chosen by older women.

DENIAL. Jenny had had several proposals since her husband died when she was 62. Although she was slim and had a good sense of humor, Jenny considered herself too ill and too "ugly" to be acceptable, so she chose to be invisible—as a woman. She discounted offers

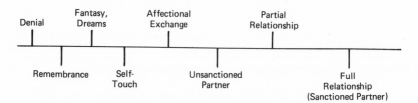

Figure 1. The continuum of sexual options.

of marriage and companionship by saying, "That doesn't interest me anymore. One marriage is enough for a lifetime." Yet Jenny openly talked about her loneliness and joked about sex a great deal, often inquiring into the sexual lives of the women she knew. She was unwilling to deal with her anger at being abandoned by her husband's death, and she channeled whatever affection she could risk toward younger women. She sometimes set herself up to be hurt when these young women did not return the emotional involvement in kind.

Anna was a lovely woman in her 80s, who attended a series of classes on sexuality and aging. She was one of the most resistant members of the class and put it very well when she said to the teacher, "You remind me of all the sexual things I can't have, so I don't like you even raising the subject!" Anna's ambivalence was apparent in her attendance of class, as well as her assumption that if the teacher didn't "raise the subject," she could then escape being exposed to sexuality in society. Her reporting of fantasies and dreams with sexual content belied her disinterest in sexual desires, thoughts, feelings, and behaviors.

Ellen, a very religious woman, combines denial of any sexual needs of her own with a great deal of affectional exchange in her church. Ellen's face glows and her eyes shine after a warm hug from the minister or many of the other men and women who cherish her presence and involvement in the church. Ellen, well into her 70s, has long since dealt with her singleness. In some ways, she considers her situation in life superior to that of her peers suffering from the loss of mates and children. While Ellen's sexual identity has taken a different hue from that of many older women, she suffers not at all from touch deprivation—a common accompaniment of denial of sexual needs. Her church not only allows but encourages physical touching and kissing, and Ellen is a very vital woman indeed.

REMEMBRANCE. Alice relives her life as a sexual partner and wife by daily verbalizing about her dead husband. She recalls what they did together and what her life as a woman meant before he died. Alice's identity emerges as she describes her relationship with her husband, her importance in the home, and her parenting role. Being a woman meant her husband's appreciation of her cooking and entertaining, her mothering, and the very private sexual life they shared. Affectionally, Alice received few gestures from her husband in public. "That wasn't nice in those days," she says. But she often repeats one story about his holding her hand in front of a large group of people. "He was very proud of me, you know," and Alice's voice takes on a sensual quality. She appreciates the warm and symbolic sexual gestures young men and women exhibit publicly today, seemingly without sadness for her own losses. Watching a couple walk arm in arm,

Alice comments, "See how he holds her. They must be in love." Although Alice sometimes bores her family members and friends with the excessive remembering, it appears to be a good way for her to remind herself that she is indeed a woman who once was a cherished partner.

Dollie's experience illustrates the relationship of remembrance to masturbation:

> I always have this picture in my mind of Fred and me, at our very best. And most times . . . when I touch myself . . . it works. I feel that he's close to me, although I miss his not being here now—he never was that good at touching anyway. So I have my memories of him, and I have this nice feeling. It seems to relieve my nervousness.

Dollie does not express the attendant guilt which many older women seem to feel when they masturbate. Her face has a relaxed, easy look about it as she talks.

FANTASY AND DREAMS. Edna, 73, speaks of her fantasy life.

> I really enjoy imagining myself doing all kinds of things with different people. Especially when I'm on the bus. I put a pleasant look on my face and daydream away. Not many people really notice older women anyway. They don't look us in the eye. So behind my glasses, I admire young men and old men, their shape, their eyes, their hands. And I admire young women and their figures.

Available to older women, as storehouses for fantasy, are strangers, neighbors, literature, their own memory banks, movies, pictures, magazines, and, of course, television. In "Media Mentors" (1978), John L. Caughey discussed the fantasy relationships that play a part in the lives of many of us, young and old. He mentioned one older woman:

> . . . an elderly suburban matron, happily married with grown-up children of her own, has spent much of her life in artificial romance with Frank Sinatra. (p. 46)

With the revival of the obsession with Elvis Presley at his death, many older women who were young or middle-aged at the inception of his career relived their earlier fantasies with Elvis. The link between sex and death is a close and deep one. Death of significant others conjures up ageless and timeless sexual fantasies that can never be experienced or reexperienced because of the ultimate loss.

Many older women who have no partners enrich their lives by vicarious relationships with television heroes and heroines, who may be more real to them than the adult children they seldom hear from. Caughey wrote,"In an era of addiction to mass media, celebrities are clearly powerful models, especially for the young" (p. 49). I believe that these dependable love objects, who may remain with us for years if the series is rerun, may be even more powerful fantasy figures for the old, who have fewer "real-life" options. If you lived alone, or with a partner who was withdrawn and seldom touched you, would you not develop a rich fantasy life with people forever young, strong, and handsome who did not abandon you through old age and death—unless the show was canceled?

Dreams are a wonderful treasury of sexual resources for older women. It is a particular joy to experience one's body as it formerly was, or as it never was, to encounter in the dream state one's own sexual energy, which may not be available, for a variety of reasons, in the nonsleep state. Barbara recounts a dream:

> I was in a department store, undressing behind a rack of clothes. I looked down, and my pubic hair was thick and very dark, as it used to be. My belly was only a little full. Suddenly this young, bearded man was there, and he was undressing too, and I noticed how white his skin was. He touched my belly, and I was not at all ashamed. We walked around the store together, and people admired us as we looked for clothes. He put his arm around my shoulders, and our hips touched as we walked side by side. I woke up feeling very much alive, and thought of things I hadn't thought of for many years. My fat hips and drooping belly didn't bother me!

In her early 60s, Barbara is still a good-looking woman by anyone's standards; but it is important that she felt more attractive and reenergized by this dream.

SELF-TOUCH. Older women do masturbate but often feel guilty about this form of getting "in touch" with their own sexual energy. Unfortunately the guilt hinders the full physical release and reduction of anxiety that masturbation can provide. Dollie's guilt-free masturbation is uncommon (see above).

Freda says, with great honesty:

> Sometimes when I touch myself a lot I feel better and can go to sleep. Other times I'm sadder, and I cry, thinking of how alone I am. When I go for a long time trying, and it doesn't help at all, I think of how angry my mother would be at me . . . she always told me I'd get a rash all over, and people would know.

Freda's mother has been dead almost 30 years now, a commentary on the timelessness of feelings and of some parental tapes.

Some women report fantasizing love relationships they wish they had had, the relationships they never had the courage to "take charge of," during masturbation. Providing a better ending to a love experience is certainly a worthy accompaniment to self-touch, and an essential part of life for a woman alone if she so chooses.

AFFECTIONAL EXCHANGE. Emma has still not let go of her husband, who died 27 years ago. She speaks of his dying in the present tense and describes the ways in which he related to her as if he were with her now. But she is able to reach out in warmth and affection to both men and women, and she enjoys the teasing she gets about what a pretty woman she is at 75. She does not initiate hugs and kisses, but she willingly receives them from one or two male friends and many woman friends. Her sexuality is expressed by the feminine way she dresses and fixes her hair, the scent she chooses to wear, and the wonderful way she has of lowering her eyes. This symbol of coquetry is dignified and age-appropriate to Emma and a totally different form of femaleness than Dody Goodman's sexist parody of a young woman described above.

Jane is 81, and although she's been single all her life, she is affectionate and open toward women and men of all ages. She reports that in her youth and middle age, she suffered from the stigma of being single and "not wanted by a man," a societal disapproval she felt keenly. But Jane extols the "blessedness" of being single now and says she feels no less a woman: "I'm not afraid to be myself, take the arm of a man, and kiss another woman. It's safer now—with my gray hair and wrinkles, no one expects bad things of me!" Jane's touching behaviors are limited to arms, hands, eyes, and cheek kissing. When asked if she is expressing herself fully, Jane says, "Yes. This is all there is—for me."

Nina is a striking woman of 78, who enjoys dressing well and for whom dining out, going to concerts, and being seen characterize being a woman. She has very clear and businesslike understandings with several men in their 40s and 50s who squire her to social functions. The public displays of male–female social behavior are important to her—taking a man's arm, being helped into a car, being helped on with her coat. Nina greatly enjoys flirting and laughing up into the eyes of her male companions. She is willing to give up lovemaking (this having depended on a near-perfect body image), but not the public social–sexual gestures that mark her as an attractive and wanted female.

UNSANCTIONED PARTNER. Betty calls herself a "man's woman." She is a well-proportioned and strong woman who values the homemaking skills that have accrued over 69 years. Since so much of Betty's identity was shaped by being a "good wife," she invites a sociable man to her home several evenings a week to eat and watch television with her. Her adult children don't trust her in this relationship and make it difficult for her to reclaim part of her female identity in this way. But Betty persists and often reassures them that she will not remarry: "I have to discourage the necking. He's a very affectionate man and wants more."

How long Betty will be able to meet her own needs for companionship is questionable, given her partner's desires and her family's disapproval of the relationship. We distrust our adolescents' sexual explorations because of *their* inexperience; we distrust our older parents' sexual explorations because of *our* inexperience—with our own aging. Remember the answer we give to our children when we want to say no to something and don't know why? "Just because." Older women are discouraged from full sexual expression "just because" *we* are afraid of sex . . . and aging . . . and death: our own.

Donna has had to separate herself from her nieces and nephews and her older sister in order to live with the woman she deeply loves. This relationship has brought her satisfaction as a woman and a sexual being, but in the event of Martha's death, she will be left very much alone. Although Donna had been married for 31 years before her husband died, she had been relieved at menopause to "give up" genital sex with her husband. She was fond of him but felt he had been insensitive to her sexual needs throughout their relationship. When Donna met Martha, their warm affectional relationship grew beyond all the bounds to which Donna had formerly imagined a marriage might grow. Both feel it hinders their relationship that they cannot share their togetherness publicly because of fear of rejection and isolation.

Lillian had been alone for several years when a young man the age of her son began showing interest in her. She was overwhelmed with the quality of their loving, for she had not experienced such wholeness and caring with a man before. She says,

> From the beginning I kept telling myself to enjoy every moment because it could not last. Yet I wouldn't have missed it for anything in the world. I grieve each night for the emptiness that's there now, and I can't tell anyone because they'd laugh at me for being a silly old fool. But I'm a fuller and richer person than I was, and I have my memories. I'm mad and sad that I was ashamed to be seen with him in public—I should have been proud that he loved me rather than worrying about what people would think!

Partial Relationship. As some of us become more disabled toward the end of life, one partner commonly precedes the other in ability to respond "in the old ways." We need to be aware that we can *choose* to be a partner to a partial relationship, or to find alternative living arrangements—if *being alone together* is too painful.

Ann's husband of 42 years is senile—or whatever garbage-can term we accept as diagnosis—but he's physically quite strong. She's chosen to carry responsibility for him 24 hours of the day. The constant monitoring to prevent him from hurting himself is less stressful for Ann than the loneliness of being with someone who has changed so much. She still strokes and touches him in the ways they formerly enjoyed, but there is often no response, or there is physical response with no recognition in the eyes or through words. The meaning for Ann is not there. We need to ask ourselves, "What does love, caring, sexual response *mean* when the *person* seems no longer to be inside the body?"

May Sarton (1977), whose companion of many years seemed to have evaporated, described poignantly the feelings elicited by loving someone who "is not there":

> Much as I love being with Judy, the fact that all holidays spent with someone no longer quite there, that there can be no real conversations, no exchange . . . ends by making me feel empty . . . We had a beautiful life together. . . . So what is unknitting now, as she grows more and more absent, had been knitted together for many years, and is still the warp and woof, the deepest relationship I have known. (p. 211)

May Sarton is in her early 60s and typifies the struggle with relationships that many face from middle age on.

In a very different way Nell, who is 69 and viewed as senile in the congregate home where she lives, searches out occasional exchanges of affection. Nell receives minimal attention because she demands so little. Wheeling slowly down the hall in her wheelchair, eating some of what is put before her, and staring for long periods of time out the window or at television, Nell is a person for whom sex has always been important. When she and another resident, Floyd, are unobserved by the staff, they wheel their chairs close by and stroke each other's chest, stomach, and thighs. So far, they have not been "caught" by staff. The look on Nell's face when she is exchanging affection with Floyd is very different from the blank stare that characterizes most of her waking hours.

As Montagu (1971) reminded us:

> . . . the rediscovery of the skin as an organ which in its own way requires just as much attention as the mind, is long overdue. . . . It is not words so much as acts communicating affection and involvement that children, and indeed, adults, require. . . . Inadequate tactile experience will result in . . . inability to relate to others in many fundamental human ways. Hence, the human significance of touching. (p. 335)

FULL RELATIONSHIP. Wilbur and Bertie have lived in the same retirement home for seven years. It was a very anxious time for them when they were deciding whether or not to marry legally. They were in the group of elderly couples who would not suffer significant financial loss if they married. But the approval of friends and family loomed large in their decision. They explored the possibility of marriage with most of the significant people in their lives prior to public announcement, and they had enough support to feel all right about their union. Now married two years, they feel they have adjusted to each other's ways. "Sometimes the bed's too crowded and I miss sleeping alone, but the minute he's gone to visit his daughter I miss him," says Bertie. "I can tell you it's just great to hold hands, and share the chores, and give backrubs! I'm less tired now, and the teasing and joking about sex are almost as much fun as the sex."

What seems crucial in envisioning a full relationship is the variety of meanings it has for each couple, depending on former life experience, health, and the current definition of a sensual–affectional–sexual partnership. An important requirement for many older women is a sanctioned partner, one whom they feel comfortable sharing with the significant family members and friends still alive. To choose a same-sexed partner might be very difficult for many older women, given the need for social sanction.

Sexual options for older women are clearly varied. Among many imminent personal losses are some that deeply affect sexuality: body loss, loss of self-image, diminished physiological functioning, loss of beloved partners and friends, and lack of societal acceptance of the aging as sexual beings. Nevertheless, a rich tapestry of sexual expression and involvement is available to the courageous older woman.

A Word to Helpers and Clinicians

Three things without which older women cannot confront their own sexuality in the fullest sense are:

1. *Self-esteem*, which defies our culture's youth-and-beauty requirements for sexual participation in life.
2. *A value system* that extols experience in loving instead of devaluing age, wrinkled skin, and changing contours.
3. *Encouragement* to initiate contact with other human beings of diverse ages, backgrounds, sex, and experience.

The latter area is one in which people in the helping professions play key roles. Many women are at war with their bodies and psyches as they grow older, and they particularly need acceptance and affirmation of their womanliness from teachers, counselors, social workers, psychologists, doctors, psychiatrists, and helpers of all kinds. They also need help in redefinition of values and behaviors and the meaning of intimacy as one ages. We who are helpers often put up the blocks to growth and change. Because of our own fears and discomfort, we may: (1) blindly accept the culture's youth-and-beauty standards for sexual eligibility and fail to respond to our clients; (2) omit the encouragement older women need because of our own inability to imagine our parents and other significant elders as sexual beings; and (3) experience distaste or repugnance toward older people who are sexually active, because of denial and fear of *our own* aging, diminishing sexual behaviors, and death.

The helper, particularly the young clinician, needs to stretch her or his imagination and range of acceptance in order to be sensitive to the affectional–sexual needs the older woman may express. Since she may be expressing these tentatively, or in symbolic language, it is the helper who must risk by checking out his or her perceptions and projections. Humor is highly useful. When a client and her helper can laugh over an obvious assumption about sex that was totally wrong, and each can learn and become more honest from that experience, they can then struggle with the real issue. The client may do a lot of "checking out" before trust develops. As one woman put it:

> In order to tell him my most personal thoughts, I told him about this friend of mine first—to see if he looked shocked. When he didn't seem upset and didn't try to change the subject, I told him a dream I'd had. It was an old dream, but I think of it a lot because it reminds me of who I used to be and what I used to do. I hoped he'd ask me some questions, and pretty soon he did. He looked awfully embarrassed for a while—but I thought, heck, he's got to grow up sometime! I think he did understand a little about how lonely I am, and his face looked soft and kind. When he said my fantasies were great, I felt a lot better. And [*laughter*] I'm having a lot more fantasies now.

See if the following dialogue reminds you of any of your own uncomfortableness in relating to older women. May is a disabled woman in her 70s:

MAY: I want to talk to you about this man who rents a room in my daughter's house. (*Pause.*)
COUNSELOR: (*Pause.*) Yes . . . uh . . . exactly what happened?
MAY: Nothing—yet. It's just that he seems to . . . well . . . he's a widower and has been alone a long time. When I go to stay with my daughter he . . .
COUNSELOR (*interrupting*): Let's see, your daughter lives in Encino, doesn't she? That must be quite a trip for you.
MAY: Yes, it is. It's painful to travel sometimes, and I wonder about living so far away from her . . .
COUNSELOR: I've been meaning to talk to you about your present housing, May. It's important that you anticipate a more protected living environment, in preparation for the time when you . . .

Needless to say, May did not bring up the incident with the widower again. Clearly, her feelings about this man were not to be part of this counseling situation. If I were May, I'd wonder if my counselor were saying, "Cool it! Forget about men and prepare for total disability."

Many professionals who don't feel comfortable talking to older women individually about sexuality do refer clients to group settings. The personal sharing in many group settings can be most valuable.

Personal growth groups, exercise and discussion groups, assertiveness classes, and many other kinds of classes for women are ideal for promoting enhanced self-image, redefinition of values, and encouragement in terms of sexual functioning. Some older women need to talk about their past sexual identities and experiences in order to lay them to rest. Others seem to become reenergized and more expansive in their socialization through the affectional warmth of a close community, the group. A minority risk new sexual behaviors through verbally exploring them in a trusting group context. Older women need to hear other women of all ages talk about their dreams, desires, and experiences in order to feel "normal."

As a group therapist, I do not allow older women to ignore the sexual side of themselves, even if the outcome of their life review is to say, "I will not risk anymore; everything I am as a woman is in the past." An honest acknowledgment like this can free life energy to be involved in areas of life other than sexuality. As long as a group leader is unconditionally accepting of where each particular woman is in her sexual development (past, present, or future) and does not program where she "ought" to be, a group experience can be helpful. There is vicarious participation in the sharing of other women, and this can be valuable to the woman who chooses not to share her own thoughts, feelings, and fantasies. The key word is *choice*. If a woman has the right to talk or not talk about her sexuality, leave the group or stay, cry or not cry, then sexual redefinition can occur. We helpers need to remind ourselves continuously that older women may have few or no outlets for the sexual expression they desire. Then, expanding the options outlined earlier in this paper becomes crucial.

One woman in her 50s who was scarred by mastectomy said, "I had to learn that there are loving men out there who care more about the feelings inside my breast than what it looks like on the outside." We are attracted to those older women who carry themselves with such joy and dignity that we respond to their inner vitality, not their outer shell! These are the women who will teach us who are helpers how to relate to fully sexual females—who will expand our horizons and diminish our fears in terms of what it means to be a woman and to be old.

Summary

To be an older woman means a variety of things: having a partner or having no partner; being accepted or being ostracized by our families for sexual behavior; colluding with or refusing to collude with our youth-oriented society in terms of what we may feel, think, and do sexually; risking relating to our bodies in sexual ways or hibernating sexually for the rest of our lives. These are not either/or's. They are simply statements to encourage you to look at where *you* are on the continuum, and how you want to help other people.

There are sexual options for women of all ages and stages, but it is particularly important for the older woman to envision all the sexual options she possibly can. These include the option of total denial of sexuality if that is the one that best meets her needs in view of personal circumstances and health. Wilhelm Reich expressed the necessity for individual choice clearly: "Each individual—child, youth, adult, and old person—[has] the right to a sex life corresponding to his or her need, when this need [does] not conflict with the right of other people to their own person" (Raknes, 1976, p. 174).

The helping person has a responsibility to look at his or her own ageism and sexism and the limitations she or he imposes on defining who the older woman may be. The helper needs to put aside the stereotypes of the aging female, which hinder affirmation and appreciation of and enthusiasm about the client's sexual–affectional goals and behaviors. These may vary widely according to the individual's definition of being "in touch" with another. As Montagu (1971) has told us:

> . . . to a very significant extent, a measure of the individual's development as a healthy human being is the extent to which . . . she is freely able to embrace another and enjoy the embraces of others . . . to get, in a very real sense, into touch with others. (p. 308)

Finally, in order to pioneer in areas of sexual thought, feeling, reading, talking, and expressing ourselves, we who are older women must defy the injunction that tells us we may have "come a long way, baby" but we're not going to make it affectionally unless we're young! In order to give ourselves permission to practice who we already are as sexual beings we need the support of professionals, volunteers, friends, and family members. Then, we may be able to broach the fearsome request to another, "Would you like to be with me—in whatever ways are pleasing to us both?" Or, at the very minimum, to say, "My body is good, what I do and have done with my womanliness is good, and I do not have to apologize for being old." Let all of us be more open to praising older women for their sexual wisdom, beauty, and depth of expression—past, present, and future!

REFERENCES

Caughey, J. L. Media mentors. *Psychology Today*, 1978, 12(4), 44–49.
Hale, J., Norman, A. D., Bogle, J., & Shaul, S., The Task Force on Concerns of Physically

Disabled Women. *Within Reach*, Planned Parenthood of Snohomish County, Inc., 1977, 4.

Kaplan, H. S., & Sager, C. J. Sexual patterns at different ages. *Medical Aspects of Human Sexuality*, 1971, 5(6), 10–19.

Mannes, M. *They*. New York: Doubleday, 1968.

Montagu, A. *Touching: The human significance of the skin*. New York: Harper & Row, 1971.

Preston, C. E. An old bag: The stereotype of the older woman. *No longer young: The older woman in America, Proceedings of the 26th Annual Conference on Aging*. University of Michigan–Wayne State University, 1975.

Raknes, O. *Wilhelm Reich and orgonomy*. Baltimore: Penguin, 1976.

Sarton, M. *The house by the sea*. New York: Norton, 1977.

Sontag, S. The double standard of aging. *Saturday Review of Literature,* September 23, 1972, 1, p. 55.

Discussion of Chapter 5

Aging and Female Sexuality

J. Robert Bragonier

In my opinion, Ms. Genevay has done a service to women by focusing attention on the traditionally scandalous and still generally embarrassing subject of sexuality in the aging woman. However, she may have added to the confusion surrounding this subject by her inconsistency in definition of the term *sexuality*. She states, for example, that "The facets of sexuality simply multiply with aging," implying that they include "all the sensory, nongenital and genital thoughts, feelings, fantasies, dreams, and behavior in [a woman's] rich life history." She then proceeds to describe, as examples of older women who choose denial as a sexual option, Anna, who reports "fantasies and dreams with sexual content," and Ellen, a "very vital woman, indeed," whose "face glows and eyes shine after a warm hug from the minister or many of the other men and women . . . in the church." If these women are denying their sexuality, the implication is that to be sexual is only to be "doing it," an implication with which I believe Ms. Genevay would heartily disagree.

I concur with the author that female sexuality includes all those aspects of personality that relate to being a women. By that definition, I would conclude that Ellen is not only a "very vital woman, indeed," but a very sexual woman as well, although one who has chosen not to express one of the many facets of her sexuality.

My reason for emphasizing this point is my concern that excessive emphasis on genital expression of sexuality is a problem for many persons, men and women, of all ages:

1. Young persons may risk unintended pregnancy, or premature intimacy, because they don't recognize that there are noncoital ways of expressing and sharing sexuality.

J. Robert Bragonier, M.D., Ph.D. • Adjunct Associate Professor, Department of Obstetrics and Gynecology, Harbor–UCLA Medical Center, Torrance, California 90509.

2. Older persons, especially those with ill health or disability, may suffer loss of self-esteem, and loss of opportunities for self-expression and intimacy, because they mistakenly believe that, without a firm, erect penis and mutual (if not simultaneous) orgasms, there is no sexual expression.
3. Persons of any age may be trapped by the need to meet ever-escalating performance goals, whether they be sexual gymnastics, multiple orgasms, or the "zipless fuck."

That having been said, my experience with older women as a gynecologist suggests that an increasing number are appreciating the genital aspects of sexuality into their later years. There are a number of reasons that they are ideally suited to do so. The fear of pregnancy, which so many women experience as a major inhibiting factor in their enjoyment of intercourse, is no longer an issue. They have had time enough for the effects of early sex-negative learning to wear off. The constant physical and emotional drain of a dependent family, a frequent factor in the chronic fatigue and "sexual anorexia" of the young mother, has diminished. And finally, although their importance is not completely understood, circulating androgens within these women's bodies are no longer opposed by high levels of estrogen. Androgens, present in both men and women, are believed to be primarily responsible for the establishment and maintenance of libido. Their relatively higher concentration with respect to estrogens may contribute to heightened postmenopausal sexual interest.

There are, however, several other factors that exert a negative influence on sexual intercourse for the menopausal woman. Health-care providers have become more knowledgeable in the management of vaginal inflammation and dryness, conditions that frequently diminish a menopausal woman's enjoyment of coitus. Better bacteriologic techniques, more accurate recognition of causative organisms, and more appropriate modes of therapy have helped to alleviate discomfort due to bacterial vaginitis. Estrogen therapy has both decreased susceptibility of the vaginal membrane to infection and increased its capacity to lubricate. In addition, estrogens may be useful in treating painful uterine cramps during orgasm.

Masters and Johnson reported spastic contractions of the uterus with orgasm in some menopausal women in 1970. These contractions may last for one or more minutes and may be experienced as lower abdominal pain, sometimes radiating to the vagina, the groin, or one or both legs. If estrogens are used for this or other signs or symptoms of estrogen deficiency, current recommendations are that low doses be used in an interrupted regimen, such as conjugated estrogens 0.3 mg or ethinyl estradiol 0.02 mg daily for three weeks out of four. Because of continuing concern about the possible relationship between estrogen and cancer of the breast and the uterus, some authorities in addition are recommending giving a progestogen, such as medroxyprogesterone acetate 10 mg, daily during the last 5–10 days of estrogen administration, to decrease the amount of unopposed estrogen to which breasts and uterus are exposed. For symptoms due to vaginal dryness, estrogen creams applied locally are the usual recommendation.

If painful uterine contractions with orgasm do not respond to estrogen administration, recent advances brought about by increased understanding of menstrual cramps may be helpful. Drugs have been identified that inhibit prostaglandins, substances released in the body that cause contraction of smooth muscle such as is found in the uterus. The woman with uterine spasms might ask her physician to prescribe one of these drugs for use prior to intercourse. They are ibuprofen 400 mg, mefenamic acid 250 mg, and naproxen 250 mg.

REFERENCE

Masters, W. H., & Johnson, V. E. *Human sexual inadequacy*. Boston: Little, Brown, 1970.

PART II

Special Circumstances

Chapter 6

The Cradle of Sexual Politics

Incest

LOUISE ARMSTRONG

EDITOR'S NOTE TO CHAPTERS 6 AND 7

Freud was ambivalent about his discovery, reported in **Studies of Hysteria** *in 1896, both that the sexual abuse of female children was more frequent than suspected and that it endangered the psychological health of the victim in later years. His own ambivalence plus the outraged criticism of his colleagues, in a culture where fathers could do no wrong, forced his continued questioning of his "seduction theory" and led to his discovery of infantile sexual fantasies (including his own) and the oedipal period in psychosexual development. The recognition of the power of fantasies and the regularity of "sexual" fantasies about the parents led to the theory that the origin of the neurosis was to be found in the repression of the conflicting desires and fears of that period. The oedipal father was vindicated, and professional enthusiasm delved ever deeper into the no-longer-innocent psyche of the child. While Freud, in a 1924 footnote to his original paper, made clear that he still believed that actual sexual abuse did take place and did cause later difficulties, his followers' pursuit of fantasies ignored the impulse-ridden father and left the victimized child unacknowledged and unprotected. Fantasies play a powerful role in psychological health and illness. However, to believe that incest is limited to fantasy is to be as provincial as those who believe that only "facts" count. If repressed incestuous fantasies were the cause of hysteria, one would expect a plethora of male hysterics, since testosterone gives such urgency and intensity to male sexuality. If sexual abuse of girls is more common than expected, then why*

LOUISE ARMSTRONG ● Author: *Kiss Daddy Goodnight: A Speak-out on Incest;* National Women's Health Network, Washington, D.C. 20008.

has hysteria almost disappeared—or is the contemporary woman's common complaint of arousal or orgasmic difficulty the hysteria of our time? Should we suspect early sexual abuse in every case of such complaints? After reading these papers, I believe that we should have that suspicion more regularly than we have in the past. Fantasies (i.e., the mental consequences of these events) may make the difference in degree and style of later neurotic difficulties.

There are some investigators who believe that incest experience can occur without bad consequence, even with occasional "good" effects (e.g., Warren Farrell, The Last Taboo, *unpublished research). This may be the fitting cover-up for oedipally driven fathers in a contemporary culture that emphasizes unrestricted sex as an ideal. Nevertheless, the oedipal theory is more than a cover-up for fathers' abuse of daughters. It is a value tool for understanding a part of early psychological experience. We do not know the consequences when the experience becomes reality. We can't know without more sophisticated and detailed research. It is hoped that these papers will provide a more balanced perspective of such little girls' sexual and psychological experience and aid in our making our research and therapy more sensitive, thorough, and compassionate.*

Remember when sexual abuse of children by fathers and stepfathers "didn't happen"? Now, the "rate of incidence is so high as to make prohibition absurd" (DeMott, 1980, p. 12).

Remember when incest was popularly thought to be a "dread taboo"? Now, it's a symptom of a "dysfunctional family."

It was only a few years ago that those of us who had been sexually abused as children by our fathers and stepfathers or older brothers began speaking out. We did so, then, with considerable and sensible apprehension. The sexual use of children had historically received overt permission (Rush, 1980). Child molestation within the family had long had tacit permission.

For centuries, the rubric of dread and horror had served to mask actual, prevalent gross male misbehaviors against the children in their care. For centuries, strong forces had held children, and women abused as children, in silence. There were terrifying threats against our speaking out: threats implicit in our total dependency as children, our property status; threats of our being excommunicated from the world of respectability—a threat to our very survival; threats of our being branded "demoralized"; threats of our being called whore, of our being blamed as seducers, of our not even being believed.

Since we spoke out, two major attitudes have emerged toward child molestation by adult male caretakers: the *treatment* attitude, and that of the *pro-incest lobby*. I want to speculate here, from a political perspective, on both these formulations insofar as they represent— obviously in very different kind, different style, different degree—new permissions for the continuing tradition of what might be referred to as the *sexually abusive parent syndrome* (SAPS).

A disclaimer is called for. I am not questioning the need for some form of treatment—particularly supportive treatment for the child-victim and for the secondary victim, the mother. Nor am I questioning the validity of family therapy theory or, in individual cases, its effectiveness.

Rather, I'd like to ask this question: What are the social–political implications of the most prevalent form of current treatment in a child-sexual-abuse context where the goal is to keep the abusive family intact? I'd like to question the social–political effects of applying an individual-illness or individual-family-illness perspective to an issue that is power-based and power-assumed in its nature and its tradition, an issue that, indeed, may be seen as the cradle of sexual politics.

The testimony of violated children, and of women who were violated in their homes as children, is now everywhere—and can be heard by any who choose to listen (Armstrong, 1978; Brady, 1979).

Those who have listened know that the primary effects of abuse were *socializing* effects. We experienced shame at being used to gratify adult male needs. We felt powerlessness and rage—an inner-directed rage. We tried to forget, to pretend it wasn't happening. We tried, during the episodes, to not-exist (Shengold, 1979).

Were this offense against us placed in a criminal law context, the charge many of us would make against our fathers would be repeated, premeditated sexual assault of a minor in trust—whether or not there was violence used, whether or not it was alleged by the perpetrator to be only "natural."

In all likelihood, our fathers' plea would be legal insanity.[1] They did not acknowledge that they were doing anything wrong. They were "teaching." They were "initiating." From a transcript of a TV show which featured an offending father in drab silhouette: "I actually in my own mind back then, I thought I was doing her a favor" (Donahue, 1979, p. 10).

---

[1] The M'Naughton test states that a man will be presumed to have behaved irresponsibly unless it is "clearly proved that at the time of committing the act, the party accused was labouring under such a defect of reason from disease of the mind as to not know the nature and quality of the act he was doing: or if he did know it that he did not know that what he was doing was wrong." (Daniel M'Naughton's case, House of Lords, 8 Engl. Rep., 1843, cited in Kittrie, 1971, p. 23)

Another father, caught, said, "I am a decent man. I provide for my family. I don't run around on my wife, and I've never slept with anyone except my wife and my daughters" (MacFarlane, 1978, p. 90).

For all the brouhaha, then, it is insupportable to assert that sexually invading one's own child is seen, or has ever been seen, by individual males as so reprehensible or horrifying as to be unjustifiable. The result of the stereotype of "dread" and the assumption of "moral outrage" has been to reinforce a widespread secondary myth: that that sort of thing doesn't happen. Universal emphasis on that public belief kept those of us who had been exploited effectively isolated. We each thought we were the only one. Collective denial, cloaked in epic language, supported the continuation of a privately assumed male "right"—a right that goes far back in history.

We can, I think, divide the history of that "right" into three periods.

The age of *permitted abuse* was that long, dark age of unexamined, uncontested patriarchal prerogative. Fathers wielded absolute power over their children's lives: they could be bartered, sold, mutilated, thrashed, starved (or raped) without recourse (Gil, 1970; Tamilia, 1971). Talmudic law decreed that betrothal and marriage could not take place before the age of 3 years and 1 day. That was not, however, a magnanimous protection of 2-year-olds. It simply said that females under 3 had no sexual validity—and therefore no virginity to lose (Rush, 1980). Even comparing the father–child relationship with that of master and servant would be inadequate, since the child had none of the rights of a servant (Giovannoni & Becerra, 1979). Within a totally patriarchal structure, sexual use of children was permitted and presumed.

With the wash of fastidious public morality in the Victorian era, the actuality of child sexual abuse went underground. Freud, listening to women tell of their having been sexually abused as children by their fathers, originally believed them. However, based on the alarming prevalence of these stories, and on introspection about his own childhood, he decided the stories could not be true; they must be fantasies originating with the child's wishes (Blumenthal, 1981; Herman, 1981; Klein & Tribich, 1979; Peters, 1976; Rush, 1980; Sheleff, 1981). We entered the age of *denied abuse.*

The Freudian theory of childhood sexuality, popularized, gave the public the understanding that "those things" did not often happen, but that children often wished they would.

This understanding had a double effect. It denied any incidence of real child molestation within the family, and it created disbelief of any child or woman who complained. And where the girl was dangerously persistent in her story, it rendered her the culprit, the seductress.

It was a recurring theme in my original 183 interviews with women who had been molested sexually as children, within the home, that when they sought psychiatric help, they were not believed (Armstrong, 1978).

Now, if present indications can be accurately read, we are entering the age of *no-fault abuse*.

It is hard to remember, given the present bloom of the incest industry, that a few short years ago, the incest taboo was publicly intact. This sort of thing did not take place, certainly not among "nice" people (although a lot of us fantasized that it happened, mind). When it did take place—by public and professional assumption—it was in places like Appalachia, among some morally defective "others."

When it was irrefutably discovered, the professional literature continued to make respectful reference to a paper written in the 1930s which stated:

> The most remarkable feature presented by these children who have experienced sexual relations with adults was that they showed less evidence of fear, anxiety, guilt or psychic trauma than might be expected. . . . The probation reports from the court frequently remarked about their brazen poise, which was interpreted as an especially inexcusable and deplorable attitude and one indicating their fundamental incorrigibility. (Bender & Blau, 1939, p. 511)

It was publicly assumed that when it was discovered, child molestation by father or stepfather would be treated as a heinous crime.

Indeed, although the past shows some isolated convictions, since the passing of the first Juvenile Court Act in Illinois in 1899, virtually all of the cases of child sexual abuse that came to light before the 1970s went to juvenile or family courts: courts that are, by their definition, nonpunitive of offenders; courts with the express goal of keeping the family intact. Their existence was originally precipitated by the pressures of social workers and child welfare reformers, far more concerned with predelinquency in children than with adult abuses of them (Platt, 1969). And it has always been to the social services that these courts have turned.

Where there were adversary criminal prosecutions, a random review of actual cases turned up these citations:

> *State* v. *Kurtz* (1917): "Where the daughter with whom defendant was accused of having incestuous relations was 16 years of age at the time the act charged was committed, and according to her testimony she and defen-

dant had been having illicit relations for a period of about a year before the date of such act, the court stated that she was an accomplice whose uncorroborated testimony was insufficient to uphold a conviction."

McClure v. *State* (1923): "Where, according to prosecutrix's own testimony, the incestuous intercourse with her father continued from the time she was 11 years of age until she was 22, being repeated once or twice a week during all the aforementioned period . . . the court said it could not believe it possible that these acts could have occurred as testified to by the prosecutrix without her consent, and that the irresistible conclusion from all the evidence was that she was an accomplice in the performance of the act, *if it occurred*" [italics added].

People v. *Oliver* (1941 Co. Ct.): ". . . the court without expressly stating whether the act was with the consent of the daughter, who was 18 years or more of age held that she was an accomplice and her evidence must be corroborated. But it is to be noted, as possibly tending to show some sort of consent on the part of the female that she testified that the father had had sexual intercourse with her during the past 8 years, and the court said that the testimony was absolutely incredible, and that it was of the opinion that the prosecutrix was a wayward girl, and was attempting to 'hang' her father for her own delinquencies." (*American Law Reports*, 1960, pp. 710–711)

As recently as 1975, a major paper in the *Stanford Law Review* advocated treating incest/child sexual abuse as noncriminal, citing as one reason questionable harm. The author stated, "I believe that such conduct may not always be harmful and therefore that the term 'abuse' may be inappropriate. While it will be used in this section, no condemnation of the behavior is intended" (Wald, 1975, p. 985n). He cited further "the likelihood of a criminal prosecution against the parents" (p. 1026) and took it as a given that "criminal prosecution will often result in the father's imprisonment" (p. 1027).

In a 1979 paper in the *Saint Louis Law Journal*, M. Leahy endorsed the need for corroboration in incest cases, suggesting that juries would be more sympathetic to a child-sexual-abuse victim than to a rape victim, and taking full account of children's alleged fantasies (Leahy, 1979).

As Leahy perceived the problem:

The typical incest situation involves at least three people. . . . At minimum it entails the unconscious participation and/or sanction by a parent who is not overtly involved in the sexual activities. . . . The non-participating member will sometimes deny the existence of incestuous behavior to herself even after having observed the incestuous pair holding hands or sleeping in the same bed. . . . A sexual relationship between father and daughter usually arises when the mother who has become physically estranged from her husband pushes the daughter forward as a substitute to preserve the family. (p. 750)

Referring to young girls' well-publicized tendencies to fantasize, Leahy said,

Even presuming that there is an incestuous relationship occurring in the home, there may be some inherent difficulty in ascertaining beyond a reasonable doubt that it was the complaining witness who was involved. Sometimes, nonparticipant siblings have seen or are aware of the acts of incest. Such knowledge can cause premature stimulation of the child's sex drives. . . .

. . . One can well imagine the situation in which the offspring shares his [sic] fantasy with a friend who in turn reports the story to law enforcement authorities. Zealous inquiries by authorities may change dream into reality. (p. 760)

As for the use of psychiatric testimony by way of corroboration: "There is no doubt that psychiatric evaluations are less reliable than even polygraphy results" (p. 761).

Moreover,

the prosecuting witness can always present a believable account of the relationship. As long as the witness can describe a sex act, regardless of whether it occurred with the defendant, her accusations can be considered credible. (p. 762)

After all, then, despite the "familiar clichés" that "characterize children as honest, pure and truthful," the author of the cited paper supports the need for corroboration which, he tells us, was originally "intended to avoid baseless accusations, neutralize possible jury sympathy for the victim, and place the complaining witness's motives under close scrutiny." This was necessary because it was

believed that many females file false charges of sexual assaults out of malice, amorality or hostility, shame or bitterness after having given consent, a desire to shield pregnancy caused by another, a yearning for notoriety, a confusion, or a tendency to fantasize. (p. 753)

Although some version of child sexual abuse by male caretakers is on the books as a crime in every state, it is, in most states, a crime without a criminal. Indeed, fewer than 15% of *all* child abuse and neglect cases ever enter the "legal/law" system—that is, either the criminal justice or the juvenile court system (American Humane Association, 1979). In those few places in the country where criminal convictions are sought, the goal is often to sentence the offender to therapy.

All that can be said for a law's existence under a nonprosecution policy is that (1) it offers a clear, but minimal and eventually transparent, threat to the caught offender—that he'd better "volunteer" for therapy, and (2) it allows us to think of ourselves publicly as possessed of virtue, while within the home it's business as usual.

Yet, with public awareness, a crisis arose—not of conscience, but of more practical concern. With the news that incest "cut across all socioeconomic lines," it was inescapable that we were talking about bankers and burghers, as well as busboys. The *assumed* reality—that men were likely to do jail time for child molestation—caused serious concern when it seemed to threaten some of our most solid citizens.

A social policy toward dealing with this now visibly widespread behavior had to be formulated. Justification for that policy had to be made.

Neatly, sexual abuse was slotted into a preexisting policy structure: the identification and treatment, by mental health professionals, of family disorders. The social work concern with child welfare issues had begun in the nineteenth century. However, its most recent and solid mandate came with the discovery and the national acknowledgment of the extensive nature of physical child abuse in this country.

It's interesting that when Henry Kempe delivered his research findings on child battering, he renamed the issue the *battered child syndrome*. This label played down the deviant aspects and played up the medical ones; it played down the legal liability and played up the need for treatment intervention (Nelson, 1978).

With the National Child Abuse Prevention and Treatment Act of 1974, the social goal for our response to child sexual abuse was sealed: it was the identification, treatment, and prevention of child abuse. The purpose of treatment was to keep the families intact. Indeed, 30 of the 50 states and the District of Columbia have "purpose clauses" that contain a "preserve-the-family" statement (American Humane Association, 1979).

And so incest, that recent monolithic bugaboo, found a snug and ready-made home. The family-treatment model, retooled for incest families, had won the franchise (Sherman, 1977). Justifications for this approach were easy.

Preserving the family continues to exceed even balancing the budget as a promise certain to win popular support—whether in spite of or because of an escalating divorce rate and an ever-rising number of single-parent households.

Specters were raised. The mothers would all go on welfare if the abusive provider were to be removed to jail. Or the *child* would be removed (a common solution, still, when dealing—as family–juvenile court mainly does deal—with the poor).

And so the punitive stance that was the publicly assumed stance on child molestation when we thought it happened only among the lower classes and degenerates was unacceptable when we discovered the prevalence of this mischief among the proper.

Given child welfare history, we could certainly have foreseen this (Coll, 1977; Leiby, 1977). What we could not have foreseen was just how the one major wrinkle of the treatment model would be ironed out. Whose is the illness to be treated?

Unlike clearly pathological acts with implications of overwhelming, out-of-control rage, sexual abuse of one's child requires remarkable planning, forethought, and care. Mommy has to be out of the house. Siblings have to be sent to the movies. Where Daddy resists using out-and-out coercion, he has to think about negotiating at least minimal accession on Susie's part.

One woman described this early experience to me not long ago:

> I was playing in the corner. Daddy was lying on the couch. He said, "Sally, come here." I said, "I don't want to, Daddy. I'm playing." And he said "Come here and play with my mousie." And I said, "I don't want to, Daddy. I'm playing with my dollie." And he said, "Well, bring your dollie. She can watch you play with my mousie."

Trouble arose as it quickly became apparent that these men did not see that they had done anything wrong. The majority, caught playing doctor with their kids, were not sociopathic, or "ill," in any previously conceived sense. They were the "pillars of the community." (That, with the "tip of the iceberg," became the paradigmatic cliché of incest.)

In any case, the anomaly had to be faced that to be ill to the degree that you are not accountable for child molestation is, in the public mind, to be very ill indeed.[2] An answer had to be found to the question: Why would an otherwise solid citizen "do such a thing"? The answer from the family systems theorists printed out: It was not entirely, or even mostly, his doing. The entire family was dysfunctional before the abuse. Mother was collusive, invariably. She always knew *on some level*.[3]

The beauty of this explanation, politically, was that it played on a mitigating underlying assumption that is so prevalent and so deeply ingrained that it cannot be questioned: It is the wife's job to control her husband's behavior; she is the causative factor—whether he drinks, plays around, or diddles his daughter; men are not equally responsible as parents; men are children.

---

[2] No amount of evidence that wife batterers and child molesters are frequently "pillars of the community" seems to stem the search for some kind of pathological trigger; nor divert the need to find "widespread deviance." Stress and alcohol continue to be major contenders. Even though "most existing research seems to support the conclusion that alcohol does not cause marital violence, that the link is not cause and effect" (Hindman, 1979), "research projects still attempt to show that it does" (Langley & Levy, 1978, p. 72).

[3] This attitude is so prevalent, it seems whimsical to cite one or five sources for it. It can be found most baldly stated in Greene (1977).

Now, by emphasizing her involvement, his has been gracefully diminished. There is no criminal, no crime victim, no ill male adult. There is a "dysfunctional family" with interacting problems, a male adult who exhibits "inappropriate behavior," and a "domineering, cowardly, passive, manipulative" mother (Kempe & Kempe, 1978; Schultz, 1965; Greene, 1977; Cooper, 1978).

Incest is not the problem. It is only the symptom.

The political effect of this actual, if not literal, decriminalization is once more tacitly to exonerate the adult male who molests his own child and to trivialize totally repeated acts of sexual invasion of a minor in trust.

The fact that the mother is implicated in the therapy suggests to the community that she was indeed a significant partner in the abuse. The effect of this "enlightened" approach is to *refuse any genuine repeal of permission.*

There is a further political effect. It is the lesson in sexual politics learned by the child. One clear message she gets is that her future role will be to accept culpability for what men do, and that it is necessary to do this—or *anything*—to keep the man of the house in the house.

What of the women who refuse this path? What happens to them? Given the number of studies completed, studies in progress, and studies planned, this population has received a degree of inattention commensurate with the need to believe that it doesn't exist.

Yet all over the country, I have heard from women who, on discovering the abuse of their child by their husband, do not choose to keep the family intact. Typically, the woman kicks the man out. She prosecutes. He is remanded to three months' counseling. She sues for divorce. In the divorce proceedings, he is awarded weekend custody of the child.

One woman, in Louisville, went back to court after the child consistently affirmed that the abuse was continuing. A psychiatrist saw the child and verified by affidavit that the abuse was actual and ongoing. The judge then removed total custody from the mother, gave custody to the child's father, and enjoined the mother from seeing or communicating with the child in any way.[4]

Roland Summit, psychiatrist at Harbor–UCLA Medical Center and author of chapter 7, has written:

> Mothers who leave a sexually abusive husband may go bankrupt trying to buy testimony that will challenge the father's demands for child custody. If a woman allows [sic] sexual abuse to go on under her roof she is accused

---

[4] A partial transcript of this case is on file at the National Center on Women and Family Law in New York City.

for setting up the abuse. If she separates with her children, she is accused
of inventing prejudicial stories to block her estranged husband's legitimate
access to his children. (Summit, 1981, unpaginated)

I also have testimony from women who, on discovering their
child's molestation, went to the police—only to find themselves charged
with neglect. This can happen when the report is made to child protective workers as well (Davidson & Bulkley, 1980, p. 7).

How often do these things happen? More research is needed. It is
unlikely that I have heard the only such stories in the country.

We were right, it would seem, to fear speaking out, to be apprehensive. We were right, as were our mothers, and their mothers, and
their mothers, about the powerful underground forces that work to
permit child sexual molestation by fathers, forces that would lash back
if we spoke out.

But look at what we could not have foreseen—the backlash with a
Barnum & Bailey tone: Step right up, ladies and gentlemen, and watch
the incest taboo dive from 3,000 feet into 2 inches of water and explode. This, truly, was a new and unanticipated act, performed by
"well-known researchers and a few allies in academe" ("Attacking the
Last Taboo," 1980).

In the name of sexual enlightenment, and vaunting the straw man
of "taboo"—newly unveiled as "moralistic" superstition—these
professionals march through the crowd selling "positive incest."

And their alleged goal? Preserving the family (DeMott, 1980).

One expert asked whether the lack of "touching" and "affection"
in families may not be contributing to family instability. (And here
it's interesting to note the therapeutic professionals' estimation that
incest is a symptom of family instability, as well as the permissivists'
estimation that it is the absence of "expressive gestures of feeling"
that is a *cause* of family instability.)

So what seemed, in 1977, like the lunatic fringe—the René Guyon
Society, for instance, with its slogan "Sex by year 8 or else it's too
late"—had huddled with experts and reappeared in the 1980s with a
new marketing strategy.

And a scary one. They are selling as "new" and "improved" a
behavior that has existed as a popular though low-profile product for
centuries; therefore, they must be taken as a serious threat. Whether
or not they get their package marketed, they are giving overt endorsement to a behavior that now has no serious penalty.

They are selling something a significant number of men have always bought on the sly. Now these men are offered the opportunity
to purchase it nicely packaged, over the counter, with a scientific im-
primatur for its use.

The "pro-incest lobby" trades on an assumption that adult–child sexual involvement represents progress, and on an assumption that there's a public attitude "that no matter how benign, any adult–child interaction that may be construed as even remotely sexual qualifies, a priori, as traumatic and abusive." (Money & Williams, *Traumatic Abuse and Neglect of Children,* cited in "Attacking the Last Taboo," 1980) Yet, in another argument, they claim that the rate of incidence is so high as to make prohibition absurd (DeMott, 1980).

Which ring are you watching?

They say, "It is time to admit that incest need not be a perversion, or a symptom of mental illness" ("Attacking the Last Taboo," 1980), but, except for lip service, it never has been seriously seen that way. Child molesters have always been thought of as people who molest *other* people's children. For the fathers who initiated the sexual intrusions on their own children, it has simply always been an assumed, just-don't-get-caught prerogative, with minuscule risk of significant penalty. And the only reason that it's "time to admit" anything is that we have only now increased the risk of their getting caught, only now begun to expose the cover-up of the "taboo," only now begun to threaten that we might get word to the children that it is their right to say no.

So, as in a western film, we have driven them out into the open. The only trouble is that in real life the bad guys often win.

Further, the permissivists say, "Incest between children and adults . . . can sometimes be beneficial." Take two children every four hours and call me in the morning.

They place a call for research by scientists who "possess the guts to find out what is really happening" (DeMott, 1980, p. 11).

The fact is, of course, that we have begun to find out what is really happening. (And they must know, too, in order to claim that the incidence is so high it's not worth bothering about.) What is really happening is that fathers are sexually violating their daughters, often starting when the children are 3, 4, or 5 years old. They are using them repeatedly, often for years, for their own gratification. They are frightening them into silence. They are justifying their behavior.

In other words, what's really happening is what has always happened. The only radical departure is our speaking out about it, against it. That is radical. And that takes "guts." The only news in the new permission is that it is overt. There is nothing either radical or gutsy about an attempt to institutionalize the status quo.

In any case, what it takes to find incidences of "positive" memories of sexual violation among women is not guts. One way is to accuse us of misremembering. Another is to apply thumbs judiciously to our palpable, generational fear of being found defective, "dis-honored," "scarred forever." Just ask the wrong question. Women who have found their way to survival from paternal sexual betrayal are going to be reluctant to say that they feel damaged beyond repair. This could surely elevate the "nontraumatic" sample (Ramey, 1979).

Dr. Roland Summit has said:

> The one area of the "patient literature" that is most often reflected in the permissivists is the one most ardently rejected by modern research. That is the persistent notion that if girls were seduced by their fathers and claimed that they didn't like it, they must either have brought it on them-selves and been disappointed in their wish-fulfillment or else they remem-bered it wrong.
>
> This kind of reluctance to accept a woman's discomfort at face value and the insistence that girls really want to sleep with their fathers trace back to an early fascination with the Oedipus complex in post-Freudian literature. The early psychoanalytic literature tends to characterize the girls in incestuous experiences as seductive and provocative, as well as empha-sizing the distortions and overtones of wishful fantasy in children's recol-lections of incest. Such literature is seldom quoted anymore except by die-hards trying to discount the realities of paternal seduction and by defense attorneys seeking to discredit a daughter's testimony. (Personal communi-cation)

A surer way to find "positive" incest is to mix in a goodly number of consenting-age cohabiting first cousins with a smaller amount of adult–child involvement.

Dr. Summit said:

> Common sense anticipates that a sexual relationship between two consent-ing adults who happen to be related (as with cousins) will tend to have different consequences than sexual needs visited by a father on his five-year-old child. In the latter instance any relevance of the blood relationship is clearly secondary to the issues of authority, responsibility, and the stew-ardship of the child. (Personal communication)

Yet what is clear is not seen clearly.

One researcher asked, "Who knows whether one result [of bend-ing over backwards to avoid any possibility of incestuous involve-ment] may not be the present rash of feverish adolescent sexual activ-ity with its undeniable results?" (Ramey, 1979, p. 7).

Its "undeniable results," if I read between the lines correctly, are the rate of teenage pregnancy. This argument plays on the myth that we are talking, primarily, about child molestation that begins at ado-lescence. The statistics are strikingly at odds with that assumption. It also, amusingly, assumes that Daddy, with his position of adult au-thority, would see to it that Susie remembered to use her diaphragm, something none of her rash and feverish peers could be trusted to do.

"How many adolescent girls have not said," Ramey went on, " 'It's the only time I feel someone really loves me'?" (p. 7).

I don't know how many girls have not said that, but to equate sexual exploitation with love is apparently, in their minds, a good thing, and to teach this lesson early will surely save later males a lot of time and trouble.

As Florence Rush (1974) has said:

> Sexual abuse of girl children is permitted because it is an unspoken but prominent factor in socializing and preparing the female to accept a subordinate role: to feel guilty, ashamed, and to tolerate, through fear, the power exercised over her by men. . . . The female's sexual experiences prepare her to submit later in life to the adult forms of sexual abuse heaped on her by her boyfriend, her lover, and her husband. In short, the sexual abuse of female children is a process of education that prepares them to become the wives and mothers of America. (pp. 73–74)

A further argument as we watch the "taboo" plummet toward the puddle is that it is guilt about the act that causes more damage to those involved than the act itself (DeMott, 1980).

As we have learned, the men who sexually abuse their children do not feel guilty; they do not, of course, call it abuse. Men who repeatedly slug their wives do not call it battering. Abuse and battering are what other people do. "Teaching" and "initiating" are what these men see themselves doing as generous and loving fathers.

So it must be *our* guilt they are trying to obviate.

Indeed, many of us did experience guilt. But it came from Daddy, from fear he instilled:

"Don't tell Mommy," fathers will say. "She'll blame you."

Or, as Maggie's father said, "Do you know what happens to little girls if they do this sort of thing? They'll lock you up for the rest of your life."

We were *not* guilty about enjoyment. We did not enjoy sexual violation. There was little to be found enjoyable in being exploited, used, "conquered." Perhaps this is why wisdom has it that incest is ruinous for boys.[5] It is a social shame indeed for them to be similarly sexually conquered. And we knew we were being used and coerced in a most gratuitous way.

Dr. Summit said:

> In our experience, the greatest loss of self-worth comes not from the guilt of engaging in forbidden sexual activity but from parental betrayal and abandonment of the child to the status of a sex object. The guilt comes far

---

[5]Ramey (1979) said Kinsey's data suggest that "some practitioners of incest have not been horribly damaged by their experience" (p. 1).

less from having "taken part" in the relationship than it does from the child's sense of being so bad that her father would do such a thing to her and that her mother would allow it to happen. (Personal communication)

It was certainly an error to assume that child sexual abuse within the family, like child battering, would be what is referred to in political science as a valence issue, one of those issues that "elicit strong, fairly uniform effective responses and thus do not have an adversarial duality, in contrast to position issues for which there are at least two alternative sets of preferences" (Nelson, 1978) Obviously, it is our preference as children *not* to be violated by our fathers. And it is their preference to violate us.

It was perhaps an error as well to use the word *incest* for the *problem* of incest: sexual abuse of a child by a needed and trusted parent, stepparent, or older sibling (not a cousin of consenting age). Perhaps something would be gained, politically, by beginning to speak of the sexually abusive parent syndrome. While (based on the precedent of the battered child syndrome) this would have the drawback of minimizing the legal implications, it would at least point the medical spotlight on the question of why otherwise normal men were and are so sick with the longing to molest their own children.

It has certainly been part of the permissivists' strategy to make child-sexual-abuse permission a rider on the bill touting a who-cares attitude toward adult family romance.

How worried should we be? Very worried, I think.

The pro-incest lobby serves a dangerous permission-giving function in the absence of serious social–legal restraints on sexual abuse.

It took less than overt permission in the past; often it just took Daddy's reading about some tribal practices in a nature magazine.[6]

What (the reader may by now be wondering) is this author advocating? I am advocating that serious attention be given to enforcing legally effective restraint of men who molest their children. There is every evidence that when we strongly disapprove of violations against persons or property, this disapproval is reflected by active attempts to enforce laws. Surely, the concept that we are allowed to do things to members of our own families that we would be arrested for doing to strangers bears scrutiny, as does the reality that these permissions are largely accorded to the male.

Perhaps more than any other issue, incest illuminates the real and continuing nature of the power game that is sexual politics, and the

[6]See Armstrong (1978). Two of the women in the book said their fathers read in a magazine that it was "natural" among some tribes for fathers to "initiate" their daughters.

tremendous, frightening stamina that the vested-interest players have in the game.

More research is certainly needed, but not on why individual fathers do this, nor on the profile of the incestuous father, nor on the profile of the incestuous family—not on whether *we* all become prostitutes or drug addicts, but on the core, dramatic issue: What is the nature of the powerful need on the part of so many men to preserve the permission to exploit their children sexually?

Dr. Summit said to me recently during a phone conversation:

> When I read about [mass child molesters/killers like] Gacey, the teenagers murdered in California, the statistics on child molestation in the family—when I realize the numbers victimized by rape—when I look at any aspect of sexual perversion and the sexualization of violence—when I watch thousands in the justice system and in the professions scapegoating the victims, then I have to wonder why we don't look at the inescapable fact that these are activities engaged in almost exclusively by men. Why do we take this thing one-at-a-time: one-at-a-time in a law, one-at-a-time in treatment? Why don't we look at the common questions: What is it about men? What is there about the condition of being male that demands exclusive domain and preserves an open season for crimes of sexual violence?

Were we to look at that question, we might discover the size and the shape of the cradle of sexual politics. And this paper could be regarded, joyously, as obsolete.

REFERENCES

American Humane Association. *Child protective services entering the 1980's.* Englewood, Colo.: Author, 1979.

American Law Reports (Annotated ALR2d). 1960, 74, pp. 710–711.

Armstrong, L. *Kiss Daddy goodnight: A speakout on incest.* New York: Hawthorn, 1978.

Attacking the last taboo. *Time,* April 14, 1980, p. 72.

Bender, L., & Blau, A. The reaction of children to sexual relations with adults. *American Journal of Orthopsychiatry,* 1939, 7, 500–518.

Blumenthal, R. Did Freud's isolation, peer rejection prompt key theory reversal? *The New York Times,* August 25, 1981, pp. C–1, 2.

Brady, K. *Father's days.* New York: Seaview, 1979.

Coll, B. Social welfare: History. In N. N. Saunders *et al.* (Eds.), *Encyclopedia of Social Work,* 17th issue, Vol. 2. Washington, D.C.: National Association of Social Workers, 1977, pp. 435–440.

Cooper, I. K. Decriminalization of incest—New legal-clinical responses. In J. M. Eekelaar & S. N. Katz (Eds.), *Family violence: An international and interdisciplinary study.* Toronto: Butterworths, 1978, pp. 518–528.

Davidson, H. A., & Bulkley, J. Child sexual abuse: Legal issues and approaches. Monograph by the National Legal Resource Center for Child Advocacy and Protection, American Bar Association, Young Lawyers Division, Washington, D.C., September 1980.

DeMott, B. The pro-incest lobby. *Psychology Today,* March 1980, pp. 11–16.

Donahue, P. Transcript #11099, November 9, 1979, WGN–TV, Chicago.

Gil, D. *Violence against children: Physical child abuse in the United States.* Cambridge, Mass.: Harvard University Press, 1970.

Giovannoni, J. M., & Becerra, R. M. *Defining child abuse.* New York: Free Press, 1979.

Greene, N. B. A view of family pathology involving molest—From a juvenile probation perspective. *Juvenile Justice,* February 1977, pp. 29–34.

Herman, J. L. *Father-daughter incest.* Cambridge, Mass.: Harvard University Press. 1981.

Hindman, M. H. Family violence: An overview. *Alcohol Health and Research World,* 1979, 4 (1).

Kempe, H. C., & Kempe, R. *Child abuse.* Cambridge, Mass.: Harvard University Press, 1978.

Kittrie, N. *The right to be different.* Baltimore: Johns Hopkins Press, 1971.

Klein, M., & Tribich, D. On Freud's blindness. *Colloquium,* 1979, 2(2) pp. 52–59.

Langley, R., & Levy, R. C. *Wife beating: The silent crisis.* New York: Dutton, 1977.

Leahy, M. United States v Bear Runner: The need for corroboration in incest cases. *Saint Louis Law Journal,* 1979, 23, 747–767.

Leiby, J. Social welfare: History of basic ideas. In N. N. Saunders *et al.* (Eds.), *Encyclopedia of Social Work,* 17th issue, Vol. 2. Washington, D.C.: National Association of Social Workers, 1977, pp. 1512–1529.

MacFarlane, K. Sexual abuse of children. In J. R. Chapman & M. Gates (Eds.), *The victimization of women.* Beverly Hills, Ca.: Sage, 1978, pp. 81–109.

Nelson, B. K. Setting the public agenda: The case of child abuse. In J. V. May & A. Wildevsky (Eds.), *The policy cycle.* Beverly Hills, Ca.: Sage, 1978, pp. 17–41.

Platt, A. *The child savers: The invention of delinquency.* University of Chicago Press, 1969.

Peters, J. J. Children who are victims of sexual assault and the psychology of offenders. *American Journal of Psychotherapy,* 1976, 3(3), 398–432.

Ramey, J. Dealing with the last taboo. *SIECUS Report,* 1979, 7(5), 1–7.

Rush, F. Sexual abuse of children: A feminist point of view. In N. Connell & C. Wilson (Eds.), *Rape: The first sourcebook for women.* New York: New American Library, 1974.

Rush, F. *The best kept secret: The sexual abuse of children.* Englewood Cliffs, N.J.: Prentice-Hall, 1980.

Schultz, G. D. *How many more victims? Society and the sex criminal.* Philadelphia: J. B. Lippincott, 1965.

Sheleff, L. *Generations apart: Adult hostility to youth.* New York: McGraw Hill, 1981.

Shengold, L. Child abuse and deprivation: Soul murder. *Journal of American Psychoanalytic Association,* 1979, 27, 533–559.

Sherman, S. M. Family services, family treatment. In N. N. Saunders, *et al.* (Eds.), *Encyclopedia of Social Work,* 17th issue, Vol. 1. Washington, D.C.: National Association of Social Work, 1977, pp. 435–440.

Summit, R. Recognition and treatment of child sexual abuse. In C. E. Hollingsworth (Ed.), *Providing for the emotional health of the pediatric patient.* New York: Spectrum, 1980.

Tamilia, P. R. Neglect proceedings and the conflict between law and social work. *Duquesne Law Review,* 1971, 9, 579–664.

Wald, M. State intervention on behalf of "neglected" children: A search for realistic standards. *Stanford Law Review,* 1975, 27, 985–1040.

Chapter 7

Beyond Belief

The Reluctant Discovery of Incest

ROLAND SUMMIT

As recently as 1962, there was no climate of belief for the fact that children are at substantial risk of injury at the hands of their parents. While the reality of child battering has emerged as inescapable, a corollary discovery is still largely ignored: children, especially girls, are at substantial risk of sexual exploitation at the hands of their parents and trusted caretakers. As Suzanne Sgroi (1978) wrote after years of frustration as a physician trying to encourage protective intervention:

> Sexual Abuse of Children is a crime that our society abhors in the abstract, but tolerates in reality . . . those who try to assist sexually abused children must be prepared to battle against incredulity, hostility, innuendo, and outright harassment. Worst of all, the advocate for the sexually abused child runs the risk of being smothered by indifference and a conspiracy of silence. The pressure from one's peer group, as well as the community, to ignore, minimize, or cover up the situation may be extreme. (p. xv)

If adult society can learn to believe in the reality of child sexual abuse, there is opportunity for unprecedented advances in the prevention and treatment of emotional pain and dysfunction. If adults cannot face the reality of incestuous abuse, then women and children will continue to be stigmatized by the terrors of their own helpless silence.

Louise Armstrong documents in the companion chapter, "The Cradle of Sexual Politics: Incest," the incredible reluctance of court systems to give voice to abused children. She makes clear also the

ROLAND SUMMIT, M.D. • Assistant Clinical Professor, Community Consultation Service, Harbor–UCLA Medical Center, Torrance, California 90509; Department of Psychiatry, University of California at Los Angeles School of Medicine, Los Angeles, California 90024.

vested interest of male society in maintaining secrecy and disbelief. What is not so clear is that the victim of child sexual abuse faces disbelief, retaliation, and revictimization at each level of disclosure within the world of adults. It is not only the court and a community of men that are so incredulous of sexually exploited children. The basic reason for disbelief is *adocentrism*, the unswerving and unquestioned allegiance to adult values. All adults, male and female, tend to align themselves in an impenetrable bastion against any threat that adult priorities and self-comfort must yield to the needs of children.

The child is trapped in a private, impossibly confusing world that gives no validation to the incest experience. The incestuous intruder into the child's private world is something like a monster that inhabits her[1] closet. He threatens her only when she is alone, and she must find her own ways of coping with his overpowering presence. She knows without question and learns through painful experience that nobody will give serious credibility to her fears. Her mother may be the most incredulous and punishing, not because she is indifferent to the child but because she must first protect her trust in the basic decency of her husband and the fundamental security of adult society. Since an adult assumes that other decent adults don't commit incest, and since it is generally believed that children wishfully imagine incestuous experiences or fabricate groundless accusations of sexual assault, it is predictable that most women will reject any hint of incest given by their children. Only an unusually free and perceptive mother can reward a child for sharing with her the bad news of an incestuous relationship.

Across the country and through the years, victims report the same litany of terror: *nobody* could believe. *Nobody* could care. Teachers, doctors, mental health specialists, police investigators, prosecutors, judges, juries, *everyone* in the adult world finds some logical reason to defend the adult against the distress of the child. The monster in the closet doesn't really exist.

"You made him up. You lied. It's *your* monster. All this trouble is your fault. Don't bother us with your childish make-believe world. We have more important things to do in the real world." There is no room for monsters in the grown-up world.

---

[1]The use of the feminine pronoun does not assume that victims of sexual abuse are necessarily female. Emerging evidence indicates that boys are at least as likely to be sexually exploited as girls, and that they are even more frequently trapped in silence. Boys, like girls, are most often victimized by trusted men. Unlike girls, boys are more likely to be victimized by someone outside the immediate family. In keeping with the general theme of these volumes for women, this chapter is directed especially to the implications of incest for female children. In many cases, the use of a feminine pronoun can be considered generic for boys as well as for girls.

This nightmarish isolation and sequential rejection reinforces what becomes for the victim the most painful reality of incest: "It's my fault. I brought it on myself. I'm so bad I invite trouble and make trouble for others. I'm not worth caring for. There's no place for me in the world of reasonable, decent people. I'll never be reasonable or decent. I'm crazy. I'm nothing but a whore."

Such a victim is likely to live out a life of self-fulfilling prophecies, deprived of a confident core identity and stripped of any capacity for trust and intimacy. If she presumes to be worthy of professional help, she will probably not trust her counselor to share the shame of her childhood. The secret goes unchallenged. If she does claim to be a survivor of incest, she may be told by her therapist that her memories are only distorted traces of old wishful fantasies. Some therapists may recognize the reality of the incest experience yet fail to appreciate the significance of related symptoms. The splitting of self-perception and the need to restructure contradictory relationships, mechanisms that are necessary survival skills of the child entrapped in incest, may be treated as indicators of intractable mental illness. These problems beg for specialized, empathic attention. Women who have considered themselves hopelessly ill through years of conventional therapy often discover redeeming self-worth and self-confidence after only a few months of contact with other survivors within a specialized incest treatment program. It can be estimated that some 5 million[2] women in the United States were sexually victimized as children by a male relative. How many such women might benefit from a chance to discover that they were not alone and not at fault?

There is a compelling urgency for all of society to discover incest. Unilateral sensitivity in any segment of the population without concomitant support at other levels only increases the crippling pain and frustration for those who must struggle for belief. Enlightened mothers offer their children the most profound alliance for protection and recovery. But a woman fights an uphill battle unless she is afforded credibility and power within the child-protective, justice, and treatment response systems. And no amount of enlightened agency response can undo the disbelief and disapproval of the extended family and the general public.

The purpose of this chapter is to help establish a climate of belief for the realities of incest. Any woman who can believe that incest happens and who can be confident that children are normally trapped into silence through no fault of their own is empowered to be a new change-

[2]This figure is a rough but conservative estimate derived from David Finkelhor's data (1980), assuming approximately 10% of women are survivors of child sexual abuse contact with an adult male relative, and assuming an adult female population of 50 million.

maker for prevention and immunity from the most crippling stigmas of incest. Such a woman can be a loving resource to her daughter, to her sister, to her friend, to her neighbor, and, so often most needed, to herself.

Every reader has the capacity to make a difference in the equilibrium of silence. Most people who insist they have never known anyone involved in incest discover the experience among friends and family, and sometimes in themselves, when they are willing to suspend their disbelief. The discovery of incest seems overwhelming only within the habitual stigmas of secrecy, helplessness, and shame. While anyone is understandably reluctant to rediscover the painful helplessness of childhood, the process carries with it also the excitement of a new understanding and empathy. Now that the monster is coming out of the closet as something tangible and physically intimidating, we can use adult systems of investigation, description, and active resolution to reduce the monster to human dimensions.

The following sections provide a map of typical incest experiences, first as statistical data, then as a synthesis of normal patterns of accommodation. Finally, we will examine the implications of these patterns for more effective recognition, prevention, and recovery.

FREQUENCY

For years, incest has been dismissed as statistically trivial, something that is too exceptional for serious concern. Official figures have been drawn from court records in the naive belief that incest is subject to report and prosecution. Not surprisingly, the official incidence of father–daughter incest remained constant for 50 years at 1–2 per million. In Santa Clara County, California, where the Child Sexual Abuse Treatment Project has invited better identification and coordination of services for incestuous families, annual incidence is approaching 1,000 per million!

Several retrospective surveys of college-age females have identified a 20%–30% rate of child sexual victimizations (Landis, 1956; Gagnon, 1965; Finkelhor 1979). These are not all incestuous or ongoing experiences. The data included one-time-only assaults by strangers. One striking finding, consistent in each of these studies, is that strangers were involved in only 25% of the experiences. A girl had a 3-to-1 chance of being molested by an adult male whom she had been taught to trust. About half (44%) of the molesters were relatives, one-quarter (22%) resided within the child's home, and about 6% were fathers or stepfathers (Finkelhor, 1979). Projecting these figures to the general population, at least 1.5% of all women could be expected to have experienced sex with their father or stepfather, with 9% of the female population having a background of victimization by relatives.

These are average figures drawn from a sample of relatively well-adjusted, high-achieving college students. High-risk subgroups show even higher rates. College girls in Finkelhor's sample who were stepdaughters experienced even odds of victimization: 50%. Surveys of foster children, runaways, drug addicts, and prostitutes show an incestuous background in the 60%–70% range. Perhaps most significant is the apparent correlation between child sexual abuse and a later tendency toward abusive parenting. Mothers in treatment centers for child abuse report an 80%–90% prevalence of incestuous abuse in their own childhood. Some abusive mothers report that their mothers and their grandmothers were also sexually abused. Yet these most damaged women are often the first to yield power to abusive males and to condemn their daughters as intrinsically evil and deserving of abuse.

What is the power of the incestuous experience to stigmatize generations of women so severely? What are the threats that achieve such perfect secrecy and victim self-condemnation? Why do so few victims seek help, and why are those few so relentlessly ignored? Is there, as Dr. Michael Rothenberg (1980) suggested, a conspiracy against children in the United States?

No single system and no simple conspiracy explains the reluctant discovery of incest, but understanding can be gained from a closer evaluation of the dilemmas faced by the child as she tries to survive on the uncharted solo voyage through the tempest of incest. Each wave of involvement in the secret realities of the experience carries her further from the mythical, commonsense "truths" or adult truisms about incest. The more normal the child is in her reactions, the more she will discredit herself. And the better she adapts to the experience, the more she will be condemned.

THE CHILD SEXUAL ABUSE ACCOMMODATION SYNDROME

Five factors define the progression of adjustment for the most typical victims of incest. These same conditions contradict much of the mythology and misunderstanding that adults apply to their perception of incest. Children's normal reaction patterns defy popular, commonsense, and professional dogma about how children *should* behave in response to incestuous assault. And the unwillingness of key adults to accept the child's behavior leaves the children all the more trapped in a sense of total isolation and self-condemnation. The cycle of disbelief and rejection serves to maintain adult comfort and to reinforce child helplessness until the child learns to behave "normally" and to present the adult world with a credible account of her experience. The first four factors of the sexual abuse accommodation syndrome are secrecy, helplessness, accommodation, and delayed, unconvincing disclosure. The fifth is retracting the complaint and reassuring the world in its insistent belief that the child only imagined the experience, or that she deliberately lied.

1. SECRECY. Children rarely tell anyone, especially when they are first molested (Finkelhor, 1979; Burgess & Holmstrom, 1975). The child typically feels ashamed and guilty. She fears disapproval or punishment from the mother (most of the girls in Finkelhor's sample who told their mother found their worst fears justified); retaliation or loss of love from the offender; and, most profoundly, loss of acceptance and security in the home. These fears are often suggested and reinforced by direct threats from the offender.

The emphasis on secrecy and the fearful isolation from the mother define the sexual activity as something dangerous and bad, even when the child is too young to understand the societal taboos involved. Even if the child is carefully and affectionately seduced without fear or pain, the conspiracy of silence stigmatizes the relationship.

2. HELPLESSNESS. The child feels obligated and overpowered by the inherent authority of the trusted adult, even in the absence of physical force or threats. Helplessness is reinforced by the sense of isolation, secrecy, and guilt, as well as the child's inability to make sense out of her father's behavior or to find any acceptable way to describe the bizarre relationship to others.

Helplessness is often expressed by immobility. If a young girl is molested during sleep, she typically "plays possum." She does not resist or cry out, even though her mother may be in the next room. A sibling in the same bed may also feign sleep, afraid to become involved.

The natural inability to cry out or to protect herself provides the core of misunderstanding between the victim and the community of adults, as well as providing the nidus for the child's later self-reprisals. Almost no adult seems willing to believe that a legitimate victim would not react with kicks and screams. Attorneys for the offender easily humiliate and confuse the child victim–witness and prejudice the jury with demands for a "normal" protest. Expert testimony on these points is crucial, both to validate the credibility of the child and to help prevent self-condemnation.

With repeated intrusions, the victimized child may lie awake in fright long into the night. Yet, if approached, she remains motionless in a pathetic attempt to protect herself, much as she has learned to hide beneath the covers from imaginary monsters.

Violation of a person's most secure retreat overwhelms ordinary defenses and leads to disillusionment, severe insecurity, and a process of victimization. Well-adjusted adults report lingering terrors and loss of basic well-being after rape or even a robbery within their bedrooms. Children, who have few defenses at best, are even more vulnerable than adults to invasion of their beds.

Finally, it must be remembered that the normal child has no real power or voice apart from the enfranchisement given by her parents. These are not older children or adolescents with strong institutional or peer-group support. The average age of incestuous initiation is 8, with a range from birth to age 16. The mean clusters sharply in the middle, with as few teenage initiates as infants. How can a third-grader feel anything but helplessness in confronting a sexually insistent father or stepfather? And how can she blame herself for inviting his attentions or for her failure to forcibly abort his intentions? For a child of 8 (or 3, 5, or 11, as the case may be), self-blame is intrinsic in the accommodation process unless her mother or some alternate caretaker can give her the power to stop the sexual entrapment.

3. ENTRAPMENT AND ACCOMMODATION. The process of helpless victimization leads the child to exaggerate her own responsibility and eventually to despise herself for her weakness. The child is confronted with two apparent realities: either she is bad, deserving of punishment, and not worth caring for, or her parent is bad, unfairly punishing, and not capable of caring. The young child has neither preparation nor permission to believe in the second reality, and there would be no hope for acceptance or survival if it were true. Her inevitable choice is to embrace the more active role of being the one responsible, and to hope to find a way to become good and worthy of caring. This self-scapegoating is almost universal in victims of any form of parental abuse. It sets the foundation for self-hate and what Leonard Shengold (1979) described as a vertical split in reality testing:

> If the very parent who abuses and is experienced as *bad* must be turned to for relief of the distress that the parent has caused, then the child must, out of desperate need, register the parent—*delusionally*—as good. Only the mental image of a good parent can help the child deal with the terrifying intensity of fear and rage which is the effect of the tormenting experience. The alternative—the maintenance of the overwhelming stimulation and the bad parental imago—means annihilation of identity, of the feeling of the self. So the bad has to be registered as good. This is a mind-splitting or a mind-fragmenting operation. (p. 539)

The sexually abusive parent provides explicit example and instruction in how to be good: the child must be available without complaint to his sexual demands. There is an explicit or implicit promise of reward: if she is good and if she keeps the secret, she can protect her siblings from sexual involvement (or have Daddy all to herself, as the case may be), protect her mother from disintegration ("If your mother ever found out, it would kill her"), protect her father from temptation ("If I couldn't count on you, I'd have to hang out in bars and look for other women"), and, most vitally, preserve the security of the home ("If you ever tell, they could send me to jail and put all you kids in an orphanage").

In the classic role reversal of child abuse, the child is given the power to destroy the family and the responsibility to keep it together. The child, *not the parent*, must mobilize the altruism and self-control to ensure the survival of the others. The child, in short, must secretly assume many of the role functions previously assigned to the mother.

There is an inevitable splitting of conventional moral values: maintaining a lie to keep the secret is the ultimate virtue, while telling the truth would be the greatest sin. A child thus victimized will appear to accept or to seek sexual contact without complaint. As Ferenczi (1933/1955) discovered almost 50 years ago, "The misused child changes into a mechanical obedient automaton" (p. 163).

Effective accommodation, of course, invalidates any future claims to credibility as a victim. It is obvious to adults that if the child *were* sexually involved, as she claims, then she must have been a consenting and probably a seductive partner. If she is not lying in her eventual complaints, she certainly lied and conspired with her "lover" in her earlier cover-up. In either event, she has no credibility in a criminal court. Again, only expert testimony can translate the child's behavior into concepts that other adults can accept.

Since the child must structure her reality to protect the parent, she also finds the means to build pockets of survival where some hope of goodness can find sanctuary. She may turn to imaginary companions for reassurance. She may develop multiple personalities, assigning helplessness and suffering to one, badness and rage to another, sexual power to another, love and compassion to another, and so forth. She may discover altered states of consciousness to shut off pain or to disassociate from her body, as if looking on from a distance at the child suffering the abuse.

If the child cannot create a psychic economy to reconcile the continuing outrage, the intolerance of helplessness and the increasing feelings of rage will seek active expression. For the girl, this expression is most often self-destructive and reinforcing of self-hate: self-mutilation, suicidal behavior, promiscuous sexual activity, and repeated running away are typical. She may learn to exploit the father for privileges, favors, and material rewards, reinforcing her self-punishing image as whore in the process. She may fight with both parents, but her greatest rage is likely to focus on her mother, whom she blames for driving the father into her bed. She assumes that her mother must know of the sexual abuse and is either too uncaring or too ineffectual to intervene. The failure of the mother–daughter bond reinforces the young woman's distrust of herself as a female and makes her all the more dependent on the pathetic hope of gaining acceptance and protection from a male.

Substance abuse is an inviting avenue of escape. As Barbara Myers (1981) recalled:

> On drugs, I could be anything I wanted to be. I could make up my own reality: I could be pretty, have a good family, a nice father, a strong mother, and be happy; . . . drinking had the opposite affect of drugs. . . . Drinking got me back into my pain; it allowed me to express my hurt and my anger. (p. 100)

All these accommodation mechanisms—domestic martyrdom, splitting of reality, altered consciousness, hysterical phenomena, delinquency, sociopathy, projection of rage, even self-mutilation—are part of the survival skills of the child. They can be abandoned only if the child can be led to trust in a secure environment that is full of consistent, *noncontingent* acceptance and caring. In the meantime, anyone working therapeutically with the child (or the grown up, still shattered victim) will be tested and provoked to prove that trust is impossible and that the only secure reality is negative expectation and self-hate.

The following was written in the midst of transient despair by Stephanie, a 36-year-old woman trying to cope with the apparent caring of her therapist and peer group despite her expectation of rejection. After some 20 years of escape within the role of a psychotic child, she had for the prior year achieved a kind of adolescent adjustment free of delusions and hallucinations. Just a month before writing this statement, she had first recalled graphic images of forcible oral and anal rape by her father. While these acts were entirely consistent with the brutal and humiliating punishments she had learned to expect from this man, remembering the repressed sexual experiences made her all the more fearful of hurt and punishment as a natural consequence of the inherent badness of her participation. For this polyabused child–woman, the omnipotent father's assertion that the child asked for and deserved the sexual punishment was tantamount to reality. In every instance, the labels she applied to herself were the names habitually used by her father some 30 years before:

> I am a filthy, sick animal trying to act like a human being and doing a pretty poor job. I'll never be anything but sick and inhuman. I am covered

with green slime that can be seen by all.[3] I am scum. I am a slut and a whore. People get nauseated when they look at me because of my ugliness. I belong in a hole where decent people don't have to associate with me. I am shit. I destroy everything I care for. My soul either kills off or chases away everyone who comes in contact with me, especially those that become dear. I make myself sick.

I deserved to be screwed in the mouth and I deserved to be fucked in the ass. I asked for it and I got what I deserve. It was my fault and I take responsibility for it. I deserved to be beaten; I was bad; I still am. I deserved to be molested; I am a whore. I deserved the verbal abuse I received; I am a stupid ass. I deserved to be shocked and locked up alone for weeks; I was crazy and still am and always will be.

I am not deserving of love or respect or comfort. I do not deserve caring. I do not deserve softness or tenderness. I do not deserve to feel warm and good. I do not deserve life.

I am disgusting. I am repulsive. I am useless. I am worthless. I am responsible for the unhappiness of all. I am the scum of the earth. I hate the very thought of me.

It is all too easy for the would-be therapist to join the parents and all adult society in rejecting such a child, looking at the results of abuse to assume that such an impossible wretch must have asked for and deserved whatever punishment has occurred, if indeed the whole problem is not a hysterical or vengeful fantasy.

4. DELAYED, CONFLICTED, AND UNCONVINCING DISCLOSURE. Most ongoing sexual abuse is *never* disclosed, at least not outside the immediate family (Gagnon, 1965; Finkelhor, 1979). Reported, investigated cases are the exception, not the norm. Reporting is an outgrowth either of overwhelming family conflict, incidental discovery by a third party, or sensitive outreach and community education by child-protective agencies.

If family conflict triggers disclosure, it is usually only after some years of continuing sexual abuse and an eventual breakdown of accommodation mechanisms. The victim of incest remains silent until

[3] Throughout the years of psychotic adjustment, Stephanie's delusional system was dominated by the belief that she was filled with malodorous slime that oozed from her mouth and from beneath her skin. It had become obvious through her associations during psychotherapy that this was a childhood concept of semen, contaminated also by traumatic exposure to the decomposing body of a beloved pet her father had unfairly blamed her for killing. With the reacquisition of oral rape memories, the actual source of the seminal incorporation became clear. Stephanie reacted to the memory with an inability to swallow any food. When she was encouraged to swallow again through positive conditioning, she experienced a sense of shame and massive defeat, remembering that her last-ditch protest for survival as a child had been her determination not to swallow the semen. Despite all her adult logic to the contrary, Stephanie used this memory to further condemn herself for her weakness and to return to the belief that anyone who refused to see the slime or to be alienated by her evil and destructiveness was only conspiring to confuse her.

she enters adolescence, when she becomes capable of demanding a more separate life for herself and of challenging the authority of her parents. Adolescence also makes the father more jealous and controlling, trying to sequester his daughter against the "dangers" of outside peer involvement. He may become harshly judgmental and punitive in a belated attempt to recapture authority and control. The mother, who has come to resent the favored position of the "spoiled" daughter, is likely to applaud the shift in discipline and reinforce the need for harsh punishment and restrictions. The corrosive effects of accommodation seem to justify any extreme of punishment. What parent would not impose severe sanctions to control running away, drug abuse, promiscuity, rebellion, and delinquency?

After an especially punishing family fight and a belittling showdown of authority by the father, the girl is finally driven to let go of the secret. She seeks understanding and intervention at the very time she is least likely to find them. Authorities are put off by the pattern of delinquency and rebellious anger expressed by the girl. Most adults confronted with such a history tend to identify with the problems of the parents in trying to cope with a rebellious teenager. They observe that the girl seems more angry about the immediate punishment than about the sexual atrocities she is alleging. They assume there is no proof to such a fantastic complaint, especially since she did not complain years ago when she claims she was forcibly molested. They assume she has invented the story in retaliation against the father's attempt to achieve reasonable control and discipline. The more unreasonable and abusive the triggering punishment, the more they assume the child would do anything to get away, even to the point of falsely incriminating her father.

Unless specifically trained and sensitized, average adults, including mothers, relatives, teachers, counselors, doctors, psychotherapists, investigators, prosecutors, defense attorneys, judges, and jurors cannot believe that a normal, truthful child would tolerate incest without immediately reporting it, or that an apparently normal father could be capable of repeated, unchallenged sexual molestation of his own daughter. The child of any age faces an unbelieving audience when she complains of ongoing incest. The troubled, angry adolescent risks not only disbelief, but scapegoating, humiliation, and punishment as well.

Contrary to popular myth, most mothers are not aware of ongoing sexual abuse. Marriage demands considerable blind trust and denial for survival. A woman does not commit her life and security to a man she believes capable of molesting his own children. That basic denial becomes pathological the more the woman herself has been victimized and the more she might feel helpless and worthless in the absence of a protective, accepting male. The "obvious" clues to incest are usually obvious only in retrospect. Our assumption that the mother "must have known" merely parallels the demand of the child that the mother must be in touch intuitively with invisible and even deliberately concealed family discomfort.

So the mother typically reacts to allegations of sexual abuse with disbelief and protective denial. How could she not have known? How could the child wait so long to tell her? What kind of mother could allow such a thing to happen? What would the neighbors think? As someone substantially dependent on the approval and generosity of the father, she is in a mind-splitting dilemma analogous to that of the abused child: either the child is bad and deserving of punishment or the father is bad and unfairly punitive. One of them is lying and unworthy of trust. The mother's whole security and life adjustment and much of her sense of adult self-worth demands a trust in the reliability of her partner. To accept the alternative means annihilation of the family and a large piece of her own identity. Her fear and ambivalence are reassured by the father's logical challenge:

> Are you going to believe that lying little slut? Can you believe I would do such a thing? How could something like that go on right under your nose for years? You know we can't trust her out of our sight anymore. Just when we try to clamp down and I get a little tough with her, she comes back with a cock-and-bull story like this. That's what I get for trying to keep her out of trouble!

Among the small proportion of incest secrets that are shared, most are never revealed outside the family. Now that professionals are required to report any suspicion of child abuse, increasing numbers of complaints are investigated by protective agencies. Police investigators and protective service workers are now more likely to give credence to the complaint, in which case all the children may be removed immediately into protective custody pending the hearing of a dependency petition. In the continuing paradox of a divided judicial system, the juvenile court judge is likely to sustain out-of-home placement on the "preponderance of the evidence" that the child is in danger, while the adult criminal court takes no action on the father's crime. Attorneys know that the uncorroborated testimony of a child will not convict a respectable adult. The test in criminal court requires specific proof "beyond reasonable doubt," and every reasonable adult juror will have reason to doubt the child's fantastic claims. Prosecutors are reluctant to subject the child to humiliating cross-examination, just as they are loath to prosecute cases they cannot win, so they typically reject the complaint on the basis of insufficient evidence. Defense counsel can assure the father that he will not be charged as long as he denies any impropriety and *as long as he stays out of treatment.*

The absence of criminal charges is tantamount to a conviction of perjury against the victim. "A man is innocent until proven guilty," say adult-protective relatives. "The kid claimed to be molested, but there was nothing to it. The police investigated and they didn't even file charges."

As outrageous as it might seem, there is an open season on children for the sexual predator. Unless children can be encouraged to seek immediate intervention and unless there is expert advocacy for the child in the criminal court, the child is abandoned as the helpless custodian of a self-incriminating secret that no responsible adult can believe.

Health-care professionals have a critical role in both early detection and expert courtroom advocacy. Professionals can help mobilize skeptical caretakers into a position of belief and protective intervention. And only strong clinical expertise asserting the reality of the accommodation syndrome can compete with the "reasonable doubt" of other adults in the court process. Obviously, the professional must first be capable of a strong position of belief. The professional who can believe in the reality of incest and who has learned to acknowledge the secrecy, the helplessness, the accommodation patterns, and the delayed disclosure may still be alienated by the fifth level of the accommodation syndrome.

5. RETRACTION OF COMPLAINT. *Whatever a child says about incest, she is likely to reverse it.* As a small child, she may deny incest when questioned, yet in later years, she may make criminal complaints when moved by anger. Beneath the anger remains the ambivalence of guilt and the martyred obligation to preserve the family. In the chaotic aftermath of disclosure, the child discovers that the bedrock fears and threats underlying the secrecy are true. Her father abandons her and calls her a liar. Her mother doesn't believe her, or she decompensates into hysteria and rage. The family breaks up, and all the kids are placed in custody. The father is threatened with disgrace and imprisonment. The child is blamed for causing the whole mess, and everyone seems to treat her like a freak. She is interrogated about all the tawdry details and encouraged to incriminate her father, yet the father remains unchallenged, remaining at home in the security of the family. She is held in custody, with no hope of returning if the dependency petition is sustained.

The message from the mother is very clear, often explicit:

> Why do you insist on telling those awful stories about your father? If you send him to prison there will be no one to provide for us and we won't be a family anymore. We'll end up on welfare with no place to stay. Is that what you want to do to us? Forget all this foolishness and come back home so we can be a family again.

Once again, the child bears the responsibility of either preserving or destroying the family. The role reversal continues, with the "bad" choice to tell the truth, or the "good" choice to capitulate and restore a lie for the sake of the family.

Unless there is special support for the child and immediate intervention to force responsibility onto the father, the girl will follow the "normal" course and retract her complaint. The girl "admits" she made up the story:

> I was awful mad at my dad for punishing me. He hit me and said I could never see my boyfriend again. I've been really bad for years and nothing seems to keep me from getting into trouble. He had plenty of reason to be mad at me. But I got real mad and just had to find some way of getting out of that place. So I made up the story about him fooling around with me and everything. I didn't mean to get everyone in so much trouble.

This simple lie carries more credibility than the most explicit claims of incestuous entrapment. It confirms adult expectations that children can't be trusted. It restores the precarious equilibrium of the family. The children learn not to complain. The adults learn not to listen. And the authorities learn not to believe rebellious children who try to use their sexual power to destroy well-meaning parents. Case closed.

IMPLICATIONS FOR RECOGNITION AND TREATMENT

The first priority for active response to incestuous abuse is recognition. Dr. Suzanne Sgroi (1975) defined recognition of incest as the last frontier of child abuse:

> Recognition of sexual molestation of a child is entirely dependent on the individual's inherent willingness to entertain the possibility that the condition may exist. Unfortunately, willingness to consider the diagnosis of suspected child molestation frequently seems to vary in inverse proportion to the individual's level of training. That is, the more advanced the training of some, the less willing they are to suspect molestation. (p. 20)

The adult who responds to the needs of an incest victim can no longer hide in the reassurance that incestuous behavior is beyond belief. The supportive adult, whether parent, investigator, physician, or psychotherapist, must first be capable of belief and then be willing to move beyond belief to responsible advocacy and intervention.

The discovery of incest as a cause of emotional problems is not unique to the 1980s or even to the twentieth century. That discovery was documented by no less an authority than Sigmund Freud in 1896! In that year, Freud (1896/1953) reported in "The Aetiology of Hysteria" that the hysterical problems presented by a series of female patients were caused by early childhood sexual seduction by adult caretakers.

He also wrote to his friend and confidant, W. Fliess, "I have come to the opinion that anxiety is to be connected not with a mental, but with a physical consequence of sexual abuse" (Rush, 1977, quoting Bonaparte, Freud, & Kriss, 1954, pp. 79–80). Such a theory was greeted with professional outrage in Victorian Vienna, and Freud spent years trying to rationalize his own discomfort about believing that so many respectable fathers could victimize their children. As he wrote to Fliess in 1897, he was perplexed by the tendency of patients to block or to abandon analysis at the level of incest discovery:

> Then there was the astonishing thing that in every case . . . blame was laid on perverse acts by the father, . . . though it was hardly credible that perverted acts against children were so general. . . . Thirdly, there is no "indication of reality" in the unconscious, so it is impossible to distinguish between truth and emotionally charged fiction. (This leaves open the possible explanation that sexual fantasy regularly makes use of the theme of parents. . . .). (Rush, 1977, quoting Bonaparte et al., 1954, pp. 215–217)

That "possible explanation" became the basis for one of the major tenets of psychoanalytic theory. In 1924, Freud renounced his earlier belief in the seduction theory and suggested the Oedipus complex instead. The Oedipus complex assumes a universal attraction of children toward the parent of the opposite sex, with inevitable conflicts, jealousy, and fear directed toward the parent of the same sex. Freud postulated that successful emotional maturation depended on the resolution of those conflicts and that neurotic problems could be traced to the child's unsuccessful resolution of that fantasied family romance:

> Almost all my women patients told me that they had been seduced by their father. I was driven to recognize in the end that those reports were untrue and so came to understand that the hysterical symptoms were derived from fantasy and not from real occurrences. (Freud, 1933/1966, p. 584)

Freud apparently came to this recognition through analysis of his own dreams and childhood experiences (Rush, 1977), as well as a continuing refinement of psychoanalytic techniques with patients. Whatever the basis for the shift to the Oedipus complex, it offered a fortuitous, adult-reassuring alternative to the seduction theory. Children, not their fathers, were responsible for the allegations of sexual abuse. It was the perverse needs of the child that scapegoated adults with undeserved accusations. Finally, whatever children (or adults) chose to say about sexual experiences with their parents must be assumed to be wishful fantasy unless proven otherwise.

Freud's early discovery was therefore an idea ahead of its time. Neither Freud nor the adult-protective world of that era was ready to explore or to validate the implications of the seduction theory. Not only was the theory discredited; worse than that, the adult-protective reaction served to discourage and delay any subsequent reappraisal of that discovery. Freud's precocious, outrageous early speculation led him and many of his followers to arm themselves with a dogma of disbelief. The messenger of incest not only risks provoking ordinary, commonsense denial but also invites charges of heresy among the most highly trained and sophisticated professionals.

As psychoanalyst Joseph Peters (1976) has written:

> After 1924 the notion that hysterical symptoms were based upon actual events, real sexual assaults upon children, fell increasingly out of favor. Psychoanalysts abandoned the search for a distinction between actual childhood sexual trauma and children's fantasies. In the Freudian theory of psychoneurosis, the fantasies became as important as real events. Since Freud's thinking developed in this way, his earlier followers were relieved from facing the fact that patients sometimes had been real victims of sexual assault. . . . It is my thesis that both cultural and personal factors combined to cause everyone, including Freud himself at times, to welcome the idea that reports of childhood sexual victimization could be regarded as fantasies. This position relieved the guilt of adults. In my opinion, both Freud and his followers oversubscribed to the theory of childhood fantasy and overlooked incidents of actual sexual victimization in childhood. (p. 401)

> In their aversion to what are often repulsive details, psychotherapists allowed and continue to allow their patients to repress emotionally significant, pathogenic facts. . . . In addition, it is important to note that because the reported offender was frequently the patient's own father, in order to avoid the fact of incest, my colleagues seized upon the easier assumption that the occurrences were oedipal fantasies. (p. 402)

> Relegating these traumas to the imagination may divert treatment into a prolonged unraveling of natural developmental processes in which fantasy is a component. Furthermore, unsuccessful psychotherapeutic evaluation opens the way for prescribing . . . antipsychotic drugs and electroshock. The treatment may compound the patient's original psychologic problems. Ascribing these events to psychological fantasy may be easier and more interesting for the therapist, but it may also be counterproductive for the most efficient resolution of symptoms. (pp. 407–408)

> An immediate supportive response by parents, criminal justice personnel, doctors and nurses is crucial to preserve the emotional integrity of the child. Particularly when the offender is a member of the family, care must be taken by service personnel to insure that the child's needs are put first. (p. 421)

Dr. Peters drew on the experience of a private psychoanalytic practice as well as extraordinary social awareness as director of the Philadelphia Sex Offender and Rape Victim Center. The Philadelphia center is one of a dozen or so specialty centers that have defined new clinical priorities for sexual abuse victims and their families. Child abuse centers, rape crisis networks, women's consciousness-raising groups, incest survivors' self-help groups, and increasingly specialized clinical research and treatment models have led the way to a growing professional and public awareness of the hazards of child sexual abuse.

Many concerned advocates for women and children fear that the issues of sexual abuse will again be submerged by ideological standoffs and adult-protective, male-dominant smoke screens. Children, after all, still have no power, and women may be sidetracked into such adult-oriented issues as equal rights in the work force. This is hardly the time to encourage women to stay home to protect their children or to devote more energy to saturating their mates with preventive flattery and loving attention.

It *is* a time to discover that men have many needs that they are too proud and too insecure to acknowledge, and that apparently normal men slip rather easily into exploiting whatever potential sexual object is most available and most easily subordinated. It is a time for better clinical and theoretical research to understand the wide diversity of offender rationalizations for incestuous abuse of children, ranging from chronic obsessive desire to apparently thoughtless opportunism. Listening to victims gives a fairly clear and consistent synthesis of common risk factors (Finkelhor, 1980). Listening to infinite numbers of offenders gives infinite variations of contradictory motivations and choices, with few common denominators except that these men were born of women and determined to express much of their individuality, power, and dependency needs through the exercise of that one appendage no woman can claim (Summit & Kryso, 1978).

I believe the time is right for a real and permanent shift in public and professional protective responsibility for children. We are not living in Victorian Vienna. We are no longer unmindful of the realities of parental misuse of children or the helplessness of children to recognize any condition of well-being outside parental sanctions. We understand that successful therapy depends on a creative balance between theoretical expectations and individual behaviors. And the word *incest* is no longer either unthinkable or unspeakable. Perhaps most importantly, women as a group will no longer defer to the unilateral powers and privileges of men. Women are today less impressed by the rhetoric of sexual intimidation. *Virgin, whore, mother, old maid, prick teaser,* and *bitch* are words that are losing their power to stigmatize and confine women within restrictive definitions of sexual behavior.

With a coalition of support from protective agencies, the justice system, treatment agencies, and self-help alliances, adult survivors are no longer condemned to a lifetime of shame and fearful silence. Mothers of present and potential victims are better empowered to make self-protective and child-protective decisions in their choice of adult sexual partners and/or adult living companions. Children, who are assaulted with all sorts of blatant and confusing media images of adult sexuality, might as well be enlightened in this age of sexual candor with honest messages about their own sexuality and their right and power to protect themselves from adult intrusions into their most personal worlds.

PREVENTION. We can start by telling children of both sexes that their bodies are uniquely their own and by acknowledging that they have the right to discover and to express their own limits of intimacy. Kids recognize rather consistently what doesn't feel right in the attentions of adults: tickling or wrestling that doesn't stop on time, "sloppy" kisses, hands poking, rubbing, and probing under clothing. Too often their expressed objections are silenced by parents urging them to be more accepting of adults' affection: "You have to be nice to grandfather, dear, that's just his way of showing how he loves you."

Several good films have been produced for classroom use to empower young children to break intimidating secrets and to say no to unwanted intrusions (*Who Do You Tell?* and *Child Molestation: When to Say No*). Others define the problems of incestuous abuse for parents and secondary-level students (*Incest: The Victim Nobody Believes* and *Shatter the Silence*). Schools need strong parental support to take rape prevention programs beyond the violent-stranger concept to address the 3-to-1 chance that children will be approached instead by a trusted adult. The helplessness of those encounters thrives on naiveté and silence.

Specific preventive efforts can be directed to high-risk families. Alcoholism, interspousal violence, child abuse, religious insularity, sexual rigidity in one or both parents, or a marked disparity in power and mobility between husband and wife have all been linked to increased risks of sexual victimization for children. A single mother searching for a new mate and a good father for her children is easy prey to a variety of opportunists who are less interested in her than in her children. Of the 50% of molested stepdaughters in Finkelhor's sample (1980), most were victimized not by their stepfathers but by some friend of their parents.

In view of all the unknowns in trying to identify potentially abusive males, there must be more support of the vital role occupied by the mother both in protecting a child at risk and in providing support if incest has occurred. Women who have been sexually abused deserve the opportunity to resolve old conflicts, to avoid the risk of stigmatizing their children with projections of fault, and to reduce the likelihood that they or their daughters will select an overpowering and intrusive male as a mate. That is not to say that all sexually abused women endanger their children or that all survivors should be forced to have treatment.

What is needed is greater availability of survivors' groups and other specialized programs for women that invite resolution of any residual conflicts without unnecessary stigmatization. Victim adjustment patterns should not be labeled as mental illness or character pathology.

Many women assume without question that they are bad or sick or crazy because of the assumed guilt and helplessness of their childhood experiences. They view their internalized rage as evil and dangerous, and they tend to live in fear of losing control of their feelings or of losing touch with reality. Those who are not aware of disturbed feelings or thoughts may still have problems with trust and intimacy or inhibition of sexual fulfillment. Finally, survivors who are sure they are free of any stigma of incest may find themselves uncomfortable in their role as parents. Now that these patterns are so well recognized and potentially so effectively resolved, it seems a tragic waste not to provide more effective community education and more assertive outreach through specialized treatment groups.

TREATMENT. Treatment groups for adult survivors are sometimes contained within the more comprehensive specialty programs for all members of currently incestuous families. Mixing these two generations of experience in discussion groups can have mutually beneficial results. The adult survivor finds a focus for her rage and a new assurance of her initial blamelessness in confronting firsthand the power differentials and coercive dynamics in newly discovered incestuous families. And the protests of the incest survivor within the parents' group give adult power to the needs of the child. Fathers and mothers preoccupied with the adult survival issues surrounding incest disclosure need continuing, insistent reminders of the needs of their children and the reality of child discomfort.

These interactions presume a model of treatment where the participants are afforded substantial peer-group contact. I believe that peer-group confrontation and support are vital to the treatment of incest and other forms of child abuse (Summit, 1978). These groups can be organized within a self-help model such as Parents United and Daughters United (Giaretto, 1976, 1978) or within a professional model or peer-group therapy. The child, especially, needs the inspiration of a peer group to offset her concept of being uniquely despised and damaged. She also needs to share the support of those who have experienced the entire progression of the accommodation syndrome to fortify herself against the temptation to retract her complaint.

I believe that proven treatment networks are vital also for the effective involvement of protective agencies in holding the adult responsible for his action. Only the combined encouragement and intimidation of experienced therapists and peers can lead an offender to accept responsibility for his actions and to hope for compassionate sentencing. Without immediate and coercive treatment intervention, the offender will usually deny his role and bluff his way through the court process by shifting responsibility to the victim. Finally, the availability of a responsible, cooperative treatment resource allows the courts to impose treatment as a condition of sentencing, often with work furlough and other considerations that encourage continuing responsibility to the family.

I believe there is a therapeutic benefit to criminal conviction for crimes against children, whether the crime is committed within the privacy of the family or on the street, and whether the child is 4 years old or 15. With conviction, the primary responsibility of the offender is clearly defined, bringing what Giaretto (1976) called "the hard edge of society" against the man rather than the child. Conviction also challenges the power of the offender to act as if he is above the law and immune from the discomfort of the child. He can be forced to vacate the home in deference to the child, and he can be forced to remain in treatment and under probationary supervision to guard against future victimization of children. For incest offenders who have not been habitually attracted to children and who have not shown any capacity to victimize children outside the family, the Santa Clara County model of coordinated treatment has proved very effective (Giaretto, 1978). For habitual child molesters, there is little optimism for treatment but all the more need for effective sentencing and societal controls. In either case, the man will not be convicted on the strength of the child's testimony without strong and immediate professional and peer-group support of the victim and her mother (Berliner & Stevens, 1979). The younger the child and the more closely dependent she and her mother are on the offender, the less likely it is that the offender will be charged with a crime unless there is close cooperation between courts and treatment resources.

As Dr. Sgroi (1978) has written:

> Perhaps the greatest lapse of societal concern for sexually abused children lies in the failure to link punishment of the convicted offender to treatment. . . . the track record in persuading perpetrators and families to undergo voluntary therapy for incest is abysmal. Although referrals to a psychiatric or counselling agency may be eagerly accepted at the outset, perpetrators of incest rarely remain in an effective treatment program when the pressure to participate slackens.

> Why do we ignore compelling evidence that an authoritative incentive
> to change his or her behavior is absolutely essential for the adult perpetra-
> tor of child sexual abuse? Why are we so slow to establish a network of
> family sexual abuse treatment programs patterned after the highly success-
> ful Child Sexual Abuse Treatment Program in San Jose, California? It has
> been demonstrated that there *is* a humane alternative to separation, family
> breakup, and incarceration for incest. It required concern, caring, skill, and
> an authoritative "or else" to insure family participation. . . . Leadership
> will have to come from the very therapeutic community that has worked
> so poorly with the criminal justice system in the past and tends to be so
> uncomfortable with authoritative incentives for treatment. However, we
> will tolerate sexual abuse of children as long as most of us live in states
> and communities where no family treatment programs for sexual abuse
> exist. (pp. xx–xxi)

Every child of incest deserves a mother who can understand her
daughter's position without feeling betrayed or resentful. Every child
deserves a mother who can make a clear choice for protection of her
child without prejudice, even if that means severing an otherwise re-
warding adult relationship. Every woman who discovers that her husband has taken her daughter as a sexual partner deserves help in sort-
ing out her own reactions to such an assaultive discovery. And every
mother who has been a partner to incestuous assault, no matter how
passive or unwitting her role may have been, should be evaluated by
professionals who are sensitive to the dynamics of child abuse before
it is assumed that she is ready to assume protective responsibility for
her children, with or without the assistance of the designated offender.

These considerations for the mother are not only minimal requirements for the safety and growth of the children but minimal services
for the needs of the mother as well.

There are philosophical differences among treatment programs, of
course. Some feel that conviction and punishment of offenders is
countertherapeutic. Others wish for conviction but will not involve
themselves in witness preparation, testimony, or reports to the courts.
Some feel that conviction and removal of the male offender offer the
only hope for enfranchisement of the child and her mother. Some demand institutionalization of the father but avoid treatment of child or
mother for fear of stigmatizing them with labels of mental illness or
culpability. Some insist that all members of the incestuous family are
linked in a shared vulnerability and must be treated as a unit, carefully avoiding any assignment of independent or individual problems.
In the extreme, such an emphasis on family dynamics can obscure the
basic understanding that the offender alone had the knowledge and
power either to initiate or to avoid the incestuous relationship.

Typical models with contrasting philosophies have been selected and funded as training centers by the National Center of Child Abuse and Neglect, U.S. Department of Health and Human Services. Further evaluation of program effectiveness should lead to increasing availability of reliable treatment programs throughout the United States.

I feel that the trends are already clear and irreversible. We are committed as a society to intervening on behalf of the children we discover to be abused. We are moving toward the discovery of increasing numbers of sexually abused children, as well as increasing numbers of adult women who can acknowledge a history of childhood sexual abuse. Knowledge gained from these disclosures gives us a better definition of the risks as well as more clearly defined patterns of entrapment and accommodation. Emerging treatment networks provide mechanisms for more effective intervention, using the power of the courts to challenge abusive parental style as well as to motivate parents to take the risks of exploring and resolving their conflicts in parenting.

I hope that the treatment programs given this power to act on behalf of the courts will draw on the most client-empathic models currently available to foster maximum self-esteem, self-confidence, and self-control in every member of the family. I hope they will be child-protective as well as adult-supportive. And I hope they will be as endorsing of loving and caring and touching as they are alert to role reversing, possessing, and intruding. I hope that the designated helpers will be selected and trained to be genuine and open with clients and to welcome client participation in treatment planning. If these second-generation treatment resources have learned from the best of the current programs, they will offer resocialization of parents and reparenting of victims. This current rediscovery of incest carries with it a new potential for belief and new guidelines for moving beyond belief to achieve a better climate of nurturance and trust between adults and children.

Some of the joy and hope of that nurturing relationship can be seen in this letter from Stephanie to her therapist, Carmen, who with a peer group of incest survivors showed Stephanie the beginnings of noncontingent caring:

> Your hugs are warm: When you hold me I feel warm and good; most importantly warm.
>
> Your hugs are caring: They prove a person is cared for. Who can willingly hold someone they dislike or hate? When you hold me I feel cared for.
>
> Your hugs are respectful: They start and stop on time, allowing respect for someone's choice. When you hold me I feel I have the right to say what happens to my own body. Not duty bound or forced. I can say *No.*

Your hugs are deeply satisfying: When you hold me the pain in my chest stops and the longing is fed. They last long enough to fill the whole with your goodness.

Your hugs are free: There are no payments expected or obligations attached to them.

Your hugs are precious: I feel I've been given something precious with each hug; and indeed I have. One of the most precious things in my life.

Your hugs are full: Arms surrounding completely and just tight enough to hold the goodness in and keep it from escaping. Close enough to really feel cared for.

Your hugs are encouraging: They make me feel that the dirt doesn't show. Who could put their arms around a mass of green slime? If it doesn't show and can't be felt, perhaps there is a slight doubt that it exists.

Your hugs are strong: They come from someone strong. I seem to be able to gain strength from them. Things don't look so bad when there's someone more than just yourself to back you up; there's someone there telling you that whatever you decide is okay.

Your hugs are sincere: There's no doubt that every hug you give away is given with true warmth and caring to back it up.

Your hugs are supportive: They make me feel worthwhile and make me want more than ever to get well, not only for myself but for you because you're taking the time and effort to try. Thank you.

Your hugs are clean: They sparkle and they look, feel, and smell as clean and fresh as you do. No amount of scrubbing could make them any brighter.

Your hugs are comforting: In the dark when I'm scared I pretend a hug from you and the dark is not so very frightening anymore.

Your hugs are mine: The hugs you choose to give to me are mine. No one can take them from me or steal their memory. They're mine forever and don't have to be shared with anyone.

Your hugs are special: Just because they come from you they're especially special.

Your hugs are everything a hug should be.

Thank you for your *hugs*.

REFERENCES

Berliner, L., & Stevens, D. Special techniques for child witnesses. In L. G. Shultz (Ed.), *The sexual victimology of youth*. Springfield, Ill.: Charles C Thomas, 1979.

Bonaparte, M., Freud, A., & Kris, E. (Eds.). *The origins of psychoanalysis*, Letters to Wilhelm Fliess, Drafts and notes: *1877–1902*, E. Mosbacher & J. Strachey (Trans.). New York: Basic Books, 1954.

Burgess, A., & Holmstrom, L. Sexual trauma of children and adolescents: Pressure, sex and secrecy. *Nursing Clinics of North America*, 1975, *10*(3), 551–563.

Ferenczi, S. Confusion of tongues between adults and the child. In *Final contributions to the problems and methods of psychoanalysis.* New York: Basic Books, 1955, pp. 155–167. (Originally published, 1933.)

Finkelhor, D. *Sexually victimized children.* New York: Free Press, 1979.

Finkelhor, D. Risk factors in the sexual victimization of children. *Child Abuse and Neglect,* 1980, *4,* 265–273.

Freud, S. The aetiology of hysteria. *Collected papers,* Vol. 1. London: Hogarth Press, 1953. (Originally published, 1896.)

Freud, S. *The complete introductory lectures of psycho-analysis.* New York: Norton, 1966. (Originally published, 1933.)

Gagnon, J. Female child victims of sex offenses. *Social Problems,* 1965, *13,* 176–192.

Giaretto, H. Humanistic treatment of father–daughter incest. In R. E. Helfer & C. H. Kempe (Eds.), *Child abuse and neglect: The family and the community.* Cambridge, Mass.: Ballinger, 1976, pp. 143–157.

Giaretto, H., & Giaretto, A. Coordinated community treatment of incest. In A. W. Burgess, A. N. Groth, L. L. Holmstrom, & S. M. Sgroi. *Sexual assault of children and adolescents.* Lexington, Mass.: Lexington Books, D. C. Heath, 1978, pp. 231–240.

Landis, J. Experiences of 500 children with adult sexual deviants. *Psychiatric Quarterly Supplement,* 1956, *30,* 91–109.

Myers, B. Incest: If you think the word is ugly, take a look at the effects. In K. MacFarlane, B. Jones, & L. Jenstrom (Eds.), *Sexual abuse of children: Selected readings.* Washington, D.C.: National Center on Child Abuse and Neglect, Department of Health and Human Services, U.S. Government Printing Office, 1981, pp. 98–101.

Peters, J. Children who are victims of sexual assault and the psychology of offenders. *American Journal of Psychotherapy,* 1976, *30*(3), 398–432.

Rothenberg, M. Is there an unconscious national conspiracy against children in the United States? *Clinical Pediatrics,* 1980, *19*(1), 10–24.

Rush, F. The Freudian coverup. *Chrysalis,* 1977, *1*(1), 31–45.

Sgroi, S. Sexual molestation of children: The last frontier in child abuse. *Children Today,* 1975, *4,* 18–21, 44.

Sgroi, S. Introduction: A national needs assessment for protecting child victims of sexual assault. In A. W. Burgess, A. N. Groth, L. L. Holmstrom, & S. M. Sgroi, *Sexual assault of children and adolescents.* Lexington, Mass.: Lexington Books, D. C. Heath, 1978, pp. xv–xxii.

Shengold, L. Child abuse and deprivation: Soul murder. *Journal of the American Psychoanalytic Association,* 1979, *27*(3), 533–559.

Summit, R. Sexual child abuse, the psychotherapist and the team concept. In H. Donovan & R. J. Beran (Eds.), *Dealing with sexual child abuse,* Vol 2. Chicago: National Committee for Prevention of Child Abuse, 1978, pp. 19–33.

Summit, R., & Kryso, J. Sexual abuse of children: A clinical spectrum. *American Journal of Orthopsychiatry,* 1978, *48*(2), 237–251.

FILMS

Child Molestation: When to Say No. Glendale, Ca.: AIMS Instructional Media Services, Inc., 1977.

Incest: The Victim Nobody Believes. Sausalito, Ca.: J. Gary Mitchell Film Company, 1976.

Shatter the Silence. Los Angeles: S-L Film Productions, 1979.

Who Do You Tell? Shiller Park, Ill.: MTI Teleprograms, Inc., 1978.

Chapter 8

Effects of Teenage Motherhood

Merle G. Church

Editor's Note to Chapters 8–11

We humans are, perhaps, evolution's experiment with the specialization of the mind. We can form symbols and therefore can think abstractly, speak about "meaning," and produce "art." An extremely early demonstration of this capacity is found in early man's manufacture of things beyond immediate use, that is, symbolic things such as the neolithic figurines of voluptuous female forms. Female fertility seems to have obsessed our early symbolic process. The Venus of Würtemberg is either grossly obese, or pregnant, or both, as are most of these fertility figures. It is a curious contradiction that while women have been prized by society for their fertility, the organ responsible has been seen as the source of danger and weakness. Quite different are the proud attributions of strength, courage, and power given to the male's procreative equipment. Perhaps awe for the female organ's capacities was too great and it was enviously driven out to wander. This wandering womb was seen as the cause of woman's infirmities and as the explanation for her inescapable inadequacies. In early America, she was not educated because it was believed her reproductive organs would shrivel and cease to function! In our more sophisticated days, she gets "the curse" monthly and is so subject to the ravages of hormonal fluctuations as to be considered unfit for public office. Motherhood was a blessing though not as blessed as virginity, which, however, if carried to extremes, could lead to pitiful spinsterhood and barenness. What a bittersweet potion of mixed messages. It is no surprise that as women have been increasingly released from a limited life and a destiny bound by their anatomy (released first by medical advances in anesthesia, antiseptics, prenatal care, and contemporary

Merle G. Church, M.A. • Legislative Advocate, former President, California Alliance Concerned with School Age Parents, Manhattan Beach, California 90266.

obstetrics, and then by contraception and safe abortion), they have had second thoughts about childbearing. We hear that a national magazine polling mothers found over 70% stating they would not become mothers if they had it to do over again! Motherhood: a lifetime contract, no pay, no training, no advancement, no insurance, a 24-hour day, and a product of uncertain quality! "Maternal instincts" have to be strong indeed for one to apply for that position. What about "maternal instincts"—are they a contrivance meant to idealize the inevitable, or something fundamental in female psychology?

One paper in this group attests to the legitimacy of interest in opting for the childless "family." The other papers demonstrate a conviction that bearing or not, woman's sexuality is symbolically connected to the potential for bearing and that the bearing processes alter her psychological and sexual status as well as her physical, economic, and social status. We are either too cynical or too wise to believe, as Freud suggested, that woman's psychological traumas in early life can be resolved by giving birth. The papers on teenage pregnancy in this series might suggest that that particular theory manifests itself as the hope of these adolescents. For the adult woman, we know the most vulnerable time for depressive illness is the six months post partum, and that women alone with children (as an increasing number of women are) are at highest risk for impoverishment and disease of all kinds.

Rachel Pape's paper makes clear the multitude of psychological tasks of pregnancy. These tasks may induce development, but they can also undermine and deplete, or they can stimulate growth and bolster the integration of the mother's past and present and prepare her for a deeper connection to human history. Can female maturation take place fully without that experience? Can other creative activities play a similiar role in women's lives? Is women's sexual culmination not orgasm, but delivery? Why does one hear in the clinical setting of the loss of a "good sex life" after the children were born? Is "mother" asexual, or does father, like the child, think she should be? What are the factors that foster the possibility that pregnancy and child care will enrich and mature a woman's psychological and sexual life? We do not have the answers. Discovering that these are real questions, as yet unanswered, can promote the appropriate inquiry.

Little mothers, bad girls, baby dolls, and children with children are all labels given to teenage mothers. While such labels serve the purpose of drawing attention to a group of women in American society who are unique, they do little to encourage the adolescent mother who is serious about being a good parent.

It is the purpose of this chapter to explore the implications of teenage motherhood in the United States. In order to do that, we must discuss teenage sexuality and pregnancy. Additionally, the special needs of adolescent mothers will be explored. And finally, some positive suggestions for change will surface.

INTRODUCTION

Teenagers in the United States are sexually active as well as sexually ignorant. While society cannot realistically prevent teenagers from being sexually active, it certainly can eliminate sexual ignorance on the part of its youth.

Teenagers are conceiving and giving birth to children, whom they keep to raise themselves, in record numbers. The challenge to professionals to help these young people be effective parents is tremendous.

Teenage mothers are a high-risk group educationally, socially, and medically. If current trends are to be reversed, all three areas must be seriously addressed.

Over a decade ago, professionals from the fields of education, social service, and medicine who came in contact with pregnant teenagers in the course of their jobs began to realize the extent and impact of teenage pregnancy in the United States. Early efforts focused on keeping pregnant girls from being excluded from public schools, on including the girls in the social service system to assure some financial support and medical care, and on increasing the awareness within the medical community of the tremendous dangers faced by young mothers in delivering children. Professional groups were formed, and government agencies began to become aware of the special problems of teenage mothers.[1]

THE SITUATION TODAY

It is estimated that of 21 million young people in the United States between the ages of 15 and 19, more than half, or 11 million, are sexually active (U.S. Bureau of the Census, 1975). In addition, of the 8 million 13- and 14-year-olds, one-fifth, or over 1.5 million, are believed to have had intercourse. (Vener & Stewart, 1974). Annually, more than 1 million 15- to 19-year-olds become pregnant—one-tenth of all

[1]The National Alliance Concerned with School-Age Parents (NACSAP), with affiliates in California, Florida, Louisiana, Michigan, Ohio, Oregon, Washington, and Wisconsin, was formed in 1971 to act as an advocate organization for school-age parents and sexually active youth in the United States. NACSAP disbanded in 1978. Current national organizational efforts are being carried out by the National Organization on Adolescent Pregnancy and Parenting, Inc. (NOAPP), headquartered in Evanston, Illinois.

State organizations continue to grow. The strongest regional organizational attempt is being made by the Teen Age Pregnancy/Western Regional Educational Comthe young women in this age group. Additionally, more than 30,000 girls younger than 16 conceive (Guttmacher Institute, 1976). These statistics indicate that teenage sexual activity is an actuality that cannot be ignored.

Teenage sexual activity, viewed in conjunction with the fact that teenage childbearing rates in the United States are among the highest in the world, presents quite a challenge to members of the helping professions. Recent studies show that one-fifth of all the births in the United States are to teenagers. Of the over 600,000 teenagers who give birth each year, 38% are married (28% marry after learning they are pregnant), 21% give birth out of wedlock, and 27% terminate their pregnancies by abortion. The remaining 14% miscarry (National Center for Health Statistics, 1974).

Concern is growing for the girls younger than 15, who face all of the problems that their older sisters face, but whose situations are compounded by their early adolescence. Generally, teenage birthrates have declined since the beginning of the 1960s, but the decline has been restricted to older adolescents. Among girls 14 to 17, birthrates have remained constant, and among girls younger than 14, birthrates have actually risen (Guttmacher Institute, 1976, pp. 12–15).

The implications of these figures can be viewed from three vantage points: education, social service, and medicine. The three areas invariably overlap in a discussion of teenage motherhood. In fact, a separation of the disciplines leads to only a fragmentary approach when teenage mothers are really in need of comprehensive and integrated services from many areas. For purposes of discussion, however, the separation will be maintained.

EDUCATIONAL IMPLICATIONS OF TEENAGE MOTHERHOOD

Although many public school systems now offer special classes and programs for pregnant adolescents and teen mothers, school at-

---

mittee (TAP/WREC). This group grew out of the efforts on the part of the California, Oregon, and Washington Alliances Concerned with School Age Parents (CACSAP, OACSAP, and WACSAP). To date, 10 western states have joined in the effort to organize on a regional basis.

The Child Welfare League of America sponsors the Consortium on Early Childbearing and Childrearing, which collects, develops, and disseminates information to serve the needs of school-age parents.

The Office of Special Programs and Early Childhood Education, U.S. Department of Education, is engaged in efforts to encourage parenthood education in the public schools.

The Office of Adolescent Pregnancy and Parenting (OAPP), U.S. Department of Health and Human Services, focuses on providing comprehensive services in local communities for pregnant teens and teen parents.

tendance continues to be a significant problem. Often, pregnant girls are subtly counseled out of the public school by school personnel. Examples of such "counseling" include the high school counselor who fails to inform a pregnant girl that she does not *have* to attend the special school if she would rather stay in her regular high school, an assistant principal who informs the girl's parents that she is pregnant before she has the chance (or the courage) to tell them herself, and a physical education teacher who makes a girl run extra laps around the track when she discovers the girl is pregnant.[2] It is true that favorable legal decisions[3] and affirmative action programs prohibiting sexual discrimination in public schools (Summary of the Regulations for Title IX Education Amendments of 1972, 1976) have assured the right of the pregnant adolescent to continue in school. But the attitudes of many school personnel continue to discriminate against these girls.

An entirely new question is raised when one considers the right of the teenage mother to continue in public school after her baby is born. There is no question that the teenage mother faces discrimination. Gone are the days when a girl who "got in trouble" was sent off to live with "Aunt May" until the baby was born and could be placed for adoption. The fact is, rather, that almost all (94%) of teenagers who become pregnant and give birth keep their babies and bring them home. The figure drops a little (87%) for babies born to teenagers out of wedlock, but it is still a significant number of very young mothers at home with their babies (Zelnick & Kantner, 1974). A recent study (Church, 1974) showed that while many teenage mothers were interested in continuing their education, the lack of care for their infants prevented them from returning to school after delivery.

The tendency of almost all teenagers who give birth to keep their babies has increased the awareness of a few educators of the tremendous need for infant care in order for teenage mothers to finish high school, perhaps continue in college or a job training program, and gain the skills that will make them employable. While infant day-care centers do exist on a few high school campuses and in a few communities across the country, the reality is that 80% of the existing day-care centers in the United States will not allow children under 2 to enroll. (Pierce, 1975). What choice does a teenage mother with no one to care for her child have other than to drop out of school?

Another immediate educational concern is the need to help teen-

---

[2]Much of the information in this chapter has been obtained from confidential counseling sessions with pregnant adolescents and teenage parents by the author. Hereafter, such information will be noted as "counseling session."

[3]*Perry* v. *Granada Municipal Separate School District*, 300 P. Supp. 748 (1969) and *Ordway* v. *Hargraves*, D. Mass, 323 F. Supp. 1155 (1971) both upheld the rights of pregnant teenagers to remain in public schools.

age mothers become effective parents. It has been estimated that about half of teenage pregnancies that result in birth are unplanned (Zelnick & Kantner, 1974). An unplanned pregnancy and birth mean unplanned parents. The question of what kind of mothers teenagers make must be addressed.

It is healthy that concern for helping adolescent mothers become good parents seems to be running parallel with a national belief that *all* age groups could use some help in becoming effective parents. Awareness by such organizations as the PTA and the March of Dimes that parenthood education is a necessary part of the public school curriculum helps focus attention on the immediate needs of teenage mothers. Also, the emergence of private groups that exist solely for the purpose of training parents to be more effective certainly cannot harm the plight of very young mothers.

Another area where public attention is being focused can also benefit the school-age parent population, that is, the problem of child abuse. While no significant data exist that show that the incidence of child abuse is greater or less in the the teen parent population than in any other group, it is still important that the implications of, and the facts surrounding, the emotional and physical abuse of children are being brought into the open. Additionally, child abuse is a subject that greatly interests most teenage mothers. Many remember being abused physically by their parents and do not want to do the same to their own children. When presented with information regarding the emotional aspects of abuse, many teenage mothers are able to relate quite clearly to the more subtle behavior of their own parents or stepparents (Guttmacher Institute, 1976, p. 26).

Yet public education remains woefully negligent in responding to the needs of teenage mothers. At one time, special programs in public schools were often presented under the umbrella of special education, which, while it gave the girls yet another label, *physically handicapped,* did provide administration and funding for programs.

Recent federal legislation (Public Law 94-142), however, does not include pregnant minors in special education. The fate of the existing special school programs is up to the discretion of state legislatures and departments of education. While such programs do tend to resemble putting a finger in the dike, they have merit and should continue to exist. Often, special school programs are the key factor in the expansion of educational services for school-age mothers.

Additionally, special programs serve as a starting point for the organization of other services for teen mothers. Educators involved in special programs for teen mothers do not ignore the need for the organization of comprehensive services for the girls. Often, they are the initiators of the contacts that pregnant girls and teen mothers make with social workers, counselors, ministers, nurses, and doctors. Unfortunately, such educators are too few in number to provide adequate services to all teenage mothers.

SOCIAL IMPLICATIONS OF TEENAGE MOTHERHOOD

Teenage motherhood also has a profound effect on the social-service delivery system in the United States. Teenage mothers are much more likely to be unemployed and to rely on welfare than are older mothers. Statistics from a study done in New York City show that 91% of women who had their first babies between the ages of 15 and 19 were unemployed, and 72% were receiving welfare payments (Guttmacher Institute, 1976). A recent California study shows that 90% of all single women who head households and who are receiving Aid to Families with Dependent Children (AFDC, or welfare) did not finish high school. As a group, they were categorized as "substantially underschooled, untrained and underskilled" (The Rand Corporation, 1977).

Attitudes of teenage mothers toward the public welfare system vary from resigned acceptance to outright refusal to apply for assistance because they are "too proud." Some girls see their welfare grants, which can be over $200 a month in some parts of the country, as a windfall. It certainly is more money than they had been used to receiving before they became pregnant. It is not very long before adolescent mothers realize how difficult it is to live the type of life they would like for themselves and their children on what welfare grants provide. In reality, however, most school-age mothers must depend on public welfare as the provider of food, shelter, and medical care (counseling sessions).

Seen from the point of view of the frustrated taxpayer, the public welfare system has often been categorized as a bureaucratic monster, a hopeless maze, and a never-ending nightmare. Seen from the point of view of the recipient, whom it is meant to benefit but whom it sometimes victimizes, the public welfare system, with its waiting, endless questions and delays, and complex rules, often leads to feelings of alienation and despair (Foster, 1977). Adolescent mothers who are not used to dealing with "the system" are often frustrated by procedures they do not understand and by personnel who do not understand them.

Intake workers and social workers, who admittedly are often overburdened with heavy caseloads, sometimes have a difficult time sep-

arating their own value systems from those of their clients. While carrying out their duties, in the strictest sense, they manage to transmit
negative and unsympathetic feelings to pregnant adolescents and adolescent mothers. At times, however, it does seem that there is a group
who are "welfare-wise," whose families and friends have been using
public assistance for several generations, and who now feel it is "their
turn" to "be their own case" (counseling sessions).

Suggestions for tying social services to required attendance in
school or a job-training program seem to make a great deal of sense in
the case of teenage mothers. Statistics relating poverty to teenage
motherhood reveal that the younger a woman is when she gives birth
to her first child, the more likely she is to be poor (U.S. Bureau of the
Census, 1976). Requiring positive and responsible actions on the part
of teenage mothers receiving public assistance may well ensure that
they will not give up and drop out and will be able to escape poverty.

Another factor that makes these mothers socially different from
other mothers is the fact that they are adolescents. In general, adolescence is a time for growth and change. It is also a time of stress, when
adolescents often find themselves in conflict with their parents and the
world around them (Howard, 1975). When pregnancy, with all of the
ensuing rapid decisions, is added to adolescence, an explosive situation exists. It is imperative that social agencies recognize and deal with
this dual phenomenon.

Divorce statistics also separate teenage mothers from older mothers. If the pregnant adolescent makes the decision to marry before the
birth of her child, she is three times more likely to separate from or
divorce her spouse than are older married women (Ross & Sawhill,
1975). A Baltimore study showed that three out of five premaritally
pregnant mothers aged 17 and under were separated or divorced within
six years of marriage. One-fifth of the marriages were dissolved within
12 months, which is 2½ times the proportion of broken marriages
among the classmates of the adolescent mothers who were not pregnant when they married. Interestingly enough, those teenage mothers
who married the father prior to the child's delivery were more likely
to stay married than those who did not marry until after the birth of
the child (Furstenberg, 1976).

While the public welfare system plays an extremely important role
for teenage mothers, it must be realized that it does not have the sole
responsibility for educating and training teenage mothers to be productive citizens. Rather, the responsibility must be shared by all public agencies to ensure that teenage mothers receive adequate educational, social, and medical services.

Medical Implications of Teenage Motherhood

The medical statistics relating to teenage motherhood are frightening. They reveal that, as a group, teenage mothers and their children are at very high risk indeed. Statistical variables describing teenage mothers include birth weight, infant survival, maternal complications, and long-term developmental consequences for the child (Stickle & Ma, 1975).

Babies born to teenagers are much more likely to be premature and of low birth weight than are babies born to older mothers. Adolescent mothers, who bear 19% of all of the infants in the United States, have 26% of all low-birth-weight babies. Low birth weight has been shown to be not only a major cause of infant mortality but also a cause of many childhood illnesses and birth injuries, such as neurological defects, which may involve lifelong mental retardation (National Center for Health Statistics, 1973, 1974).

In addition, teenagers are much more likely to lose their babies soon after birth than are older mothers. The younger the mother, the more likely it is that her baby will die. In fact, about 6% of first babies born to girls under 15 die in their first year. This is a rate 2½ times higher than for women who give birth in their early 20s (National Center for Health Statistics, 1973, 1974).

Not only is the infant of a teenage mother at a greater risk of death, defect, and illness than the infant born to an older mother, but the teenage mother herself is more likely to suffer illness or injury or to die than is an older mother. The death rate from complications of pregnancy, birth, and delivery is 60% higher for girls who become pregnant under the age of 15 than it is for mothers in their early 20s. In the 15- to 19-year-old group, the risk is 13% higher than for mothers in their early 20s (National Center for Health Statistics, 1973, 1974).

The "special hazard" of pregnancy among the younger group of teenagers is toxemia. The incomplete development of the endrocrine systems of early adolescents, coupled with the emotional stress of the pregnancy, poor diet, and inadequate prenatal care, contributes to toxemia. In very young pregnant teens, the pregnancy itself depletes nutritional reserves needed for their own growth and thus places them at a higher risk for a variety of ills (Guttmacher Institute, 1976, p. 23).

The medical community also has its share of personnel who pass judgment on pregnant teenagers and very young mothers. (It is probably the same percentage as is found in the educational establishment and the social service agencies!) Consider the doctor who schedules all of his patients who rely on welfare for the same day and then regularly cancels appointments on that day because of an "unexpected" emergency; or the doctor who makes snide and insulting remarks while giving pregnant teenagers their first pelvic examinations; and the nurse who offers the girls unsolicited advice and directives regarding abortion and adoption. Unfortunately, such individuals are practicing today and are treating pregnant teenagers (counseling sessions).

USE OF CONTRACEPTIVES AMONG TEENAGERS

When confronted with some of this information related to teenage motherhood, many hitherto-uninformed individuals reply with statements like "Why, in this day and age of sexual freedom, don't they take the pill?"

Whether or not a sexually active teenager uses contraceptives depends on many factors. Many are simply ignorant and feel that they cannot become pregnant because of the time of the month, their age, or the infrequency of intercourse (Shah, Zelnick, & Kantner, 1975). Even though some states have liberalized the laws concerning the ability of minors to obtain contraceptives without parental consent, many young people simply are not aware of their rights. Most are unwilling to go to their parents to ask for contraceptive information (counseling sessions).

Other reasons for the nonuse of contraceptives by teenage girls are fascinating, if somewhat unrealistic. They can be identified with certain cultural or ethnic groups. White middle-class girls tend to view "taking the pill" as planning to be promiscuous; in their eyes, intercourse is a result of "love" and should be "spontaneous." Black teenage girls may have been told that "taking the pill" is a form of black genocide on the part of the white community, and they are mistrustful. Contraception and the Latin population are historically at odds with one another, and this shows in the number of teenage mothers in the Latin community (counseling sessions).

Some teenagers simply want to have a baby. For some, especially the younger adolescents, a baby represents "something that's mine, that I can love and that will love me back." These girls are sorely disappointed when they discover the tremendous and constant needs that infants and young children have. The demands of motherhood are often more than they can bear and are certainly not what they expected while pregnant. The percentage of teenagers who do not use contraception because they consciously want to become pregnant is small (1 out of 5 in one study; Guttmacher Institute, 1976, p. 30). But it does reflect a part of the value system of American society that views childbirth and child raising in a frighteningly unrealistic manner.

WHAT CAN BE DONE?

Obviously, from what has been said before, the problems associated with teenage pregnancy and motherhood are not going to disappear without a great deal of concerted effort by the American public as a whole. Solutions to the problems created by such young parenting are both short- and long-range.

Immediately, teenage mothers need comprehensive educational, social, and medical help. At the present time, services are fragmented, and agencies are often out of touch with each other. Professionals from all fields must work together to ensure that services will be readily available to teenage mothers. They must work together to ensure that such services will be delivered in nonthreatening and humane settings and will be administered by caring professionals who are aware of the teenage mothers' problems, both actual and potential.

More permanent solutions, which should, in effect, eliminate unwanted teenage pregnancies and births, are much more complex than the short-range solutions. They involve tremendous changes in the attitudes of a great number of Americans. When punitive, judgmental, and unsympathetic attitudes exist among the professionals who are working directly with pregnant teenagers and teenage parents, it takes little imagination to discern what uninformed individuals might have to say on the subject of adolescent sexuality and teenage motherhood! In short, professionals working with teenagers and teenage parents not only need to educate their less caring associates, but also share the enormous responsibility of educating the public in general.

To suggest immediate solutions to the problems of teenage mothers, however, is to return to the question of the parenting skills possessed by teenage mothers. Two thoughts come to mind: what are good parents, teenage or otherwise? and how do you teach parents, teenage or otherwise, to be good ones?

One of the primary requisites of a good parent is a positive feeling of self-worth. Constructive interaction between parents and children can occur only when the parents feel good about themselves. As many teenage mothers have very poor self-concepts, this is an important point to remember. Programs designed for teenage mothers must include components that concentrate on values and self-awareness (Church, 1977).

Being a good parent is not a static thing. It is, rather, an ongoing process that involves constant reevaluation and change. Effective parenting involves constant and continual questioning of values and relationships. Relating these concepts about parenting skills to adolescents may at times seem monumental, but it can be done effectively.

In addition to poor self-concepts, teenage mothers frequently have very poor models for parents. Here is where the professional is of vast importance in shaping the parenting skills of teenage mothers. Professionals working with teen parents must be able to provide that lacking model. An interesting study in progress seems to be showing that a high number of teenage mothers were born to mothers who were teenage mothers themselves (Merle G. Church, study in progress in the Glendale Unified School District, Glendale, California).

A very effective way to supply this substitute model is through an infant day-care center that is used as a laboratory in which the young parents and professionals can interact with babies. The young mothers bring their babies to the center for care wile they attend school or work. Built into the program is the requirement that the young mothers spend time at the center interacting with the professionals as they care for their children. The young parents not only learn from each other, both positively and negatively, but they have a chance to observe trained people at work with their babies.

Just imagine the possibilities if such an infant day-care center existed on every high school campus in the country! Not just teenage parents but the community as a whole could benefit. Other mothers, in addition to teenage mothers, could take advantage of such centers. Think of all potential "grandparents" in the senior-citizen age group who would be fantastic aides or volunteers in such centers. Also, consider the impact on the teenagers who are not yet parents, but who probably will be someday. The educational aspects of such centers for helping *all* age groups learn to be effective parents seem almost endless.

It must be remembered, however, that teaching parenting skills to teenage mothers is a very delicate process. Even though professionals may consider the parenting models to which teenage parents have been exposed inadequate, they must proceed cautiously so as not to give undue criticism of a parent (a grandparent, by now) who is loved by the teenage parent and who may have been abusive.

A classic example is that of a teenage mother who was teaching her 16-month-old daughter not to bite other children at the day-care center by biting the child herself! When a professional intervened and suggested that she isolate the child and firmly tell her not to bite, her reply was "My mother bit me back. I'm seventeen years old, and I don't bite people anymore, so that must be the right way." It took some time, not to mention a very patient professional, to get the young mother to realize that she was, indeed, reverting to an abusive technique that her own mother had used on her. It certainly is a great challenge to help teenage mothers develop parental skills and value systems for themselves and their children.

Probably, the most important long-range solution to unwanted teenage pregnancy is realistic sex education that is available to all young people. It sounds so very simple, but the fact is that at the present time only 7 of 50 states *require* sex education in the public schools (Castile, 1976). The high degree of ignorance displayed by teenage mothers regarding contraception and birth should be message enough that the present system is not working.

Sex education that is honest and pertinent should be the number one priority for professionals working with pregnant adolescents and school-age parents. They should organize to ensure that legislation mandating sex education in the public schools will be enacted. Additionally, public pressure should be brought on churches, youth agencies, and the media to offer information about sexuality and human reproduction as well as contraception. Educational programs are also needed for parents so that they can better understand their children's needs, and how to help them.

Other suggestions include expanding the network of preventive family-planning programs designed especially to reach adolescents. Coverage in a national health insurance of all services related to adolescent pregnancy is a possibility as long as there is a particular emphasis on mechanics that will ensure the protection of the privacy of the teenagers. Expansion of biomedical research to discover new, safe, and effective contraceptive techniques better suited to the needs of young people also seems desirable (Guttmacher Institute, 1976, pp. 55–56).

WHY ISN'T IT BEING DONE

It is amazing to realize that the expertise for implementing all of the aforementioned ideas already exists within American society. The data concerning the high risks of teenage mothers and their children to society exist. The costs of implementing programs to make teenage mothers more responsible citizens and to ensure that their children will be healthy and happy are really not particularly high when compared with the cost that society is already paying for the epidemic of teenage births. Lack of necessary resources certainly does not explain why teenage mothers are only fragmentarily included in American help services.

Probably the most "comfortable" reason for the lack of attention being paid to the plight of teenage mothers is that many Americans do not know, or choose to ignore, the extent of the problem of adolescent pregnancy and childbearing. Certainly there are many other more pressing problems with which society must concern itself than those related to teenage motherhood! Even though the facts indicate that millions of people annually are affected by teenage sexuality, pregnancy, and childbirth, much of society chooses to ignore the situation.

A less popular, and much more insidious, reason for not facing the problems of teenage mothers is the still-prevalent opinion that adolescents must be punished for their sexual activity in the false hope that they will be so fearful that they will stop this activity. Such attitudes seem to reflect an inhibited and unhealthy view of sexuality on the part of many adults. So disturbed are they by adolescent sexuality that they prefer to avoid facing it. Yet the facts show that ignoring what exists only compounds the effects of the problem.

Several techniques have been effective in persuading some reluctant and judgmental adults to consider positive programs for teenage mothers. One is to give up on a person who is deemed uneducable on the subject and to move on to another person or group, rather than wasting time on someone whose ideas cannot be changed. Several years ago, when explaining why a pregnant girl could not remain in the regular high school, a school administrator commented, "We can't have a pregnant girl here. She might transmit oral sex information in the bathrooms."[4] Obviously, the time spent trying to educate or inform such an individual about teenage mothers is better spent elsewhere!

However, when confronted with the inevitable raised eyebrows, it sometimes is helpful to remind one's listener that hardly a family in the United States has *not* had to face the problem of a pregnant teenager at some time or another. Suddenly the cobwebs clear, and what happened to "poor cousin Lucy" is remembered. If a family situation is not to be admitted, it can be suggested that surely a friend must have gone through the experience.

Also, calling attention to the high risks that the babies of teenage mothers face can be useful. Again, some individuals are bent on condemning the pregnant adolescent, but when it is pointed out that to deny services to the teenage mother is also to deny services to her child, sometimes attitudes soften. After all, in five years the child of that pregnant teenager will be knocking on the door of a public school somewhere in the United States as a child ready for kindergarten. By providing adequate educational, social, and medical programs for the mother of that child, society is helping ensure that the child will be

---

[4]This statement was actually made to the author. She thought it so "classic" that she committed it to memory.

physically and emotionally healthy instead of being a handicapped child requiring added attention (and funds) from society.

Many individuals who oppose social programs to help those less fortunate than themselves do so on the basis of cost. The costs of special school programs, welfare grants, and medical facilities and services are deplored. Yet, persuasive arguments can be made that in the long run, it is much cheaper to provide educational, social, and medical services for pregnant teenagers and teenage mothers than to risk the expense of caring for a child that is born with handicaps.

Summary

Educationally, teenage mothers often suffer because they are forced to drop out of school in order to care for their infants. Socially, because of lack of education and training, teenage mothers are forced to rely on public assistance to exist. Medically, teenage mothers face high risks of complications associated with childbirth, and their children face a high risk of being born with defects.

Comprehensive educational, social, and medical programs are a must if American society wants to reduce the incidence of unwanted teenage pregnancy and childbirth, to reduce welfare dependence on the part of teenage mothers, and to ensure the physical and emotional health of both the mothers and the babies.

Opposition to such comprehensive programs for teenage mothers comes from ignorance of the situation, refusal to acknowledge the situation, and punitive attitudes based on personal values. In order to overcome such attitudinal opposition, professionals working with school-age parents must wage a full-force campaign. Through information disseminated by professionals, the American public must be educated about the problems associated with teenage motherhood and the solutions to those problems. Only in this way will attitudes be changed and adequate programs implemented.

Instead of the earlier-mentioned labels for teenage mothers, it is, indeed, a happy thought that an author recently writing about teenage pregnancy and parenthood labeled teenage mothers "only human."

References

Castile, A. S. *School health in America*. Kent, Ohio: American School Health Association, 1976.

Church, M. G. School-age parents express their concerns about their educational needs. *CACSAP Newsletter*, March 1974, pp. 2–5.

Church, M. G. Perspectives on parenting and child development: Young parents must feel good about themselves. *NACSAP Newsletter*, Winter/Spring 1977, pp. 6–8.

Foster, S. A short guide to welfare. *CACSAP Newsletter,* September 1977, pp. 4, 7–9.

Furstenberg, F. F., Jr. *Unplanned parenthood: The social consequences of teenage child-bearing.* New York: Free Press, Macmillan, 1976.

Guttmacher Institute. *11 Million Teenagers.* New York: Planned Parenthood Federation of America, 1976.

Howard, M. *Only human.* New York: Seabury Press, 1975.

National Center for Health Statistics. Natality. *Vital Statistics,* 1973, 1974.

National Center for Health Statistics. Department of Health, Education and Welfare. Natality. *Vital Statistics of the United States,* Washington, D.C.: U.S. Government Printing Office, 1974.

Pierce, W. L. Child Welfare League of America. Child Care Arrangements in the U.S. in 1974. Testimony before the 94th Congress; February 21, 1975.

The Rand Corporation. *AFDC caseload and the job market in California: Selected issues* (R-2115-CDOBP), April 1977.

Ross, H. L., & Sawhill, I. V. *Time of transition: The growth of families headed by women.* Washington, D.C.: The Urban Institute, 1975.

Shah, F., Zelnick, M., & Kantner, J. F. Unprotected intercourse among unwed teenagers. *Family Planning Perspectives,* 1975, 7, 32.

Stickle, G., & Ma, P. Pregnancy in adolescents: Scope of the problem. *Contemporary ObGyn,* 1975, 5 (6), 85–91.

Summary of the Regulations for Title IX Education Amendments of 1972. *Peer,* NOW Legal Defense and Education Fund, 1976.

U.S. Bureau of the Census. *Current Population Survey.* Unpublished tabulations of 1975.

U.S. Bureau of the Census. *Characteristics of the Population Below the Poverty Level, 1974* (CPR, Series P-60, No. 102). Washington, D.C.: U.S. Government Printing Office, 1976.

Vener, A. M., & Stewart, C. S. Adolescent sexual behavior in middle America revisited: 1970–1973. *Journal of Marriage and the Family,* 1974, 36, 728.

Zelnick, M., & Kantner, J. F. The resolution of teenage first pregnancies. *Family Planning Perspectives,* 1974, 6, 74.

Chapter 9

Does Motherhood Mean Maturity?

Max Sugar

Articles abound on the pregnant adolescent or the one who obtains an abortion, while the adolescent mother has received less consideration. This chapter focuses on whether, in adolescence, motherhood is a sign of maturity or helps in the teenager's development toward adulthood. Although the focus is on the adolescent, this question may also apply to those in their majority.

The Pregnant Adolescent

Before discussing motherhood, some remarks about its antecedents for the adolescent may be useful. Mothering is not an innate or inherited trait, but a learned one. It begins with childhood doll play and fantasy, to which is added the experience of the first pregnancy and the first child, and which is modified by later experience and subsequent children. The pregnant teenager has been described as a girl who has "a syndrome of failure—failure to fulfill her adolescent functions, remain in school, limit her family, establish stable values, be self-supporting, and have healthy infants" (Webb, Briggs, & Brown 1972). Probably, in three-quarters of the cases in the United States at present, this girl is black and in the low socioeconomic class; there is a 2-to-1 likelihood that she is on welfare and a 9-out-of-10 chance that she is not married and that she will have repeated pregnancies during her adolescence (Sarrel & Davis, 1966). One-third of these girls are from one-parent families, while another third have repeated family dislocations encompassing numerous substitute parents (La Barre, 1972).

Max Sugar, M.D. • Clinical Professor, Department of Psychiatry, Louisiana State University Medical Center, New Orleans, Louisiana 70112.

This group of girls has intercourse earlier than white girls of a comparable age and socioeconomic group; they experience pregnancy sooner, have a lower ideal age for marriage, and are less likely to use contraception. The black adolescent mother has a three times greater chance of becoming pregnant than her white teenage counterpart, and when pregnant, she is usually out of school or soon drops out (Zelnick & Kantner, 1972). If she is in school, she has about a one-third chance of not being up to grade level (Foltz, Klerman, & Jekel, 1972).

There are variable and numerous psychological descriptions of the pregnant adolescent. Schaffer and Pine (1972) found a recurring theme of conflict in the pregnant girl about mothering and being mothered. On learning of the pregnancy, she reacted with gross denial which seemed connected with a lack of cognitive appreciation of her body and its functions. There were regular fantasies by the pregnant teenager about being a better mother to the baby than her own mother had been to her, along with marked feelings of disappointment and anger toward her own mother.

Pregnancy Complications in Adolescence

There may be more complications for the pregnant adolescent than for the adult woman, but if she has access to a counseling program, the rate of complications may be reduced (La Barre, 1972). Compared with pregnant adults, pregnant teenagers have a three times greater chance of toxemia, prenatal and perinatal morbidity, hypertension, neonatal death, and perinatal and maternal death (Aubry & Pennington, 1973; Grant & Heald, 1972; Ruppersberg, 1973; Webb et al., 1972). Some contributing factors are race, marital status, unsuspected infection, self-induced abortion attempts, anemia, malnutrition, increased blood pressure, endocrine disorders, Rh-negative mother, and reproductive tract abnormalities, as well as the psychological and socioeconomic state.

Frequently, the pregnant teenager is unwed or becomes divorced. The likelihood of her marrying depends on the program to limit pregnancies that she might be in, but generally, without special help, about two-thirds remain unmarried. Of the 36% who do marry in adolescence, prior or subsequent to the pregnancy, about three-fourths are not living with their husbands after five years (Sarrel & Davis, 1966). Oppel and Royston (1971) noted that in the cases of 86 teenage mothers, only 24 fathers were there six to eight years after the birth of the baby, in contrast to 86 mothers over age 18 who still had the father of the baby there in 50% of the cases six to eight years later. To avoid a one-sided picture, the recent increase of father absence should be noted: in all nonwhite families, it has increased from 18% in 1950 to 30% in 1972, in contrast to father-absence rates in white families of 8% in 1950 and 9% in 1972 (Sciarra, 1975).

The emotional development of the teenager's ego and superego structures is incomplete (Jacobson, 1961). While an adolescent may rebel against parental direction, she may accept that provided by her boyfriend. One youngster said, "It's funny; I do what he wants even though the things he tells me are just like what my parents say, such as going on with school or not coming in late. I do it now to avoid hassles with my parents." Her capacity for abstract thinking may not have been reached, and circumstances may prevent her reaching it (Piaget, 1972). She has not satisfactorily settled the question of her mothering needs or her wish to be mothered, which is related to her second individuation development; nor has she settled her negative oedipal conflicts (Blos, 1962). She has been thrust into the mother-to-be role with little preparation, thought, or plan. She may become severely depressed and may attempt self-induced abortion or suicide. She has not completed her education and has little likelihood of doing so for many years to come, if ever. Her chance of getting married is much less than that of her nonpregnant teenage counterpart. She has a greater chance of divorce if she does marry, and if divorced, she will very likely live on welfare in a polymatric family.

The pregnant teenager consciously states that is is "no big deal" to have a baby, but getting married is a big event, even if she has been a mother for some time (Williams, 1974). This attitude appears to be denial, since several studies have indicated regrets or mixed feelings about the pregnancy in a large percentage of cases (Adler, 1975; Presser, 1974). The conscious attitude and the actual behavior leading to pregnancy seem connected with a lack of "fidelity"—distancing instead of intimacy (Erikson, 1968). The girl feels a very intensified rivalry with her own mother, since the teenager's sexual maturity is self-evident and may pose a threat to her mother, who is now nearing or facing the end of her own reproductive life. Rivalry may be brewing between them over the maternal role, and this will be focused on the questions of whose baby the girl is actually having, and who will care for it after delivery.

Among adolescent mothers, 22% have complications in labor or delivery, which are based to some extent on the complications of pregnancy (Webb et al., 1972), along with an 18% neonatal mortality rate. In a study of maternal deaths in Ohio over a 16-year period (Ruppersberg, 1973), adolescents accounted for 9% of the maternal death rate. In this group, 37% had infants who weighed 2500 grams or less, and only 49% had live births.

Pregnancy may help the adolescent mother to effect a separation from her own mother, but she remains dependent on her or on someone else for financial and other support if she is unmarried. Thus, the pregnancy may initiate a round of self-defeating behavior, instead of leading to a successful separation from home, a development of self-sufficiency and self-acceptance, and a healthy environment for the adolescent mother and her baby.

PROBLEMS IN MOTHERING

Brain-damaged, blind, or premature infants are at greater risk for poor mothering or becoming battered children than normal infants (Robson & Moss, 1970; Klein & Stern, 1971). Frommer and O'Shea (1973) found that mothers who had problems managing their infants were very depressed, had many physical complaints, and were polarized: either they were perfectionist in their pursuits and had a great deal of accompanying anxiety or they did not care for the infant. The authors felt that the basis for this was the common feature among these mothers of having had a permanent separation from one or both parents before age 11 (Frommer & O'Shea, 1973).

In a study of failure-to-thrive children by Evans, Reinhart, and Succop (1972), 50% of one group of mothers were depressed adolescents who had experienced a severe object loss within four months of the baby's hospitalization. Mothers in the second group had received very poor mothering in their own childhood, while those in the third group were victims of failure to thrive themselves.

CRISES IN THE PREGNANCY

Holmes and Rahe (1967) rated various life events as stresses for their weight in having some "etiologic significance as necessary but not sufficient cause of illness and [accounting] in part for the time of onset of disease" (p. 213). From my study of premature and full-term infants[1] I have tabulated these events during the pregnancy of their mothers, which occurred in 1969–1975. They were seen at the outpatient clinic of a large municipal hospital and at a city health clinic. Of the total group seen, 90% were black and 10% were white; 91% were in the lowest socioeconomic stratum. Adolescent mothers made up 52% of both the group of mothers whose infants' birth weights were 1250

[1] I am grateful to William Johnson, David Taylor, and Larry Webber for help with the statistical analyses.

Table 1. Comparison of Crises in Pregnancies of Adolescent and Adult Mothers by Infants' Birth Weight

Infants	Birth weight in grams		Crises in:		χ^{2a}	df	p^b
			Adolescent mother	Adult mother			
Premature	≤2500	Number	154	142			
		Percentage	56.5	35.6	12.33	2	0.002
Full-term	≥2501	Number	61	122			
		Percentage	55.7	33.6	8.41	1	0.004
All infants		Number	215	264			
		Percentage	56.3	35.2	20.74	3	<0.001

[a]If $\chi^2 \geq 3.84$, the percentages are significantly different.
[b]If $p < 0.05$, the percentages are significantly different.

grams or less and the group with infant birth weights over 1250 grams; they made up 33% of that group of mothers whose infants' birth weights were over 2501 grams. From anova, analyses of covariance, factor analyses, and t tests for the groups, the data indicate that the younger the mother, the greater chance she has of having a low-weight baby and one who will have a lengthier hospital stay than the infant of the adult mother ($p < .01$). Table 1 lists the crises or emotional stresses in pregnancy, except for the pregnancy—as outlined by Holmes and Rahe (1967)—for each of the different groups of mothers by birth weight of the infant and by the mother's age (i.e., adolescent, 19 or under; or adult, 20 or older). The difference between the adolescent and adult groups of mothers is notable. Only singleton births were listed.

There may be constitutional, genetic, environmental, nutritional, or metabolic factors, but the development of crises is partly self-arranged, and particular emotional patterns or dynamics are involved.

As indicated in Table 2, in the first six months, the adolescent mother also gave significantly less stimulation to the infant than the adult mother. The rate of stimulation was tabulated from the data from routine monthly visits resulting in an assessment of the mother's knowledge of and interaction with the infant, consisting of knowing what the baby does day to day, such as onset date of thumbsucking, the social smile, recognition of the mother's voice and face, following, reaching, rolling over, and cooing, as well as knowing its eating, sleeping, and play patterns intimately. The percentage of adequate stimulation for all adolescent as opposed to adult mothers was 76% versus 89%. But the percentage of adequate stimulation for adolescent

Table 2. Comparison of Adequate Stimulation of Infant by Mother's Age and Infant's Birth Weight

Infants	Birth weight in grams		Adequate stimulation by:		χ^{2a}	df	p^b
			Adolescent mother	Adult mother			
Premature	≤2500	Number	154	142			
		Percentage	73.4	85.2	6.72	2	0.035
Full-term	≥2501	Number	61	122			
		Percentage	83.6	94.3	4.38	1	0.036
All infants		Number	215	264			
		Percentage	76.3	89.4	11.10	3	0.011

[a] If $\chi^2 \geq 3.84$, the percentages are significantly different.
[b] If $p < 0.05$, the percentages are significantly different.

mothers of premature infants versus adult mothers of premature infants was 73% versus 85%. This finding supports the possibility of special problems in mothering premature infants.

DISCUSSION

The large number of crises in adolescent pregnancies may be related to the adolescents' incomplete education and emotional development, ambivalence, unsettled life situation, and lack of experience. Also, it would appear that the adolescent with a crisis in pregnancy may have a greater risk of a premature birth. In general, as Table 1 shows, adolescent mothers have about a one-third greater risk of having crises in pregnancy than adult mothers. This finding coincides with the findings by Holmes and Rahe (1967) and Heisel, Ream, Raitz, Rappaport, and Coddington (1973). Many of the crises are beyond the individual's control (e.g., death of a loved one or being laid off). The idea that more crises are to be expected with increasing age does not take into account that the individual makes a decision or has some input into the making of crises (e.g., dropping out of school, unemployment due to quitting a job, marrying, moving, resuming school, or taking a new job).

The adolescent mother's stimulation of her infant in the first six months is significantly less than the adult mother's. Two reasons for this appear to be the adolescent's narcissism and inadequate preparation for motherhood. These seem to be related to the adolescent's ambivalence about commitment to motherhood and her inexperience and lack of education.

The relationship of an adolescent mother with her own mother determines much of the girl's mothering behavior. The mothers of these girls seem to have been unable to provide for them satisfactorily, and perhaps some disturbance or deprivation occurred in the adolescent's rearing. The effect of early parental loss and of educational, cultural, and socioeconomic deprivation needs consideration in assessing the development of motherhood in adolescence.

Conflicts about mothering and the wish to be mothered seem to be regularly unresolved and may have contributed to the girl's acting out by becoming pregnant. The oedipal conflict may be the focal point, but perhaps less intensely than, or not exclusive of, a symbiotic state or other pregenital conflicts.

The adolescent's need for infantile objects and the conflict about detaching herself from them leads to a state of normal adolescent mourning (Sugar, 1968), and there are many varied responses to the loss of an object that may be intermingled with pathological defenses and maladaptation. Hetherington (1972) noted the effects of father absence on the daughter's heterosexuality. Singer (1975) described three defensive coping styles involved in adolescent promiscuity: (1) the girl may hate men but uses heterosexuality as a defense against regression to the preoedipal mother; (2) promiscuity is used as a defense against the oedipal defeat by a cruel or absent father, and the girl picks men with glaring personality defects; (3) the girl identifies with a rejecting father, chooses the mother as a sex object, and defies any man to conquer her.

Among my research group of mothers were some who made an unconscious ambivalent gift to the maternal grandmother in the form of the new baby for the grandmother to mother. This gift also served as a ransom for some to move out of the grandmother's home. This was particularly obvious in the 2% of the mothers who deserted their infants.

Thus, pregnancy in an adolescent may also be an unconscious effort to effect a separation, an attempt to make up for the loss of the infantile objects, a substitution and avoidance of early separation–individuation conflicts, or an attempt to avoid regression.

Laufer (1968) indicated that some adolescent suicides are related to a feeling on the youngster's part that her body does not belong to her and that it belongs to her parent. If she inflicts damage on it, it is not her body that is being damaged, but her parent's. The sense of disavowal and denial involved can reach psychotic proportions. Perhaps, in these girls who become pregnant in their teens, there is a similar sense of uncertainty about who owns the body they inhabit, so that when they become pregnant, it is not their body but the mother's body that they are experiencing as being pregnant, and they themselves are experiencing being mothered again. This attitude may be a factor in their promiscuity, drug addiction, and other self-destructive behavior.

The mother who gives up her infant for economic, psychological, or other reasons has to face some questions about her self-esteem and lack of confidence as a mother. The mother who is separated from her infant, whether because of prematurity or other complications, has a further difficulty in that she has lowered feelings of self-esteem and confidence in her ability to mother. Instead of feeling enhanced by the experience of the crucial first months, she has a possible loss to contend with and a sense of mourning for a child who may not live. If it lives, the child may not be healthy, and its lack of health results in the mother's loss of self-esteem since she could not deliver a viable or healthy child.

The unwed adolescent mother has difficulty in making a commitment. Many of these girls feel that it is a greater problem to consider marriage than it is to consider getting pregnant, which involves denial of the significance to them of both of these events. In my study, there seemed to be a connection between the infant's sleeping in the mother's bed and the mother's being very dependent on the grandmother, with whom she has had a rivalrous relationship involving maternity rights to the infant. Where a father was present, he was the target of the mother's hostility whether he resided with her or not, and she used the infant as a barrier against him. Both of these aspects of the mother's behavior seem to reflect the mother's arrested development (borderline state-symbiosis with the maternal grandmother). Frequently, the mother worked or was a student, and the maternal grandmother shared the mothering. The mother then felt part child and part mother, dependently hostile and uninterested in a commitment to any male. Some of these mothers had repeated pregnancies, and their dependency problem was quite clear and significant, but they had no wish to have a man take care of them. They seemed to prefer dependency on their own mother or the state. This condition precludes a sense of fidelity (Erikson, 1968) and commitment to a heterosexual object, which involves a further stage in adolescent development.

These particular factors have some commonality for the group of adolescent mothers, but the dynamics, defenses, and diagnoses are quite individual. Behaviorally, it may seem that a young adolescent, especially if single, who becomes a mother is "grown-up," but psychodynamically she is probably not yet in adolescence. A well-defined and well-structured arrangement would be required for treatment of such a youngster, and some such programs have described a marked improvement in the youngster's development (La Barre, 1972).

Summary

The question of adolescent motherhood's reflecting emotional maturity and its relation to the girl's further development is examined in this chapter. It appears that there are a number of antecedent experiences and psychological configurations that determine whether an adolescent becomes pregnant, and then a mother, whether wed or not, and what kind of mother and person she will be. The dynamics of adolescent motherhood seem related to oedipal conflicts, but symbiotic or other preoedipal conflicts predominate.

Complications accumulate for the adolescent mother, along with frequent crises, as well as physical difficulties before and after the pregnancy and labor. The inadequacies of the adolescent mother may be manifest in her inability to provide for herself or her infant or to relate to a mate satisfactorily, since she is in a symbiosis with her own mother. These needs, her lack of commitment, and her fantasies about her infant seem to be reflected in her relatively inadequate stimulation of her infant, in her sharing the mothering of the infant with its grandmother, in repeated pregnancies while unwed, or in her raising youngsters with serious emotional problems.

For most girls, adolescent motherhood confounds emotional development by engendering or protracting their dependency on their own mothers, which further delays their development of separation-individuation, adult psychic structures, a sense of commitment, and fidelity to a heterosexual object. From a practical point of view, this signifies an arrest in emotional development and incomplete preparation for self-sufficiency and motherhood, which perpetuates pathological dependency and self-defeating behavior. This obviously implies a delay in, or lack of, maturity.

References

Adler, N. A. Emotional responses of women following therapeutic abortion. *American Journal of Orthopsychiatry*, 1975, 45, 446–454.

Aubry, R. H., & Pennington, J. C. Identification and evaluation of high-risk pregnancy. *Clinical Obstetrics and Gynecology*, 1973, *16*, 3–27.

Blos, P. *On adolescence: A psychoanalytic interpretation*. Glencoe, Ill.: Free Press, 1962.

Erikson, E. H. *Identity, youth and crisis*. New York: Norton, 1968.

Evans, S., Reinhart, J. B., & Succop, R. A. Failure to thrive. *Journal of the American Academy of Child Psychiatry*, 1972, *11*, 440–457.

Foltz, A., Klerman, L. V., & Jekel, J. F. Pregnancy and special education: Who stays in school? *American Journal of Public Health*, 1972, *62*, 1612–1619.

Frommer, E. A. & O'Shea, G. Antenatal identification of women liable to have problems in managing their infants. *British Journal of Psychiatry*, 1973, *123*, 149–156.

Grant, J. A., & Heald, F. P. Complications of adolescent pregnancy. *Clinical Pediatrics*, 1972, *11*, 567–570.

Heisel, J. T., Ream, S., Raitz, R., Rappaport, M., & Coddington, R. D. The significance of life events as contributing factors in the diseases of children. *Journal of Pediatrics*, 1973, *83*, 119–123.

Hetherington, E. M. Effects of father absence on personality development in adolescent daughters. *Developmental Psychology*, 1972, *7*, 313–326.

Holmes, T. H., & Rahe, R. H. The social readjustment scale. *Journal of Psychosomatic Research*, 1967, *11*, 213–218.

Jacobson, E. Adolescent moods and the remodeling of psychic structures in adolescence. *Psychoanalytic Study of the Child*, 1961, *16*, 164–183.

Klein, M., & Stern, L. Low birth weight and the battered child syndrome. *American Journal of Diseases of the Child*, 1971, *122*, 15–18.

La Barre, M. Emotional crises of school-age girls during pregnancy and early motherhood. *Journal of the American Academy of Child Psychiatry*, 1972, *11*, 537–557.

Laufer, M. The body image, function of masturbation, and adolescence. *Psychoanalytic Study of the Child*, 1968, *23*, 114–137.

Oppel, W. C., & Royston, A. B. Teen-age births: Some social, psychological and physical sequelae. *American Journal of Public Health*, 1971, *61*, 751–756.

Piaget, J. Intellectual evolution from adolescence to adulthood. *Human Development*, 1972, *15*, 1–12.

Presser, H. B. Early motherhood: Ignorance or bliss? *Family Planning Perspectives*, 1974, *6*, 8–14.

Robson, K. S., & Moss, H. A. Patterns and determinants of maternal attachment. *Journal of Pediatrics*, 1970, *77*, 976–985.

Ruppersberg, A. Maternal deaths among Ohio teenagers: A 16 year study. *Ohio State Medical Journal*, 1973, *69*, 692–694.

Sarrel, P. M., & Davis, C. A. The young unwed primipara. *American Journal of Obstetrics and Gynecology*, 1966, *95*, 722–725.

Schaffer, C., & Pine, F. Pregnancy, abortion and the developmental tasks of adolescence. *Journal of the American Academy of Child Psychiatry*, 1972, *11*, 511–536.

Sciarra, F. Effects of father absence on the educational achievement of urban black children. *Child Study Journal*, 1975, *5*, 45–55.

Singer, M. *The value of a group modality for treating promiscuous adolescent girls*. Paper presented at American Society of Adolescent Psychiatry meeting, Los Angeles, 1975.

Sugar, M. Normal adolescent mourning. *American Journal of Psychotherapy*, 1968, *32*, 258–269.

Webb, G. A., Briggs, C., & Brown, R. A comprehensive adolescent maternity program in a community hospital. *American Journal of Obstetrics and Gynecology*, 1972, *113*, 511–523.

Williams, T. M. Childrearing practices of young mothers. *American Journal of Ortho-psychiatry,* 1974, 44, 70–75.

Zelnick, M., & Kantner, J. F. Some preliminary observations on pre-adult fertility and family formation. *Studies in Family Planning,* 1972, 3, 59–65.

Some Developmental Aspects of Adolescent Mothers

MIRIAM TASINI

This discussion addresses itself to the developmental and psychological factors in adolescent girls that contribute to conception and to the decision to bear a child.

Any investigation of pregnancy in adolescence must be approached with an attempt to evaluate the relationship to normal adolescent development. Adolescence and pregnancy are both developmental transitions (Bibring, 1961). As such, both are accompanied by multiple physical, psychological, and social changes. These changes lead to revival or intensification of previously unresolved conflicts. The resolution of these conflicts requires intrapsychic reorganization and assumption of new interpersonal relationships.

The prepubertal girl is preoccupied with the acquisition of physical, intellectual, and social skills. For her emotional and physical needs, she remains largely dependent on parental figures. With the onset of puberty, the young girl is faced with rapid changes in body size and shape. The new capacity for sexual activity and the increase in sexual drive bring to the fore questions of sexual role. The dependent relationship to the omnipotent adult is modified, eventually to be given up.

The turmoil of the new internal conflicts and external demands must be faced without external support from parental figures. Confronted by these new, seemingly dangerous situations, the adolescent longs for the tranquility and safety of childhood. To be a baby again, with all needs instantly fulfilled, is an ever present, though unconscious, wish.

MIRIAM TASINI, M.D. ● Assistant Clinical Professor, Department of Psychiatry, University of California at Los Angeles School of Medicine, Los Angeles, California 90024.

To resist this regressive pull, the adolescent must find new sources of need gratification. She searches for peer-group support, develops new skills for mastering the environment, and forms a relationship with a heterosexual love object. The ability to mobilize these supports is compromised by earlier developmental failures. Defeat may result in the use of deviant behavior as a defense against the onslaught of adolescent turmoil.

Pregnancy may serve as one form of such behavior (Deutsch, 1944). Typically, adolescent girls who conceive and choose motherhood have experienced maternal deprivation in infancy and early childhood (Blos, 1962). Descriptions of developmental histories and family constellations of adolescent mothers (Abernathy, 1974; Barglow, 1968; La Barre, 1968, 1972) reveal lack of constant adequate care by their own mothers or mother substitutes. The girl does not perceive any single individual as the major source of nurturance during childhood. She is often the product of an unwanted pregnancy of a young mother or one burdened by a large family. Her care has been shared by relatives, babysitters, neighbors, foster homes, and older siblings. At a very young age, she assumed responsibility for the welfare of younger siblings. A 92-pound 14-year-old girl informed a nurse who questioned her ability to care for her newborn son, "I have diapered babies since I was six years old." Fathers are either absent or emotionally unavailable; they are seen as unapproachable or threatening.

Development of her social skills and intellectual curiosity was not encouraged by her parents; scholastic achievement was never valued. Parental approval meant, "I did my chores and stayed out of my mother's way." School records indicate escalating impairment of academic achievement. At the time of pregnancy, the testing average is two or three grade levels below the age-appropriate level.

These girls are peripheral members of the adolescent peer group. As passive followers, they conform by involvement in activities that will provide approval by the group. They are depressed and lonely and perceive themselves as unwanted. Drugs, alcohol, or heterosexual activity may be used to relieve the chronic sense of inadequacy and isolation (Blos, 1957).

Heterosexual involvement is a result of the desperate search for closeness and acceptance. It is not a product of unrestrained passion. Intercourse is rarely enjoyed, and these girls view sexual activity with condemnation (Schaffer & Pine, 1972). The physical contact of "being held" is described as the most pleasurable aspect of sexual activity. The male is seen as a protector and a caretaker rather than as a lover. A pregnant 15-year-old married to a man 12 years her senior described her relationship in this way: "He takes care of me, gives me everything I need."

The pregnancies are not consciously planned but are usually welcomed by the girls as well as by their mothers. A striking example was recently seen in one of our medical clinics when a childlike 14-year-old was seen for evaluation of repeated nausea and vomiting. When the examining physician sheepishly informed the mother and the girl that she was pregnant, the overjoyed mother and the bewildered daughter threw themselves into an ecstatic embrace. The pregnancy always provides either real or fantasized closeness to mother.

Teenage pregnancies often coincide with maternal hysterectomy or menopause or with parental separation. The baby is perceived as a gift to the mother to replace the one she is no longer able to bear. The behavior of mother and daughter indicates that there is confusion as to who is the mother of the baby. The closeness that develops is far beyond the normal feeling of comradeship of a mother and her pregnant adult daughter.

The girl renounces all her adult roles. She has difficulty living away from the family; is unable to care for herself or her husband, if married; often moves in with her mother; and may manifest a wide spectrum of regressive behavior. This may present as multiple somatic complaints, food fads, or sleeping with pets, with stuffed animals, or even with the mother.

Although at first glance the pregnancies of these girls may appear to be shortcuts to adulthood, their pregnancies are in fact not maturational processes but attempts to recapture an idealized relationship with a mother figure in a more satisfying way than has been previously experienced. The process of pregnancy in an adolescent bears little resemblance to the normal process of pregnancy in adult women.

Bibring (1961) described the major developmental move for a woman in becoming a mother as "The step between her being a single, circumscribed selfcontained organism, to reproducing herself and her love object in a child who will then remain an object outside of herself." If the woman is to accomplish this task, changes and shifts in identifications and relationships must occur throughout the pregnancy.

Transient heterosexual relationships are the hallmark of adolescence. Intense infatuation that may cease abruptly is a common pattern of adolescent dating. The relationship of the pregnant girl and her mate has the same superficial, tenuous quality found in her peers. When pregnancy is discovered, her interest in her mate as a sexual object wanes rapidly. At this juncture, the relationship is either terminated or restructured. In lasting relationships between adolescent parents, the boy assumes the role of the nurturing parent to the girl and their baby. The girl is unable to relinquish her wish to be mothered. She is unable to take on the mother role unless she identifies with the infant. The identification with her baby that is present throughout the pregnancy reflects further regression to an infantile position. This position remains unmodified in adolescent mothers even following delivery.

"I will get it all back; they will take care of my baby," a 15-year-old announced with glee as she took her newborn daughter home to her family. She was the oldest of eight. During their pregnancies, girls are preoccupied with fantasies of idealized, perfect mother–child relationships. In this fantasy, they describe their children as receiving "better care than I got." Often a specific aspect of child care is emphasized: protection from older children, avoidance of punishment, or careful selection of mother substitutes. This aspect invariably reflects the area perceived by the girl as responsible for her own deprivation and abuse in infancy. The plans and fantasies rarely extend beyond infancy. The baby is seen as always remaining small and attached and simultaneously providing love and care for the mother. This paradox is the result of the pregnant girl's constantly shifting identification, first with her own mother and then with her baby. This is experienced as "I am like my mother; I take care of my child," which equals, "She takes care of me. I am like my baby—I take care of my baby—I get cared for."

A consistent pattern emerges in the responses to motherhood of adolescent girls. With the birth of the baby, the girl is faced with the constant demands of a young infant. This situation does not match the fantasized expectations of constant bliss. She is unable to provide adequate care for her baby unless she delays gratification of her own needs. She feels deprived and enraged and becomes depressed. Her role as a mother is abandoned, and she withdraws from the baby, who is at best subjected to benign neglect.

This pattern is dramatically illustrated by Betty, who was 15 years old and 22 weeks pregnant when her 8-month-old baby was placed in a foster home. He had suffered a skull fracture; child abuse was suspected. Betty was tearful, despondent, and remorseful. She is the youngest of 11 children but has been left to her own devices since her baby was born. The abandonment by her family, particularly by her mother, was totally unexpected. "We were close like this," she said, crossing her fingers to emphasize her perception of the relationship with her mother. The mother has recently started to work for the first time in her life and was unwilling to become involved in child care. The girl became depressed, disappointed, and angry. Her rage was directed toward her mother and her baby, neither of whom had met her expectations.

In contrast, Kathy, who is 19, lives with her mother and her 4-year-old daughter. She feels that she has achieved a measure of stability in her life since the birth of her daughter. Kathy was 3 months old when her parents separated. Her mother was a depressed, lonely woman who worked long hours as a bookkeeper to support her family. Her children were cared for by other people. The family moved frequently, and there was no stability in their lives. At 12, Kathy ran away and was placed in a foster-care facility at the request of her mother, who was unable to control her drug abuse and promiscuity. She had not had any contact with her mother for three years. When she discovered she was pregnant, her mother took her in, and the two women have lived together ever since the reunion. The mother works, providing for Kathy and her child; she also participates in child care on a regular basis. Kathy's social life is limited to an occasional evening with a girlfriend. She feels content and does not have any plans to alter her life situation.

The previous discussion and clinical vignettes illustrate that the core conflict of adolescent mothers is the gratification of their infantile needs. Although their difficulties span a wide range of psychopathology, the single most important factor that determines their response and adjustment to motherhood is their relationship to a mother figure. In the presence of external supports that allow the girl to assume an infantile position, a period of quiescence follows the arrival of a child. It is during this temporarily stabilized situation that therapeutic intervention can be initiated to provide a framework in which growth can take place.

REFERENCES

Abernathy, V. Illegitimate conception among teenagers. *American Journal of Public Health*, 1974, 6 (7), 662–665.
Barglow, P. Some psychiatric aspects of illegitimate pregnancy in early adolescence. *American Journal of Orthopsychiatry*, 1968, 38, 672–687.
Bibring, G. Some considerations of the psychological process of pregnancy. In R. S. Eissler et al. (Eds.), *Psychoanalytic study of the child* (Vol. 14). New York: International Universities Press, 1961, pp. 113–121.
Blos, P. Pre-oedipal factors in the etiology of female delinquency. In R. S. Eissler et al. (Eds.), *Psychoanalytic study of the child* (Vol. 12). New York: International Universities Press, 1957, pp. 229–249.

Blos, P. *On adolescence: Psychoanalytic interpretation.* Glencoe, Ill.: Free Press, 1962.

Deutsch, H. *Psychology of women,* Vol 2. New York: Grune & Stratton, 1944.

La Barre, M. Pregnancy experience among married adolescents. *American Journal of Orthopsychiatry,* 1968, *38,* 47–55.

La Barre, M. Emotional crisis of school age girls during pregnancy and early motherhood. *Journal of the American Academy of Child Psychiatry,* 1972, *2,* 537–557.

Schaffer, C., & Pine, F. Pregnancy; Abortion and developmental tasks of adolescence. *Journal of the American Academy of Child Psychiatry,* 1972, *2,* 551–536.

Chapter 10

Female Sexuality and Pregnancy

RACHEL EDGARDE PAPE

In one sense, pregnancy can be thought of as an end for which all previous maturational development was necessary preparation, the culmination of successful sexual development, the outcome of biological sexuality—the last, as the poet Browning said, for which the first was made. But once pregnancy occurs, after the union of sperm and ovum, what happens to female sexuality?

This is a question about which surprisingly little has been studied or written in the past, and only in recent years has it begun to emerge as a subject for scientific investigation. As a subject, it is too large for one short article, but the purpose of this paper is to draw attention to some of the factors that influence sexuality during pregnancy and that affect the relationship between two people in the process of becoming parents of the new generation.

Sexuality involves far more than the contact of sexual organs. Biological sexual maturation is only a part of sexuality—a term that, defying definition, includes a psychological as well as a physical development and takes into account not only reality but phantasy[1] experience from some early beginning to the present. In any circumstances, mature sexuality includes, besides eroticism, loving, caring,

---

[1]The word *phantasy*, here and throughout this chapter, is used differently from the word *fantasy*, which is conscious as in daydreaming. Phantasy is intended in the psychoanalytic meaning of the ubiquitous, active, unconscious representation of a mental phenomenon which is capable of becoming conscious. The precursors of phantasy are thought to be operative from birth and accompany, affect, and are affected by reality experiences. An example would be the Oedipus complex.

RACHEL EDGARDE PAPE, M.D. ● Assistant Clinical Professor, Department of Psychiatry, University of California at Los Angeles School of Medicine, Los Angeles, California 90024.

and the ability to sacrifice, to endure pain, and to be grateful for love and care, and it is inevitably related to growth and change.

Pregnancy, as Bibring, Dwyer, Thomas, Huntington, and Valenstein (1961) pointed out, is not merely a period of growth and change but a maturational crisis that takes place within a complex set of physiological, hormonal, anatomical, psychological, and sociological conditions, which both affect and are affected by sexuality.

Factors Affecting the Pregnant Woman

The complex of factors that affects the pregnant woman includes her age, her previous pregnancy experience, her health, her education, her economic and social position, her previous personality structure, her unique psychological adjustment and methods of conflict solution, her relation to her partner—in a sense, everything she has ever been or hoped to be as well as everything she is now. But because pregnancy is a state of crisis, she does not go through a smooth transition to a new state of being; rather, she experiences far-reaching psychological change.

During the maturational crisis of pregnancy, as Bibring et al. noted, the psychological organization that a woman has achieved in adulthood undergoes a significant degree of dissolution in order to allow for a corresponding recomposition to a new psychological position different from that previously held. Childhood is truly at an end. A pregnant woman knows that never again will she be what she was before the biologically monumental experience. Her appearance and physiological factors in addition keep her constantly aware of change. Psychological conflicts of earlier developmental periods are revived.

The pregnant woman is reminded of her earlier childhood self and her earlier relation to others—to siblings as well as parents—and of feelings about parents on all levels of awareness (as part objects, early internal objects, and larger differentiated objects), specifically in relation to her mother, with whom identification as a mother takes place if the pregnant woman has previously achieved a state of psychological separateness. That is to say, if the pregnant woman has successfully progressed beyond symbiosis (i.e., that state in which she is psychologically undifferentiated from her mother in her mind) and has achieved separation–individuation, the baby allows her to become "the mother" as the new baby takes her previous place as "the baby." But if she has not completely passed beyond symbiosis to individuation, there is psychologically incomplete separation from her mother, and in phantasy, mother and baby will be confused in the mind of the new mother. The baby may then be experienced as the return of an aspect of her own earlier phantasy "mommy" relationship, from which she is not differentiated. The baby will seem to be the mommy coming back, like the return of the repressed, and what may then be experienced is the coming back of a baby–mommy who will suck her dry like a parasite.

Pregnancy can also mean the fulfillment of an oedipal wish, not only in the sense of an incestuous wish of having the forbidden baby with her father, but in the aspect that followers of English psychoanalyst Melanie Klein tend to emphasize, that both girls and boys wish to give good babies to the parent of the opposite sex as a sign of reparative wishes (i.e., giving a good baby to replace the good baby one deprived the parent of when one was the "bad" baby doing the damage one now seeks to repair). One was once a troublesome baby with one's own mother and father; now one is able to have a troublesome baby and take the trouble to be a responsible parent to the baby, out of appreciation of and identification with the good parent. This attitude is considered to be the normal, healthy outcome of what is called, in Kleinian terminology, the *depressive position*, that is, a psychological constellation of mental experiences in infancy, characterized by awareness that the prior experiences of separate and different "good" and "bad" mothers were of one and the same mother, thus awakening feelings in the infant of pain, guilt at having damaged and fear of losing as a result the attacked, ambivalently loved mother as an external and internal object.

The crisis of pregnancy, however, is also the testing ground of psychological health and tends to lead, under unfavorable inner or outer conditions, to neurotic or even psychotic responses. Becoming pregnant can be used mentally in a defensive way as a kind of cure, as it were, for undesirable feelings never resolved in earlier life. The outcome of such mechanisms, since they are magical in nature, "cure" nothing; instead, they perpetuate problems and predispose to further complications. Pregnancy, which on one level can mean one is all right inside because one can have babies, can be used unconsciously, for example, as a cure for depression, especially a depression characterized by feelings of being bad, of being shameful, of having bad things inside, or of being empty inside. The sense of being able to have babies and of being all right inside by virtue of being full may temporarily mitigate these feelings, but once the baby is delivered, the emptiness and bad feelings can return. This return may explain the predisposition to postpartum depression. In addition, one might here consider the possibility that the placental hormones that generally elicit a feeling of well-being may in a sense contribute to or even possibly act as a pharmacological stimulus to a kind of euphoria or a manic way of handling depression. In any case, once the titer of these hormones drops in the postpartum period, the patient is vulnerable to the depression she has been seeking to avoid. Some women show a kind of pregnancy addiction and cannot stand not to be pregnant.

Pregnancy can also be used mentally as a magical, omnipotent means of dealing with unwanted feelings of littleness and neediness, still present from childhood. These feelings are reactivated and intensified in pregnancy. Rather than being accepted and slowly resolved, they may be managed in a manner that attempts to avoid the slow, difficult process of growing up gradually, by becoming suddenly, in an instant, magical way, *the mommy*. Becoming *the mommy* can also temporarily relieve envy of one's mother, but using pregnancy this way effectively postpones growing up, rather than enhancing it.

From the point of view of object-relations theory, the special task that has to be solved in pregnancy and by becoming a mother lies within the sphere of the distribution and shifts between the cathexis (i.e., emotional investment) of self-representation and of object representation. In other words, any normal girl, though she might have intense wishes for a child and love the man who will be the father of this child, still must make a major developmental move in becoming a mother. This move takes place from a position of being a single, circumscribed, self-contained person to one who is reproducing herself and her love object–partner in the form of their child, who will from then on be a separate object outside herself. And a unique relationship will be established with this child that is different from any other relationship earlier or later. It will persist in the form of a synthesis of her relationship to the child in his or her own right, of her relationship to the child representing her husband, and, last but not least, of her relationship to the child representing herself.

Furthermore, on an unconscious level, the baby represents a new form of her. The new baby is replacing her as a baby; she is being pushed out of the womb of naiveté and innocence because she now has to protect and care for the new baby. A baby is taking her place, and she becomes inescapably an adult. But how she intrapsychically manages this inescapable event is another matter. She may adaptively regress—in a movement toward reexperiencing earlier problems, unresolved at that earlier time—in the progressive service of settling them into a better order (i.e., a kind of getting her act together in order to develop some useful and mature means of coping that will be necessary for the care of an actual new baby by a new self in a new relationship and set of relationships). Thus, the experience of pregnancy puts a woman into contact not only with who she is but also with who she is no longer and can never be again, as well as with who she must become and continue to be. All these factors are bound to affect her relationship with her partner as well.

FACTORS AFFECTING PARTNER

The pregnant woman's relationship with her partner is of paramount importance in her sexuality. The nature of that relationship is bound to change in the monumental circumstances of the pregnancy and postpartum period, which both affect and are affected by these circumstances, just as the partners themselves as individuals are bound to change. The male and the female are in two basically different positions. The female, once impregnated, is never again in a zero or not-ever-gravid state (a never-impregnated state). She may miscarry, elect to abort, or carry to term, but physiologically and psychologically, she can never again be a not-ever-pregnant self. This fact in itself affects her sexuality.

The male, however, never goes through the biological event of impregnation: he may impregnate, but his body never experiences impregnation or pregnancy. He can literally—biologically, physiologically, and psychologically—walk away from conception and pregnancy in complete ignorance of the event itself.

However, when the man stays around to be the mate to his pregnant partner, the pregnancy for him also, in my opinion, represents a developmental phase. The maturational crisis will not be as clear-cut as in the woman, who literally carries the pregnancy in her own body and whose attention must inexorably be drawn to the difference between her nongravid, gravid, and postgravid states, regardless of how she may handle that knowledge intrapsychically.

But the father, too, is a complex individual, meeting this time of his life in a complex manner, affected also by his environment, both external and internal, by his age and education, by his socioeconomic status, by his relationship with his work, by other people in the family, by his own personal history, by his changed and changing relationship with his wife as well as himself in the changing relationship, and by his relationship with his own internal, personal child-self (i.e., the child he, too, must give up along with his earlier relationships with his parents), all of which affect him and, therefore, what he brings to his multifaceted "sexual" relationship with his wife.

The partner's biology, too, may play a role in his sexuality. Although he does not go through the obvious physiological changes that are part and parcel of being pregnant, his psychological state may affect his physiology, possibly even his hormones, during his partner's pregnancy. (This reaction has not been studied, to my knowledge, but may be of interest.) I would like here to draw attention to the phenomenon of couvade, where the father unconsciously takes on some of the manifestations of pregnancy. Some cultures ritualistically prescribed couvade as a means of relieving the pregnant woman of some of her difficulties. For example, evil spirits are fooled into pursuing the father so that the mother and the infant are left unharmed. In our culture, we sometimes see fathers with morning sickness, "labor pains," and backache, but the father, for all his magical "help" to relieve his pregnant wife of her difficulties, is not realistically available to her.

But whether or not the father takes on some of the manifestations of pregnancy, he does not experience the physiological and biological changes. Nevertheless, although—to put it at its simplest—he wears the same size clothes throughout the pregnancy, he undergoes profound psychological stirrings, paralleling those of the woman, as psychological conflicts of earlier developmental periods are similarly revived.

The Partner Relationship

The psychological changes in both partners affect their relationship, their sexuality, and their sexual activities. For the pregnant woman in a continuing relationship, the status of the relationship is influenced by many preexisting factors.

Was the preexisting relationship loving or not? Was the pregnancy desired or not? Was there an attempted abortion? What was her previous sexual arousal and behavior in relation to her partner? Does he initiate sexual activity? Does he take her state of mind and physical being into consideration? What does sexual intercourse mean to him? His previous sexual attitudes and behavior are bound to affect his sexual relationship with his pregnant wife. What are his unconscious phantasies about (1) a pregnant woman, for example, his mother, pregnant with him or with his siblings? (2) the father's role in impregnation? (3) the baby itself? What is his attitude toward his own father as a sexual partner in relation to his own mother? Does the pregnancy so affirm his manhood that he does not "need" to perform again? Is there a threat of competition with the baby? Will that threat lead him to reaffirm his manhood again and again through sexual intercourse, or will the threat of the baby's competition cause him to reenact his own childhood, with his wife as mother? Is he too anxious or depressed in relation to fact or phantasy to desire sexual contact when she does? What consideration is she showing in response to her partner? What is the couple's belief and attitude toward sexuality in pregnancy? Cultural taboos? Fear of harm to the baby?

Confusion as to whether they should or should not have intercourse during pregnancy often causes problems in the relationship. Restraint, strain, and constraint can lead to resentment of the partner and especially of the child. Is this a form of jealousy and envy? Does it more often occur in an undesired pregnancy?

These are among the many questions that have not been explored and correlated with other factors affecting sexual responsiveness and activity during pregnancy. I have deliberately stated these few considerations in question form to open up these questions and to encourage an inquiring attitude in the mind of the reader who is interested in aiding the pregnant mother and father at this crucial time.

With very rare exceptions, humans are the only primates who engage in sexual activity during pregnancy. For other primates, the smell of progesterone is a deterrent. Is there any remnant of this response in humans? Continued sexual erotic interest in humans after conception could be thought of as progressive development, representative of the tenderness and affection present in human sexual interest, but might it not in some circumstances be considered maladaptive? Some cultures prohibit the male from engaging in sexual activity with his pregnant partner. Is this only a taboo related to an oedipal fear of a forbidding and vengeful father? Or may it not also be based on some intuitive protection of the fetus? In other cultures, repeated intercourse during pregnancy is attempted in the service of completing the fetus and nourishing the woman. In still others, fear of danger to the fetus has resulted in limiting or prohibiting sexual activity after the first, and sometimes also the second, trimester of pregnancy. Is the parents' fear related to unconscious identification with their own child-selves, thus unconsciously prohibiting parental intercourse?

These fears, valid or not, point up one of the most important psychological aspects of sexuality during pregnancy. There is now a third party involved in the sex act. Not only are the pregnant woman and her partner stirred by memories of their past selves and family relationships and concerned about their future roles as parents, they are immediately involved in the present welfare of the fetus. The one-to-one relationship has become complicated, not only because neither partner is the same "one" as before, but because each is now reacting to the third party.

Interviews with expectant parents and cross-cultural information bring into focus the universal conflict between the wish for the child's survival and the wish for his or her death during pregnancy. Unconscious destructive versus protective wishes toward the fetus influence both parents and their sexual relationship. Just as in the Oedipus story, unconscious destructive wishes toward the baby are universally experienced in both parents; so are the protective wishes (as manifested in the fact that Laius does not kill the baby himself; these wishes are further demonstrated by the shepherd who rescues the baby Oedipus and gives him to Polybus and Merope, who rear him). Anthropological observations and other studies draw attention to the father's role in protecting the mother against her fears or wishes of destroying the fetus (and later, the baby).

SOME STUDIES

Klein, Potter, and Dyk (1950) found that good marital relations counteracted typical pregnancy fears. This study of 27 primiparas was among the first and was conducted by retrospective interviews, as were most early investigations, asking the subject to recall sexual feelings and activities for time periods long before the interview or questionnaire was administered. Later, in an attempt to overcome some of the hazards of fallible memory in retrospective reporting, the use of a diary or a daily recording system was introduced. In recent years, more sophisticated techniques and laboratory methods have helped to overcome two additional hazards of investigation into female sexual arousal and response: first, self-reports are often colored by moral, religious, and other psychological inhibitions, and second, until the development of devices such as the plethysmograph, which measures changes in vaginal pressure, pulse, and vasocongestion, women could report physiological arousal only subjectively, though men could always do so with complete reliability.

In general, studies have fallen into four main categories: studies using retrospective interviews or questionnaires, daily record studies, studies of dream analysis, and studies using direct observations and physiological measurements.

It is impossible in a paper of this length to review all studies in detail, even though there is a regrettable lack of published research on the subject, but some reports bear directly on the problems of female sexuality during pregnancy. In 1966, Masters and Johnson reported on a study of 107 multiparas and primiparas, examining changes in sexuality that accompany pregnancy and the postpartum period, and found that

> . . . after an initial decrease in coital frequency and sexual desire in the first trimester, there was a marked increase in the second trimester, followed by a diminished interest in the third trimester. Half of the respondents reported low levels of sexuality at three months past postpartum.

Masters and Johnson also studied six pregnant women who agreed to engage in sexual activity in the laboratory setting; they were able to collect repeated physiological and hormonal measurements:

> Observations included the degree of vasocongestion of the labial and vaginal area, contractions of the uterus during orgasm, and time span of resolution, along with other physiological responses during coital and manipulative sexual activity. These six women who participated in the laboratory study showed a pattern of increased sexual arousal in the second trimester similar to women in the interview study. All of these women experienced multiple orgasms during this period of pregnancy, including two who had not been multiply orgasmic before.

Most other studies agree that there is a general decline in sexual activity during pregnancy, especially toward the end of pregnancy. The cause of the decline is not established, nor is the decline conclusively authenticated. Falicov pointed out in a study published in 1973 (which corroborated the Masters and Johnson findings except for the marked second trimester increase in sexual interest) that differences in findings might be related to personality characteristics in the samples involved or to the fact that the Masters and Johnson sample was drawn from women self-enrolled in a study of sexuality, with consequently possible high levels of sexual interest. Falicov also noted that "Lack of knowledge about normal sexual changes during pregnancy and postpartum caused women anxiety about the normalcy of their reactions" (p. 999). Many women mentioned that fear of harming the fetus by sexual activity caused anxiety even though they "knew better." The Falicov study concluded that "whether sexual response during pregnancy is a correlate of hormonal, metabolic or psychological changes during pregnancy, or of psychophysiological mechanisms, remains largely in the field of speculation" (p. 999).

Among the attempts to replace speculation with data is the study of McCauley and Ehrhardt (1976) on hormonal and behavioral interactions in female sexual response. They pointed out that it is difficult to assess the role of hormones in the decline of sexual activity during pregnancy:

> It is possible that high levels of progesterone in interaction with numerous other physiological and psychological factors leads to a reduction of libido. The return of sexual desire during the second trimester cannot be explained by a reduction in progesterone, however. It is more likely that the increase of sexuality at that time is due to secondary physiological effects, such as vasocongestion and sensitivity of the woman's sex organs. Other physiological changes might contribute to a decrease in sexual behavior during the early and late phases of pregnancy. The first trimester is frequently marked by constant nausea and excessive fatigue and at times a

disconcerting gain in weight. By the second trimester, many women have overcome these initial adjustment problems and are psychologically more at east with their pregnancy. A more relaxed attitude coupled with increased pelvic vasocongestion may explain the return and sometimes increased sexual arousal. Over the third trimester, physical discomfort may become advanced enough to override increases in arousal due to pelvic congestion. Sexual activity at this time may also be curbed by fears that coitus and orgasm will lead to premature labor or fetal damage. In fact, coitus itself does not seem to cause premature delivery but there is some evidence that the uterine contractions of orgasm can initiate actual labor. The risk appears to exist primarily for women who have a history of premature deliveries or who have premature cervical dilation.

All researchers have found that women who valued sexual activity before pregnancy may show a slight decline in sexual arousal during pregnancy but usually have a rapid return to pre-pregnancy levels of sexuality after childbirth. On the other hand, women who were less positive about sex before pregnancy show a more marked decline in sexual behavior during gestation, show a longer period of abstinence after delivery, and sometimes have a diminished sexual response after pregnancy. (p. 470)

McCauley and Ehrhardt concluded that

It is critical that the behavior data not only include more detail on various aspects of sexual feelings but also assess a woman's beliefs about the possible influence of pregnancy and motherhood on her sexuality and uncover her fears and anxieties related to sexual behavior during these time periods. (p. 471)

This need for a broader approach was also expressed by Tolor and DiGrazia (1976) in a study generally confirming the decline in both sexual interest and sexual activity as pregnancy progresses. They stated:

It is not known whether these changes in sexual functioning result from the varied physiological changes which occur during pregnancy, including physical discomfiture, or whether the changes result primarily from more subtle psychological changes in the woman's conception of herself as a sexually desirable or undesirable person and free from conflicting role concepts, such as the maternal role as opposed to the wife role. (p. 459)

These same investigators, finding a high incidence of a desire to be held during pregnancy, theorized that "it serves as a substitutive function for the more advanced and complex sensual response which is compromised during pregnancy" (p. 549).

It might be advisable for all investigators to temporize rather than to theorize. As investigators, we should not be too quick to develop theories from any data, especially psychological data, which are unusually difficult to gather and evaluate in any case. The need to be held, for example, which shows up repeatedly in other studies, may be substitutive or may be related to dependency. Among other reasons for this need is the fundamental one of the pregnant woman's state of mind and identification with the intrauterine baby who lacks separateness. The pregnant woman may thus need to be held to reestablish boundaries for herself.

We need a great deal more research, of a broader nature than ever before, and with more reliable data, with freedom to assess the data open-mindedly. Retrospective interviews, for example, depend on highly fallible human memory and result in an inherent flaw in method, compounded by the fact that memory may be colored by cultural or religious and phantasy beliefs about sexuality and pregnancy. In laboratory testing, investigators may not take sufficient note of observation as a factor in itself. In addition, in any method, subjects may be drawn from selected population samples. This is not to say that the studies undertaken to date have not been important. If they have accomplished verification of the need for better methods in addition to the enormous need for accurate information, they have been well worthwhile. Unfortunately, however, too many people seek to establish norms from inadequate data and, from these norms, to establish theories. We must exercise extreme caution in establishing norms or theories without reliable data.

Human behavior is such that even with better data, theorizing is fraught with peril. For all their differences in technique, the studies to date show a wide range of sexual manifestation. Human sexuality and response are highly individualistic, and during pregnancy, they are influenced by a multitude of factors, often conflicting and producing fears and anxieties.

Many of these fears and anxieties, referred to by most researchers and indicated as needing further study, may be recognized by the women themselves, who are still unable to deal with them. As one of the women in the Falicov study reported, "I'm not fulfilled right now. I think my husband and I are both concerned about harming the baby, even though we both know better" (p. 995).

In many instances, pregnant women and their partners may have been given physiological information and may be aware of the normal biological changes in pregnancy, but they are not usually well cognizant of the magnitude of the maturational crisis they are going through. It sometimes seems that the people they turn to for help are not in a position to guide and help the pregnant woman and her partner. They may not be aware, for example, that much of what is called *regression* during pregnancy, such as crying, moodiness, and so on, may in fact be adaptive, related to the feelings and memories appropriately stirred up in the woman, a stirring up that makes her unusually available for help. Unlike those therapists who believe that therapy should be discontinued during pregnancy, I believe it presents a unique opportunity for help.

HELP IN CRISIS

Long-submerged psychological conflicts come close to the surface during pregnancy, making it an important time for intervention. Husband, parents, and peers in the woman's everyday life and obstetrician and others in health-care roles (e.g. Lamaze teachers and psychiatrist) are all in a position to help the woman in the developmental aspects of pregnancy. Conversely, of course, they can also interfere, thwart, or even damage. But because the pregnant woman is unusually vulnerable and accessible and receptive to introspection, this crisis period offers an unparalleled opportunity to all who may be in a position to help her.

In addition, pregnancy is the last chance to help the pregnant woman and her partner work through old problems before they undertake the guidance of a new life. The more their psychological conflicts are resolved during pregnancy, the better their chances are for becoming good parents. After the baby is born, most help will be remedial, for both parents and child, to the extent that the child is affected by them. The child, the new generation, receives its best help before it is born, when the father and the mother are helped to understand themselves, each other, and their relationship. Psychological conflicts of parents that are not resolved before the baby's birth not only continue and may affect the child's development adversely but can contribute destructively to the relationship between partners. Though it is beyond the aims of this paper to discuss the effects of a child, after birth, on a formerly two-party relationship or to discuss the effects on a child of either a one-parent family or a warring two-parent family, the fact remains that the two-parent family is still considered the best unit for a child's development, and that the fundamental problems that will arise between partners as parents are best resolved during pregnancy.

Unfortunately, the professional or lay person seeking guidance in helping the pregnant woman and her partner finds a scarcity of material. Studies to date are mainly biological, with some theoretical considerations of psychological and physiological factors. A few, such as Bibring *et al.*'s (1961) and Gillman's (1968) studies of dreams of pregnant women, focus mainly on psychological aspects, but to date, no major attempt has been made to study the physiopsychological aspects concurrently.

Though it would be an enormous undertaking, there is a need to study the pregnant woman in relation to all parts of her life situation, the physiological aspects simultaneously with the psychological. What have been done to date can be considered pilot studies pointing a direction. Emphasis on biological, hormonal, physiological, or psychological aspects has, in most instances, led to conclusions indicating interrelationship and a need for more simultaneous correlation with observable immediate reactions.

To understand what is happening biologically concurrently with what is happening psychologically and in relation to the partner is probably the only way to gain full understanding of the pregnant woman. The need for that understanding is not only great, it is urgent.

REFERENCES

Bibring, G. L., Dwyer, T. F., Huntington, D. S., & Valenstein, A. F. A study of the psychological process in pregnancy and the earliest mother–child relationship. In R. S. Eissler *et al.* (Eds.), *Psychoanalytic study of the child* (Vol. 16). New York: International Universities Press, 1961.

Falicov, C. J. Sexual adjustment during first pregnancy and postpartum. *American Journal of Obstetrics and Gynecology*, 1973, *117*(7), 991–1000.

Gillman, R. D. The dreams of pregnant women and maternal adaptation. *American Journal of Orthopsychiatry*, 1968, *38*(4), 688–692.

Klein, H., Potter, H., & Dyk, R. B. *Anxiety in pregnancy and childbirth*. New York: Hoeber, 1950.

Masters, W. H., & Johnson, V. E. *Human sexual response*. Boston: Little, Brown, 1966.

McCauley, E., & Ehrhardt, A. A. Female sexual response: Hormonal and behavioral interactions. *Primary Care*, 1976, *3*(3), 455–476.

Tolor, A., & DiGrazia, P. V. Sexual attitudes and behavior patterns during and following pregnancy. *Archives of Sexual Behavior*, 1976, *5*(6), 539–551.

The Developmental Crisis of Pregnancy

JUDITH E. VIDA

Dr. Pape's paper attests to the increasing scientific interest in the psychological state of men and women surrounding the experience of pregnancy. This interest owes some of its legitimacy to Grete Bibring's landmark study (1959), which showed that the emotions and behavior of pregnant women in a certain clinic, which looked so alarming and pathological on the surface, were understandable manifestations of a profound developmental crisis occurring in a nonsupportive environment. It bears emphasizing that not only is the first pregnancy a major developmental crisis, but each subsequent pregnancy affords opportunity for further understanding, mastery, and psychological growth. To hear from a mother that a subsequent child is experienced more pleasurably than the first one(s) suggests that the crisis has undergone significant resolution (Brazelton, 1969).

The decade of the 1970s saw important changes in the way women perceive themselves and are perceived by men. A woman is now acknowledged to have an innate capacity for competence, autonomy, and self-determination. At the same time, there has been a veritable revolution in obstetrical practice. Klaus and Kennell's studies (1970, 1972) of mother–infant bonding have been stimulating doctors and hospitals to reevaluate policies that kept parents and babies physically separated during the immediate postpartum period. Equally significant has been the cumulative impact of growing social support for breast-feeding (La Leche League) and prepared childbirth classes (Lamaze method and others), as well as increasing consumer demand for family-centered childbirth services. Far from being banished to the waiting room,

JUDITH E. VIDA, M.D. • Psychiatrist in private practice, Pasadena, California 91101.

199

fathers have taken a vital, active role in the process of parturition, from attending preparation classes, to "coaching" the labor, to presence at or even participation in delivery, not to mention sharing in the care of the baby, once it is born.

In the not-too-distant past, a woman's role in childbearing vis-à-vis the obstetrician was stereotypically seen as that of a frightened little girl; she was told not to worry her pretty little head, to do what the doctor advised, and he would reward her with pain-dulling medication during labor and, eventually, the gift of a nice little baby. Such a view is entirely consistent with the regressed and childlike behavior that a pregnant women often presents, which is merely the manifest content of the developmental crisis going on underneath. Having her surface behavior mistaken for the whole picture robs a woman of the emotional support she needs to work optimally toward resolution.

There has been a profusion of articles in the last five years or so on the experience of pregnancy and childbirth, in professional journals and popular magazines, written by those who have done the experiencing. This is indeed an adaptive response to the developmental crisis. These writers take themselves seriously enough to write it all down. Other women can confirm some of their own feelings in these accounts and can develop a more useful perspective. No less important is the opportunity for others on whom a childbirth impinges (fathers, obstetricians, pediatricians, hospital administrators, nurses, childbirth educators, professional colleagues, etc.) to develop empathy and to discover what may be required of them in response.

We have, therefore, a rapidly increasing pool of information about the consciously introspected experience of the pregnant woman's developmental crisis. We also have some information about the less conscious aspects. Judith Kestenberg (1976) examined eight psychoanalytic case histories before, during, and after pregnancy, in hopes of identifying modes of regression and patterns of reintegration. She presented her findings as preliminary and inconclusive, but some of her observations are particularly relevant to this discussion. Kestenberg characterized the third trimester as the impetus to the new mother for giving up the now idealized inner baby in order to deal with a real outside child. During this period, the pregnant woman is becoming more clumsy and ungainly, as the baby gets heavier and more burdensome, encroaching uncomfortably on her internal organs (bladder, intestines, and diaphragm). Anger appears, directed toward this creature who is causing so much trouble, but there is often also shame at wanting to get rid of the baby. Urinary frequency and leaking stimulate a urethral-mode regression manifested by fears of losing the baby, fears of dying, and fears of losing control in general. Kestenberg noted that the women in analysis seemed to weary of introspection as delivery neared and, as a transformation of underlying aggression, became instead more involved in working out the practical details of what lay ahead. Kestenberg also observed that the three phases of stress during labor, originally described by Friedman (1975), were anticipated by the women:

> The impending separation from the fetus revives separation and stranger anxiety and evokes fears of the hospital. The second stress, which comes to a peak during the greatest stretching of the cervix, is anticipated in the fears of being injured by the baby's movement. The third stress, most prominent during delivery proper, concerns the loss of the genital that would come out with the baby. (p. 224)

In this context, we can better understand the current interest in breast-feeding, prepared childbirth, and family-centered delivery. Breast-feeding is a concrete expression of maternal capability. The manual of the La Leche League (Thompson, n.d., *The Womanly Art of Breastfeeding*), though it supports the traditional male–female role division, nevertheless emphasizes the notion that all women with breasts have the innate capacity to breast-feed, is full of practical advice for dealing with unusual as well as usual circumstances, and elaborates the real work done by a mother in caring for young children. The effect is to marshal support for a woman's newly emerging identity as a real mother, and to encounter the regressive impact of those who would discourage or disparage her bodily capacity to nurture. Classes in prepared childbirth, which are attended typically in the mid to late third trimester, teach the anatomy and physiology of pregnancy, labor, and delivery, as well as a practical method of exercise and rehearsal specifically to maintain a sense of control during parturition. What is offered, therefore, is information and a realistic method of dealing with the externalized derivatives of the anxieties described by Friedman and Kestenberg. The emotional support of the group further facilitates mastery. The various components of family-centered childbirth include fathers coaching labor and present in the delivery room, holding and nursing the baby immediately after birth, infant rooming-in with the mother, unlimited family visiting, and the uncomplicated labor and delivery taking place in a homelike setting within or near the hospital (alternative birth center) or in the home itself. Here, very clearly, we can see the environment being structured to minimize the separation and stranger anxiety that are built into the labor experience.

Kestenberg concluded that

> . . . under optimal conditions of pregnancy, conflicts regarding inner genitality and procreation have been resolved and a way has been paved for joyful acceptance of parental responsibilities. The aid of the husband makes

the conquering of stresses into an adaptive creative task for both parents.
(p. 244)

But what of those conditions that are not optimal? The current widely accepted list of indications for cesarean delivery (Hausknecht & Heilman, 1978) includes the following: cephalopelvic disproportion, failure to progress (dystocia) or prolonged labor (increased fetal and maternal risk in labor longer than 16–18 hours), fetal distress, abnormal positions, premature breech, transverse lie, hemorrhage, cord accidents, multiple gestation, fibroids or tumors, "advanced maternal age," maternal diseases (diabetes, hypertension, toxemia of pregnancy, heart disease, Rh disease, etc.), failed elective induction, prolonged ruptured membranes, herpes progenitalis, postmaturity, unusual indications (such as extensive previous pelvic surgery with fragile scars), and, of course, previous cesarean section. Marut and Mercer (1979) noted that the national rate of cesarean births reached 10% of all deliveries in 1977, with incidence nearing 25% in some hospitals, and they found considerable evidence to attribute the increase to sophisticated fetal monitoring, with a subsequent decrease in fetal mortality.

Large numbers of women, therefore, are not having "optimal outcomes" of their labor; they are having live and presumably healthier infants, to be sure, but what does this mean in their individual development? Kestenberg's data allow us to guess that an emergency cesarean delivery amounts to a realization of the third trimester's worst fears, whether necessitated by fetal distress or a nonproductive labor. Such an occurrence must seriously undermine whatever resolution of the developmental crisis had been previously under way. Factors of the cesarean delivery that would be expected to exert a major regressive pull are the unanticipated surgical intervention itself, with the woman relegated to being a passive participant (or even being unconscious, if general anesthesia is necessary); the mental confusion that accompanies the existence of multiple sites of physical discomfort (engorging breasts, incisional pain, uterine cramping, and postsurgical intraabdominal irritation and intestinal distention with gas); the absence of a familiar person in the operating room; and the lack of immediate contact with the baby, or illness in the baby.

Using 48-hour-postpartum interviews and a questionnaire measuring maternal perceptions about labor and delivery experience, Marut and Mercer (1979) [1] compared 20 primiparous cesarean mothers with 30 primiparous mothers who had vaginal deliveries. There was signif-

---

[1]Special acknowledgment to Roberta L. Berg, M.D., for bringing to my attention the study by Marut and Mercer.

icantly lower satisfaction with the birth experience among cesarean mothers, and among cesarean mothers who had general anesthesia compared with regional anesthesia. Interviews with the cesarean mothers revealed their considerable sense of confusion, emotional distress, anger, and feelings of failure and worthlessness. They tended to view the delivery as abnormal and as having social stigma. In addition, they showed greater hesitancy in naming their infants.

Cohen (1977) made the point that before education for childbirth was widespread, there was essentially no difference between a vaginal and a cesarean delivery from the parents' point of view, except for the site of physical discomfort. Cohen cited Willmuth's (1975) study of women in prepared childbirth classes who delivered vaginally and concluded that maintaining control was the one factor that made women feel positively about their birth experience. The task now before health professionals is to make the cesarean experience as indistinguishable from the prepared vaginal childbirth as possible. This approach would include informing prospective parents during pregnancy that cesarean delivery is a real possibility. Education toward cesarean delivery is now more frequently included in standard prepared-childbirth classes, but there are also classes in prepared cesarean childbirth that discuss the options for family-centered cesarean delivery that exist in a given geographical area. Cohen (1977) listed 29 components of family-centered cesarean birth that were currently available in the Boston area, largely because of the educated consumer pressure of newly formed support groups of cesarean parents.

The medical and psychiatric literature have contributed little to the subject of cesarean birth as a psychological event. Research is vitally needed if we are to understand better the indications for cesarean intervention, to document the prenatal physical and emotional circumstances of the cesarean mother, and to explore the length and characteristics of resolution of the developmental crisis complicated by cesarean delivery. Nursing journals are publishing much valuable work, which deserves the attention of their medical counterparts.

The cesarean delivery is a serious obstacle to the successful resolution of the developmental crisis of pregnancy, but the principle of family-centered cesarean care restores a sense of self-sufficiency, autonomy, and active participation, which had previously been denied to cesarean parents. Cesarean-birth support groups have much to offer distressed postcesarean parents, who ordinarily do not come to a psychiatrist's attention. Just as with the "optimal" childbirth experience, only when the developmental crisis is mastered will these new parents be free to devote themselves wholeheartedly to their baby.

REFERENCES

Bibring, G. L. Some considerations of the psychological process in pregnancy. In R. S. Eissler *et al.* (Eds.), *Psychoanalytic Study of the Child* (Vol. 14). New York: International Universities Press, 1959, pp. 113–121.

Brazelton, T. B. *Infants and mothers*. New York: Delacorte Press/Seymour Lawrence, 1969.

Cohen, N. W. Minimizing emotional sequelae of cesarean childbirth. *Births and Family Journal*, 1977, *4*, 114–119.

Friedman, D. Conflict behavior in the parturient. *Transactions of the 4th International Congress of Obstetrics and Gynecology*. Basel: Karger, 1975, pp. 373–375. (Quoted in Kestenberg, 1976.)

Hausknecht, R., & Heilman, J. *Having a cesarean baby*. New York: Dutton, 1978.

Kestenberg, J. Regression and reintegration in pregnancy. *Journal of the American Psychoanalytic Association*, 1976, *24* (supplement), 213–250.

Klaus, M. H., & Kennell, J. H. Human maternal behavior at the first contact with her young. *Pediatrics*, 1970, *46*, 187–192.

Klaus, M. H., & Kennell, J. H. Maternal attachment: Importance of the first post-partum days. *New England Journal of Medicine*, 1972, *286*, 460–463.

Marut, J., & Mercer, R. Comparison of primiparas' perceptions of vaginal and cesarean births. *Nursing Research*, 1979, *28*, 260–266.

Thompson, M. *The womanly art of breastfeeding*. Franklin Park, Ill.: La Leche League International, n.d.

Willmuth, L. R. Prepared childbirth and the concept of control. *Journal of Obstetrics, Gynecology, and Neonatal Nursing*, 1975, *4*, 38.

Chapter 11

Voluntary Childlessness

Elissa Benedek and Richard Vaughn

The editors of this book initially titled this chapter "Voluntary Childlessness: A Work Inhibition?"; however, in this chapter, the authors have discussed the conscious decision of a couple to remain childless, not a neurotic unresolved conflict leading to childlessness. Approximately 11% of the families in the population remain childless. Of this group, 10% are infertile for psychological and medical reasons. The other 1%–2% chose childlessness as a life-style, after consciously weighing both the pleasures and the problems inherent in their decision (Bram, 1976; Kaltreider & Margolis, 1977). This paper focuses on that latter 1%–2%.

After further defining the population and placing them in a historical perspective, the authors review current developmental, psychological, and sociological theories presented to explain childlessness and describe childless couples and the culture and climate of their lives. Finally, recognition is given to the need for additional research in this area, for only through an understanding of voluntary childlessness can motivations for childbearing and child rearing be fully explored.

Initially, the population of the voluntarily childless must be isolated. The Judeo-Christian ethic reflects at least two important mores regarding procreation (Veevers, 1972a): the expectation that married people will have children and the expectation that they will want to have them and will rejoice at the prospect of parenthood. Current psychological theories support the normalcy of these ideas (Benedek, 1959; Erikson, 1959). Veevers (1973c) classified all couples in the following

Elissa Benedek, M.D. • Clinical Professor, Director of Training, Center for Forensic Psychiatry, University of Michigan, Ann Arbor, Michigan 48106.   Richard Vaughn, Ph.D. • West Shore Mental Health Center, Muskegon County Community Mental Health Board, Muskegon, Michigan 49442.

fourfold typology based on these two expectations: (1) conforming couples who both want to have children and actually do have them; (2) unfortunate couples who accidentally become parents of unplanned and unwanted children; (3) involuntarily childless couples; and (4) voluntarily childless couples who are deviant from the dominant mores, in terms of both their behavior and their motivation. It is only recently that this life-style of voluntary childlessness has been the focus of social and behavioral scientists. Parenthood as a developmental phase, parenthood as a form of psychopathology (unwed mothers and fathers), and unrealized parenthood (due to psychologically or somatically induced sterility) have served more usually as the subjects of research in this area.

The voluntarily childless family arrives at their decision in at least two characteristic ways. One route to childlessness involves a conscious decision on the part of a couple during the courtship period, with a definitely and explicitly stated intention never to produce children. The second route involves the prolonged postponement of childbearing until such time as it is no longer considered desirable at all. The first route clearly involves an explicit decision on the part of both members of the couple. One or the other may proselytize his or her mate to a world view or to a theoretical commitment to this life-style; or a common desire for no children may serve as one of the features in the partners' attraction. The other route is described by Veevers (1975) and involves a group of couples who remain childless because of a series of decisions to postpone having children until a future time: "a future which never came." These couples defer procreation until it is convenient, convenience being defined by financial, social, and/or emotional criteria. The postponement pattern is described as a gradual procession through four stages (Veevers, 1973c). The first stage involves postponement for a definite period of time. It is similar to a honeymoon period, and the couple decides to have children "as soon as conditions are right." The second stage involves a shift from postponement for a definite period of time to an indefinite postponement. The couple remain committed to the idea of parenthood, but they become increasingly vague about exactly when to stop practicing contraception and to attempt conception. The third stage involves a quantum leap, a shift in orientation and thinking. The couple acknowledges for the first time the possibility of remaining permanently childless. Here, the conscious decision is made after considering the pros and cons of extending their family and deciding to "consolidate." According to Veevers (1975), at this stage in the consideration of parenting, the only definite decision is to postpone deciding until some vague and usually unspecified time in the future, but the decision now allows for the possibility that, as a couple, this dyad may choose not to have children *ever*. The fourth stage involves the definite conclusion that the couple is not going to have children, that their childlessness is a permanent rather than a transitory state. This decision may be implicit or it may be made explicit.

Voluntary childlessness, or childlessness by choice, has always been an alternative in family planning. The technology for such a lifestyle is, of course, more immediately available now and includes a host of scientifically demonstrated alternatives. In primitive societies, the connection between coitus and conception was not always grasped, with the consequence that parenthood or childlessness was less a choice than it was a state "visited" on the couple (Cautley & Borgatta, 1975). Voluntary childlessness is hardly possible if cause and effect remain mutually isolated. However, today, in most Eastern and Western civilizations, the vast majority of adults intellectually grasp this link.

Though the tools of voluntary contraception have improved dramatically over the last 20 years in industrialized societies, the availability of improved contraception alone cannot account for significant historical differences in attitudes toward voluntary childlessness. For example, the impact of socioeconomic climate on family planning is one illustration of an important variable in family planning other than the availability of contraception. The Depression period, with its social and economic hardship, discouraged couples from conceiving. Personal attitudes rather than contraceptive practice accounted for a dip in the birthrate. In an investigation of a set of fertility data collected on the Rhode Island population during the late 1960s, Rao (1974) attempted to discriminate between a proportion of married women who had never had a live birth and a proportion of married women who had never been pregnant—two classes of childless women that are quite different: one group attempting to have children and failing, another selecting childlessness. The Rao studies distinguish three birth cohorts that had different childbearing patterns: a cohort aged 50 or over, a cohort aged 30–49, and an under-30 cohort. In the under-30 cohort, 24% were childless. The explanation for the large percentage of young childless women here is that many of the identified families were in the process of family building. They would not be childless at the end of their productive period. On the other hand, the Depression cohort (i.e., women 50 or over) had a 19% childlessness and a 17% never-pregnant rate. Rao explained that these women were in their "prime reproductive years" during the Depression, a period of relatively low fertility in the United States. Moreover, in many instances, pregnancies postponed for economic reasons were never "made up," with the result that a disproportionately large number of women in the Depression cohort remained childless. A majority of the women aged 30–49 were the so-called baby boom mothers, those women who had children in the high-birthrate years of 1946–1957, a time of economic prosperity. They were characterized by high fertility and consequently approximately an 8% rate of childlessness.

A commonsense perspective suggests that the incidence of voluntary childlessness in Western society is increasing. The changing status and role of women vis-à-vis the women's movement, the availability of career options to women other than motherhood, the improvement in birth control technology, the persistent trends toward greater urbanization (and the correlative studies of smaller-sized families in urban population), and the growing awareness of population pressures ("zero population growth")—all could be expected to influence couples not to have children, and, in fact, a number of researchers have endorsed this view by insisting that voluntary childlessness is on the increase, at least in the United States (Bram, 1976; Sheldon, 1975; Kaltreider & Margolis, 1977). But Veevers (1972b) cited the reverse, that since about 1940, childlessness—and especially voluntary childlessness—has experienced a steady decline. His data relate to Canadian populations. The central point to be made would seem to be that the determinants—the intrapsychic, interpersonal, social, and cultural pressures to have children, which we discuss later—are more influential factors in the procreation equation than the women's movement. Veevers noted that with the exception of race, childlessness tends to be influenced in an expected direction by the major sociodemographic determinants known to influence fertility in general: changes—that is, increases—in education, urbanity, and socioeconomic status or less rigid religious beliefs all decrease family size.

In addition to the unexpected difficulties in predicting voluntary childlessness in relation to specific social changes, such research as exists in the area has been limited by problems in discriminating voluntary from involuntary childlessness. Demographic data, abstracted from census data, simply count the number of childless couples. They do not give the reason for this status. Self-questionnaire data suffer from built-in hazards. The voluntarily childless couple have developed a host of defenses to avoid disclosing, or defending, their choice. In contrast, those who are involuntarily childless readily explain their family status either by accepting responsibility for their infertility or by projecting it. Unfortunately, one of the strategies for defending voluntary childlessness is to claim infertility. Veevers (1972a) described a contemporary TV play, "Dear Friends," in which the couple, who do not want children, toss a coin to see which of them will pretend to be sterile and thus lessen the social pressures by providing a relatively acceptable excuse for their behavior. Other strategies involve answering questions about family status with pat and stereotypical answers that do not inform the inquirer, but that serve to satisfy his or her curiosity and thereby protect the childless from involved and potentially disruptive conversations. (Veevers, 1975).

Veevers (1972a) has attempted to determine the prevalence of voluntary childlessness in Canadian populations. His reasoning might serve as an illustration of how the voluntarily childless population was computed in one country:

> Natural sterility in Canadian populations probably does not exceed about 5% of all couples. When the prevalence of childlessness among married women is greater than 5%, it can be assumed that the difference is due to psychological factors. Although some psychological factors result in psychosomatic infertility, it seems probable that the major cause is the deliberate decision to avoid motherhood. Since the overall prevalence of childlessness in Canada is about 12% and since only about 5% of wives are unable to have children, it has been estimated that about 7% of all wives are childless because of psychological rather than physiological reasons. (p. 576)

We noted earlier the importance of the culture and society as they impinge on freedom of choice in the area of childbearing, and we commented that, with increased education and increased liberation of both women and men, the incidence of childlessness seems to be increasing, at least in the United States. It is important to look at those social factors that make our Western society a "pronatalistic" society. Veevers (1973b) observed that in our society, there is a clear and exceptionally strong consensus that married people should want to have children. There is, indeed, a "cultural" expectation of parenthood that is supported by many sociologists and psychologists. The dominant religious groups in North America—Judaism, Catholicism, and Protestantism—all expound definitions of parenthood couched in terms of moral and religious responsibility, and all support in varying degrees the biblical injunction to "be fruitful and multiply." The Bible is replete with examples depicting the glory of parenthood and the curse of childlessness, beginning with Sarah, the first Jewish mother, whose child, conceived after years of barrenness, is a reward for her hospitality to angelic visitors. The theme of producing children to continue the religious tradition is explicit. Veevers cited Jakobovits (1959): "A man has performed a biblical precept 'to be fruitful and multiply' if he has had at least a son and a daughter, yet he should seek further to augment his natural increase beyond his minimum duty" (p. 155).

The Catholic Church characteristically sanctifies marriage as a permanent union for the procreation of children and specifically endorses the position that a marriage contracted with the intent of being child-less is not valid in the eyes of God (McFadden, 1961). For the devout Catholic, the alternative of voluntary childlessness is nonexistent, as it cannot be reconciled with religious and moral obligations. Protestant ideologies accept the principle of birth control by other than natural means, but birth control does not mean the abandonment of the tra-ditional definitions associating marriage with procreation (Veevers, 1973b). Thus, it is apparent that the major religions commend a pro-natalistic perspective and condemn and abhor voluntary childlessness. The logic in their dogma is apparent. Children assure continuation of the religious sect for the future.

Even without religious expectations to "be fruitful," current eco-nomic policy in many Western nations would promote a high birthrate. For example, Americans receive a yearly rebate of $750 at tax time for each child they have. Additional behavioral incentives are readily ap-parent in the form of Aid to Dependent Mothers, welfare, and food stamps, which increase proportionately with additional children. Many women openly admit that their motivation for childbearing is finan-cial. Similar support programs are extant in Russia, Sweden, Canada, France, Germany, and other Western and Eastern societies. Pronatal-ism is made equivalent to pronationalism and, at one level, means increased manpower and womanpower for territorial defense. Thus, to seek to avoid parenthood is to seem to avoid civic responsibility; one should have as many children as one can (Veevers, 1973b).

The state, religion, and the media are for once united in doctrine and ideology. Radio, television, and the lay and scientific press sup-port a pronatalistic policy overtly and covertly. For example, childless-ness as an alternative life-style has no place in today's television pro-gramming, despite the media's endorsement of a variety of family styles: the one-parent family, the black family, the father-headed fam-ily, and the foster family. Advertising consistently portrays the mother bathed in a romantic light surrounded by hosts of clean, smiling, happy children. In a review of 122 fictional short stories that appeared in three leading women's magazines between the years of 1940 and 1950, Franzwa (1974) concluded that motherhood was presented as the ideal condition for a woman. The childless woman is portrayed as wasting her life and as being bored, guilty, unfulfilled, and unhappy. Peck (1974) observed that pregnancy is portrayed as a device for winning a desirable man: the means by which a woman becomes the center of attention, "saves a faltering marriage," and retreats from or works out unresolved conflicts. Peck observed that the underlying assumption held by the media is that the duty, glory, and destiny of every woman lies in her ability to bear children and that before a woman can fully grasp the joys of life, she must become a mother.

Unfortunately, behavioral scientists have supported this stereotypical, pejorative image of the childless couple in our society. Beginning with Freud, who observed that the childless woman is the unfulfilled woman, Erikson and other theorists have considered childlessness undesirable and symptomatic of mental health problems. While they have noted that the mature man can love and work, a mature woman can only love. It is interesting to note that even the most sophisticated clinicians consider childlessness a form of pathology and relate it to problematic development and interpersonal difficulty, if not actual psychopathology. Three hypotheses put forth by Veevers (1973b) explain this view:

> Hypothesis One postulates that a number of benefits accrue from the parenthood experience, and that childlessness (both voluntary and involuntary) will therefore be associated with social and psychological problems. Hypothesis Two postulates that for the involuntarily childless, the distress caused by their failure to achieve parenthood will aggravate the above conditions. Hypothesis Three postulates that voluntary childlessness in particular is closely associated with unsatisfactory "mental health." Three possibilities associated with Hypothesis Three are put forth. The absence of a desire for children may be taken as de facto evidence of mental abnormality. Alternatively, it may be assumed that the same factors which predispose individuals to forgo parenthood also predispose them to a number of social problems, such as neuroticism, alcoholism, suicide, drug addiction, divorce, etc. In this interpretation, it is not that childlessness causes the social problems, but rather that both childlessness and other symptoms are caused by the same underlying psychological predisposition. Yet another alternative explanation suggests that whatever the mental health of those who choose to forgo parenthood, the social pressures and stigmas associated with this deviant role will create a number of significant psychological problems. (p. 304)

It therefore comes as no surprise, since government, religion, media educators, and clinicians are united in stereotyping and condemning a childless couple, that the general public regards them as selfish, sinful, and sick. Their fantasies of the childless couple leading a totally hedonistic, self-centered, and self-indulgent life are rampant. Womb envy is considered equivalent to penis envy in psychological literature (Nelson, 1967). The male is alleged to be jealous of the procreative and creative capacity of the female, but no psychological theory yet discusses the envy parents feel for their childless colleagues. Such envy may be generated by lack of financial stress; after all, it costs the average family $60,000 to raise one child and send it to college (Veevers, 1973a), not counting the costs of the mother's labor, social freedom (one need not provide child-rearing alternatives, baby-sitting, day-care), and the freedom from responsibility for a more helpless person's life.

A wide variety of theorists have proposed rationales for remaining childless. Such rationales are based for the most part on theoretical conceptions since, as we have mentioned earlier, studies of voluntarily childless couples are limited in number, methodology, and depth. Theoretical relationships focus (1) on the couple's own family of origin and relationships with father, mother, and siblings; (2) on the couple's relationship with each other; and (3) on more sociological and conscious choices.

RELATIONSHIPS WITH FAMILY MEMBERS

Relationship with Mother. Veevers (1973b) postulated that the childless woman's relationship with her mother may be one that could categorically be either very good, very bad, or somewhere in the middle. He reminded us that the most important female example that the childless woman has had to identify with is the "mother with children," or her own mother. Of course, this example is *never* a childless one. She may have been exposed to particularly bad mothering, including such pathological conditions as depression, psychosis, alcoholism, or drug addiction, which prevented her own mother from adequately mothering her. Kaltreider and Margolis (1977) found that child-free women surveyed perceived their mothers as "cold and unresponsive" and didn't want to be like them. For these reasons, the childless woman may feel that she does not have the capacity to mother a child herself. Kaltreider and Margolis went on to cite the young daughter of a schizophrenic mother who said, "A baby would drive me crazy the way it did my mother. My mother told me many times, "You will repeat my life.' "

Relationship with Father. There is no correlation shown between the woman's relationship to her father and her desire either to have children or to remain childless. However, one could hypothesize that the woman with a very bad father (i.e., a physically or sexually abusive father) might be fearful that in her marriage she would repeat such a pattern and would be the agent of such maltreatment to her own children. Kaltreider and Margolis (1977) described their sample of child-free women as identifying with their fathers' professional aspirations. Their early identification was as achievers rather than "little mothers."

Relationship with Siblings. The childless wife may have replaced her mother at a very early age and thus learned firsthand the trials and tribulations of child care, especially as an eldest child. The mother-hood mystique may hold no mystery and the "joys of parenthood" may be fictitious to her. She has seen that many enjoyable activities were forbidden or unavailable to her in her child-care role (Veevers, 1973a). She may have had an emotionally disturbed, mentally re-tarded, or physically ill sibling who required an inordinate amount of care, either from her or from her parents, and she may have seen that the sacrifices inherent in raising such a child are the kinds of sacrifices she is unwilling or unable to make. Additionally, concerns about the hereditary aspects of such illness may play a role in the decision to remain childless.

RELATIONSHIP WITH HUSBAND. The woman may have selected—consciously or unconsciously—a mate with "childlike qualities" who demands mothering. Veevers (1972a) pointed out that the voluntarily childless couple are often seen as a domineering, masculine-identified, overambitious woman absorbed in her career and an impotent, effem-inate man who serves as a child substitute. She may recognize her limited ability to mother or his limited ability to tolerate children. For-tunately, Veevers went on to refute this stereotype. The healthier cou-ple, whose relationship fulfills less neurotic needs, may elect childless-ness for reality-oriented reasons described later in this chapter.

SOCIOLOGICAL EXPLANATIONS. This is an interesting phenomenon that while parents are very seldom placed on the defensive with re-gard to their motivations for childbearing, even when the number of children in their families might be considered excessive, the childless couple find themselves constantly asked by well-meaning friends and relatives to explain the causes of their "lamentable" state. It is likely that this questioning has been reinforced, at least partially, by the often-repeated opinion voiced by many writers and researchers, as well as the entertainment media, that childlessness is nearly always a result of unfortunate circumstances of an involuntary nature (Bell, 1971; Kal-treider & Margolis, 1977). Therefore, inquisitive friends and relatives may see themselves as merely expressing curiosity in preparation for the expression of sympathy for the couple's childless state. That the couple may have voluntarily elected to remain childless is considered so unlikely as to be impossible. It is probably assumed that if the couple offer the information that they are childless by choice, the truth is that they are simply too embarrassed to expose the real, involuntary reasons. Fortunately, this opinion is now being countered. The pos-sibility that childlessness is consciously chosen and is not solely a re-sult of involuntary factors is gaining credibility (Rao, 1974; Veevers, 1972a; Waller, Rao, & Li, 1973).

As a starting point for an investigation of the factors that may influence a couple consciously to decide to be child-free, it would be informative to examine those motivations that are perceived as being most important in the decision to become a parent. These motivations for having children, which may be conscious or otherwise, have been conveniently categorized by Rabin and Greene (1968). Nearly all parents will be able to recognize within them their own personal reasons for childbearing.

Altruistic Reasons. These are the unselfish motivations for parenthood predicated on an affection for children and concern for their needs as well as one's own needs to express love and nurturance.

Fatalistic Reasons. These are best summarized by the belief that humans were brought into this world to procreate; therefore, to do otherwise would be wrong or even sinful.

Narcissistic Reasons. These derive from the expectation that the child will reflect glory on the parents or possibly allow one or both parents to relive portions of their youth with, hopefully, a better outcome. The child will provide a sense of continuity by carrying on the family name, career, or estate and will establish a feeling of immortality or make up for a sense of loss or deprivation by acting for the parent as someone who "belongs to me." Another possibility is that children may serve as proof of masculinity or femininity or self-enhancement as a productive, fertile, useful, and sexually functional adult.

Instrumental Reasons. This sort of reason is frequently considered the least acceptable, but it remains a prominent one. This expectation is that the baby will serve as an instrument or mechanism of change or security rather than being a goal in itself. For example, consider the couple who have a child to save their marriage, to placate their parents' wishes, to "prove" they love one another, or eventually to act as security for old age.

The reasons that a couple would choose not to have a child are not as clear-cut. Even the decision-making process is frequently fraught with ambivalence. The series of events that lead to the decision are not explicit and do not involve a number of obvious choice points. Surveys of women of childbearing age who have not yet been pregnant typically illustrate a vast inconsistency of response even from the same woman at different times. This inconsistency reflects the ambivalence and ambiguity associated with the childbearing decision (Flapan, 1969; Veevers, 1973c). This ambivalence tends to continue to a greater or lesser degree throughout the couple's or, more specifically, the woman's childbearing years. Resolution seems to come with the taking of definite action in one direction or another, that is, becoming pregnant or adopting permanent contraception. For example, attitudes toward motherhood and babies among women who have had a tubal ligation—a sexual sterilization operation—tend to be more unambivalently negative than those of fertile but voluntarily child-free women (Kaltreider & Margolis, 1977).

Despite the difficulties involved, a number of explanations have been offered to investigators by the voluntarily childless to clarify their motivations. Although they are regarded here as discrete entities, the extreme likelihood is that nearly all of these reasons figure in each decision with varying impact.

First, there is a concern about the irrevocability of a child. In life, children (and death) are just about the only things that are irrevocable; many individuals prefer to avoid such a decision, especially in view of the considerable emotional risk associated with having a child without knowing how he or she will develop.

A second concern, somewhat related to the first, involves the fear, or realization, that one does not know how to be a parent. The correlation between acceptable adult behavior and acceptable parental behavior is minimal, and pregnancy certainly offers no preparation for the role of parent to either male or female. The status of parent is very abruptly thrust on one without a training or transition period, such as may be found in taking a new job or even in the engagement period prior to marriage. There is instead immediate 24-hour duty involving unfamiliar tasks during the assumption of a role that calls for a greater adjustment than any other (Rossi, 1968). Mistakes frequently live on and are magnified in the children. Unfortunately, the nuclear family is a very poor setting for parent education.

The third reason for electing childlessness is one cited more frequently during the last decade: the belief that having no children is a dramatic patriotic gesture in view of potentially dangerous population expansion (Fischer, 1972). While certainly a noble gesture and one that addresses affirmative action toward a practical solution to the problem, the association of such a belief with the expressed desire to restrict one's own reproduction suggests a mixture of rationalization and intellectualization rather than pure unadulterated altruism.

Perhaps the most prominent, and reportedly the most attractive, reason given to explain childlessness is one that will be explored in detail: the unwillingness to give up a satisfactory life-style to take on the responsibilities and problems of parenthood. The desire for wider experiences, the wish to preserve the special intimacy of the dyadic relationship, and the disinclination toward assuming 20-odd years of additional responsibility tend to steer many couples away from having children. In many cases, children are in competition with travel, the new house, and professional standing. Certainly, with the advent of major societal changes such as day-care, the working mother, and the "househusband," the necessity for a dichotomous choice between motherhood and other gratification is diminishing, but nonetheless, a woman may feel compelled to give up a career, if only temporarily, to have a child. The expense involved in having and raising a child is frequently an issue. In order to "afford" children, it is often necessary to go into debt to some extent. It is illuminating to observe that surveyed childless couples characteristically showed a greater reluctance to go into debt for any reason than couples having or planning to have children (Veevers, 1973a).

Notwithstanding the reasons given for their way of life, the voluntarily childless couple necessarily experiences an alternate, atypical life-style, if only because of the dyadic structure of the family relationship as compared with that of partners with children. For some, this life-style is attractive and figures prominently in their decision to remain childless; for others, it is not as attractive. It is, however, observable.

It is a fact of life in the United States that, with the exception of the very rich, the very indifferent, or the very innovative, most adults structure the greater portion of their adult lives in such a way as to take into account the demands of children and their needs. This emphasis obviously limits the life-style options open to most couples. The desire for children seems to act as a sort of organizing principle in the lives of even those couples who are currently childless but who are planning to have children in the future (Bram, 1975). They tend to begin to evaluate their future plans and their personal activities by the standard, "Would it be possible with children?" or "Would it be good for the children?" the implication being safe, conventional, and predictable. It would seem that many young mothers go from being children to setting an example for children without a transition period that affords an opportunity to enjoy the pleasures of adult life.

With a continuing or increasing delay in the birth of the first child, regardless of the reason, or with an overt decision to remain childless, many couples become aware of an "alternate" life-style—childlessness—which may appear quite attractive, being free from the responsibility of children or of planning to have children. Suddenly, or over a period of time, the purpose of the marriage may shift to the preservation of the enjoyments of the relationship itself. Children come to be viewed as a disruptive force that would thereafter disturb both the intensity and the quality of the husband–wife relationship (Veevers, 1974).

The aspects of this "alternate," child-free life-style, which are felt by some to be attractive, are many and varied. An investigation of these aspects offers not only an understanding of the distinctiveness of this life-style as compared with parenthood, but also an insight into the needs and priorities of those who choose it. Without question, such a way of life is not attractive to everyone and perhpas not even to many, so, hopefully, a better understanding of the person opting for childlessness may be derived from what they view as important.

One integrating concept that is central to this alternate life-style is a feeling of freedom, for example, the freedom to be mobile. First, in their social life, child-free couples report more leisure time and both the desire and the ability to act spontaneously. They enjoy increased utilization of more expensive consumer goods and services because of their affluence. Without the large, fixed expense of child rearing, their income is all profit. Coupled with less of a need to spend for household help or child care and the fact that both members of the couple are typically working full time, a financial advantage becomes readily apparent.

Professional, occupational, or geographic freedom of mobility is also a major aspect. For those individuals not intensely involved in their work, an important component of the child-free life-style is the freedom to change their employment or even their careers with less concern about financial security. But for the career-minded woman, being child-free provides a greater opportunity—at the very least, more time and energy—for pursuing career goals. Veevers's (1974) research pointed out that childless wives tend to become significantly more involved in their work than do mothers, and they are more likely to be satisfied and successful in their employment. He went on to add that it has been suggested, in contrast, that the greater achievements of child-free wives are a compensation for a feeling of unfulfillment caused by lack of children. There is no firm evidence to support this suggestion, but he stated that some voluntarily childless wives have said that they have considered having children after a serious career setback, indicating that children and a career may fill many of the same needs.

Freedom is attractive in both a professional and a social sense—in the first sense because child-free couples are somewhat more easily able to change residences in pursuit of career goals than parents, and in the second, because they are typically able to enjoy the freedom to travel and entertain more spontaneously and for longer periods without being confined to the limitations of the school year. There is, however, the problem of arranging travel around two work schedules, but it is much less likely to be restricted to a one or two-week "vacation" period.

Another freedom to be considered is the freedom to step out of traditional sex roles in favor of a more egalitarian relationship. While many modern couples start marriage with this intention, it is most often the case that with the birth of the first child, sex differences are accentuated and sex roles are more clearly defined and differentiated. Childless couples, however, have the ability as well as the tendency to lead nonconventional lives without traditional sex-role definitions. They appear to share decisions that affect the couple more than parents do and reportedly enjoy each other's companionship more and engage in more activities as a couple than parents. The lack of sex roles is also apparent in their leisure activities (Veevers, 1974). Within the child-free home, a blurring of role distinctions in the division of labor often results in a convergence of roles or even role reversal. Child-free husbands tend to do more cooking and general housework than do fathers. They also do the bill paying, whereas for the traditional couples, this chore is included in the wife's role (Bram, 1975). Interestingly, controlling for the wife's employment fails to account for this greater egalitarianism found among voluntarily childless couples. The bargaining power of the employed wife was not found to be a major variable. Even when the wife was not employed, there was a greater sharing of tasks than was found among parents (Bram, 1975). It seems that it is not so much a solution to the structural problem of accomplishing domestic tasks around the demands of the wife's job as it is a different value orientation in these couples that results in an equalizing relationship.

What sort of person is likely to choose this child-free alternative life-style? Some of the factors involved have been considered above, but in addition, Veevers (1975) delineated three factors essential both to the choice of such a life-style and to finding satisfaction with it. Other individual personality characteristics, while of importance, must be omitted in this discussion because of the overview nature of the material presented. First, there must be a genuine agreement between husband and wife regarding the undesirability of childbearing. If one member of a couple secretly wants children, that person is likely to feel martyred if denied and to be less than satisfied with the life-style. Martyrdom can also fall on a person who is persuaded to have a child against his or her desires.

Second, an awareness of the advantages of the child-free life-style is necessary, along with a recognition that adherence to conventional norms does not guarantee happiness. It is especially important that the couple, and particularly the wife, learn to view the differences associated with voluntary childlessness as worthwhile. The mere fact of being childless is not sufficient to ensure participation in or enjoyment of this life-style. One needs to recognize the advantages of being child-free and to direct one's energies into enjoying them.

Third, the couple must develop an adequate social defense of their decision and way of life to be able to cope with the previously mentioned pronatalistic pressures of friends, relatives, and society in general. These pressures have been observed to begin after about one year of marriage, after the rewards of remaining childless for the first months and of negating the possibility that they "had" to get married have diminished. The pressures and expectations subtly, but persistently, increase until about the third or fourth year of marriage, when they seem to peak out. A couple find themselves needing to be firm in their resolve as well as glib in their response to counter such pressures. Once the marriage has lasted five or six years, there seems to be a diminution of pressure and negative response from others (Veevers, 1973d). This may result from an increased ability on the part of the childless to cope with such pressures, thus making the early years of marriage seem difficult only in retrospect. It may also be that they have learned to avoid those who constantly chastise them. And, of course, there is the possibility that a change has actually occurred in the behavior of others, possibly due to resignation. A curious note was offered by Veevers (1974) to the effect that those child-free couples who have the most satisfactory marital relationship are the most likely to encounter hostile responses from society, while those couples who are least likely to be greeted with hostility are those who have a mediocre or poor relationship but who maintain extensive involvement with their community (Veevers, 1974). Apparently, civic leadership is one acceptable substitute for children, where a close marital relationship may not be, or perhaps the poor relationship substantiates society's expectation.

In order to cope with the pressure to reproduce, which is considerable, especially early in the marriage, the woman finds it necessary to defend her beliefs. Veevers (1975) described four mechanisms that facilitate the maintenance of a "variant" belief system such as voluntary childlessness.

1. *Selective perception.* This mechanism allows one to give special attention to those perceptions that are congruent with one's beliefs, to ignore those that suggest contradictory conclusions, and to interpret ambiguous evidence as confirming one's beliefs. For example, the voluntarily childless couple may view the experience of pregnancy and childbirth as unpleasant or even dangerous. Child care may be seen as excessively burdensome and unrewarding, and motherhood may be perceived as deleterious to happiness and certainly not significant or creative.

2. *Differential association and identification.* This approach leads to

limited interaction with those who do not share one's beliefs, coupled with a disparagement of those whose beliefs differ and resultant physical or psychological isolation from them.

3. *Structured social situations.* The structure includes the environment, the participants, and the activities, which are all designed so that their outcomes support the original beliefs. Evidence for this hypothesis comes also from Houseknecht (1977), who noted that voluntarily childless couples develop their own group-support systems.

4. *Capitalizing on ambivalence.* In our culture, except for a small minority, everyone is somewhat ambivalent about their choice to have or not to have children. Most parents will confess that occasionally they wonder what it would be like to be childless. By recognizing and capitalizing on this ambivalence, one's own viewpoint may be supported.

Of course, the voluntarily childless are not immune from this ambivalence. It may appear to others as though they are at times, but this is more likely a response designed to cope with criticism of their life-style. Many child-free women admit to this ambivalence, and for these women, adoption is frequently considered as a future option. In this way, the decision not to have children is never irrevocable. Seemingly, the symbolic rather than the practical meaning of adoption is what is important. It acts as a reaffirmation of the couple's normalcy regarding their views on children, as well as a continual avoidance of an irreversible decision.

Though voluntary childlessness seems to be increasing as a life choice by women and couples throughout the United States, it has not yet gained universal acceptance. The mere fact that such an exploratory paper needs to be written stands as evidence. It is a choice that goes against centuries of tradition and existing cultural expectations. It requires a considerable degree of conviction. But in exchange, it offers opportunities not readily available to the parent.

In an age of rapid social change such as this one, the future of voluntary childlessness is difficult, or impossible, to predict. As the female role in Western society continues to evolve, space travel continues to develop, and *extero-utero* childbirth ("test tube babies") becomes a reality, new questions and possibilities present themselves. For example, in an age of space travel and possibly even colonization, would overpopulation remain a problem? Or on a more basic level, is childlessness defined as not having a baby or as not rearing a child, and what will conception and development outside the womb do to our traditional mores of parenthood? These issues and more will arise well within our lifetime and will significantly alter the institution of parenthood in unpredictable directions.

Hopefully, this discussion will act to elucidate this apparently emerging option and to convey the authors' conviction that consciously chosen voluntary childlessness need not be a form of psychopathology.

REFERENCES

Bell, R. R. *Marriage and family interaction.* Homewood, Ill.: Dorsey Press, 1971.

Benedek, T. Parenthood as a developmental phase: A contribution to the libido theory. *Journal of the American Psychoanalytic Association,* 1959, *7*, 389–417.

Bram, S. Vrywillig kinderloze echt paren, anders dan anderen [The voluntary childless marriage: Two's company]. *Intermediar,* December 19, 1975.

Bram, S. Kinderer ja of nee? [To have or have not: A social psychological study of voluntarily childless couples, compared to parents-to-be and parents]. *Intermediar,* January 9, 1976.

Cautley, P. W., & Borgatta, E. F. *Role definitions and fertility orientations* (Working paper 75-36). University of Wisconsin–Madison: Center for Demography and Ecology, 1975.

Erikson, E. *Identity and the life cycle.* New York: International Universities Press, 1959.

Fischer, E. H. Birth planning of youth: Concern about overpopulation and intention to limit family size. *American Psychologist,* 1972, *27*, 951–958.

Flapan, M. A paradigm for the analysis of childbearing motivations of married women prior to the birth of the first child. *American Journal of Orthopsychiatry,* 1969, *39*, 402–417.

Franzwa, H. H. Pronatalism in women's magazine fiction. In E. Peck & J. Senderowitz (Eds.), *Pronatalism: The myth of Mom and apple pie.* New York: Crowell, 1974.

Houseknecht, S. K. Reference group support for voluntary childlessness: Evidence for conformity. *Journal of Marriage and the Family,* May 1977, 285–292.

Jakobovits, I. *Jewish medical ethics.* New York: Bloch, 1959.

Kaltreider, N. B., & Margolis, A. G. Childless by choice: A clinical study. *American Journal of Psychiatry,* 1977, *134*, 189–182.

McFadden, C. J. *Medical ethics* (5th ed.). Philadelphia: F. A. Daru, 1961.

Nelson, J. B. Anlage of productiveness in boys' womb envy. *Journal of Child Psychiatry,* 1967, *6*, 213–225.

Peck, E. Television's romance with reproduction. In E. Peck & J. Senderowitz (Eds.), *Pronatalism: The myth of Mom and apple pie.* New York: Crowell, 1974.

Rabin, A. J., & Greene, R. J. Assessing motivation for parenthood. *Journal of Psychology,* 1968, *69*, 39–46.

Rao, S. L. N. A comparative study of childlessness and never pregnant status. *Journal of Marriage and the Family,* February 1974, 149–157.

Rossi, A. S. Transition to parenthood. *Journal of Marriage and the Family,* 1968, *30*, 26–39.

Sheldon, E. *Social indicators on the status of women.* Paper presented at the meeting of the American Psychological Association, Chicago, August 1975.

Veevers, J. The violation of fertility mores: Voluntary childlessness as deviant behavior. In P. C. Whitehead (Ed.), *Deviant behavior and social reaction in Canada.* Toronto: Holt, Rinehart & Winston, 1972, 571–591. (a)

Veevers, J. E. Factors in the incidence of childlessness in Canada: An analysis of census data. *Social Biology,* 1972, *19*, 266–274. (b)

Veevers, J. E. The child free alternative: Rejection of the motherhood mystique. In M. Stephenson, *Women in Canada.* Toronto: New Press, 1973, pp. 184–199. (a)

Veevers, J. E. The social meaning of parenthood. *Psychiatry*, 1973, *36*, 291–310. (b)

Veevers, J. E. Voluntary childless wives: An exploratory study. *Sociology and Social Research*, 1973, *57*, 356–366. (c)

Veevers, J. E. The life style of voluntary childless couples. In L. Larson (Ed.), *The Canadian family in comparative perspective*. Toronto: Prentice-Hall, 1974.

Veevers, J. E. The moral careers of voluntarily childless wives: Notes on the defense of a variant world view. *The Family Coordinator*, 1975, 473–487.

Waller, I. H., Rao, B. R., & Li, C. C. Heterogeneity of childless families. *Social Biology*, 1973, *20*, 133–138.

Voluntary Sterilization in Childless Women

Lidia M. Rubinstein

Voluntary sterilization has become the most widely used form of contraception for married couples. In the past several years, sterilization by tubal interruption through laparoscopy has become the method of choice for voluntary female sterilization. Furthermore, an increased number of young, childless women are requesting and obtaining this procedure.

Although a commitment to remain childless is not new or widespread, there is certainly a striking change in society's acceptance in regard to surgical requests to achieve this goal.

As Lindenmayer, Steinberg, Bjork, and Pardes (1977) have indicated, requests for sterilization by young, nulliparous women were very rare 10 or 20 years ago and would have been considered unusual at that time. It would also have been rather unusual if not downright impossible for a young, childless woman to obtain a sterilization procedure, even if medical indications were present. The influence of changing cultural norms, overpopulation concerns, the Civil Rights Act, and the women's movement have been influencing women and society to comfortably separate reproduction from sexuality. A more subtle and perhaps underestimated reason for sterilization requests is the progressive dissatisfaction and disillusionment with the present contraceptive techniques.

Several reports, including ours (1979), have analyzed the indications and the long-term implications of permanent sterilization in par-

LIDIA M. RUBINSTEIN, M.D., F.A.C.O.G. ● Associate Professor, Department of Obstetrics and Gynecology and Family Planning Clinic, University of California at Los Angeles School of Medicine, Los Angeles, California 90024.

ous women (i.e., women who have had children). In the case of childless women, there have been scattered reports with a few anecdotal cases that have shed some light on the reasons for deciding on permanent sterilization. In a study of seven childless women ages 20–26 at the time of sterilization, Lindenmayer et al. (1977) examined factors contributing to the wish to remain childless. The women expressed fear of the responsibility of caring for children. They also felt very strongly about their ability to move about freely. The interviewers were struck by these women's expression of urgency and need to control their reproductive lives. It seemed almost a lack of confidence in their responsibility to control themselves with less radical methods.

Long-term follow-up studies after tubal sterilization in parous women have yielded conflicting data. In particular, there has been a lack of uniform opinion regarding whether disturbances of the menstrual cycle and psychosocial distress may result from the sterilization procedure. In addition, whether nulliparous women have an increased rate of menstrual and psychosocial problems is not known because long-term follow-up studies have not been available. Although not substantiated, there is the notion that nulliparous women are at a higher risk of regret than their parous counterparts.

In a study conducted at UCLA over a 3½-year period, we followed 35 childless women who were sterilized. The age at the time of the procedure ranged from 18 to 42 years, with two-thirds of the women less than 30 years of age, and a mean age of 28.3 years. At the time of sterilization, 23% were married, 48% single, and 29% divorced or separated. The proportion of married, single, and divorced women remained almost unchanged at the time of follow-up. Only 2 women indicated a change in their marital status.

None of the women in the group defined themselves as housewives, and all listed occupations outside the home. However, none of them had top managerial responsibilities.

Although by definition none of the women desired future pregnancies, their reasons for sterilization fell into three categories: (1) a strong commitment to remain childless accounted for 60% of the women; (2) inability to tolerate other contraceptive methods accounted for 23%; and (3) medical indications accounted for 17%. All of these women had used more than one method of contraception in the past. More than one-fourth of the women (28.5%) had a prior history of one or more pregnancies that were terminated by induced abortions. Prior to scheduling the surgery, the women were interviewed in individual sessions. After a complete medical and psychosocial history was obtained, questions pertaining to the reasons for wanting sterilization, the risks, alternatives, and expectations were discussed, with particular emphasis on the possibility of regret. Three-and-one-half years later, the women were contacted and asked to answer a series of questions related to their sterilization. Although some of them had had changes in their menstrual cycle, these were almost always related to discontinuation of birth control pills; none could be attributed to the sterilization procedure. The majority of these women (80%) stated that the tubal ligation did not elicit changes in either their sex lives or their relationship with their partner. Where changes were noted, they were almost always for the better. None of the women felt that sterilization resulted in a worse sex life, and only one woman felt a deterioration of the quality of the partner relationship. These findings are to be expected, since most childless women requesting sterilization have been entertaining this decision for some time. Therefore, their life-styles are not drastically altered by sterilization. Nevertheless, 11% of the women expressed unhappiness about their sterility, and an equal number of women indicated ambivalence about the results. The women with feelings of unhappiness or ambivalence about having been sterilized were distributed throughout all age groups. For the majority of them, medical reasons had prompted the sterilization. However, in spite of their negative feelings, all of these women would have been willing to repeat the operation. The fact that the women with the strongest or most justifiable indications for sterilization felt the worst regret is not a new correlation. This regret has been described in women requesting sterilization because of a large number of children—even though they would not, under any circumstances, consider continuing another pregnancy.

It is not possible to establish generalizations or meaningful correlations in regard to the incidence of regret based on whether a woman is childless or not at the time of sterilization. For each individual, there is a different combination of circumstances, personalities, and factors (including children) that lead to the same decision, that is, the request for sterilization.

It is now becoming clear that the incidence of regret following sterilization is more directly related to circumstances prompting the decision than to any other factor. Women who are sterilized at the time of an induced abortion, because of poor marital relations, or for medical reasons are more likely to be sorry about their sterility, regardless of the number of children they have had. These women usually express anxiety and complain of feelings of inadequacy and depression lasting for a few weeks to several months. One may question whether these are expressions of regret about sterilization or regret over unfulfilled goals.

Education and appropriate counseling are essential in dealing with sterilization requests. This has to be viewed as a feedback process. On the one hand, the counselor has the opportunity to explore the elements of decision making about sterilization. On the other hand, women should be made aware of the complexity and interaction of factors that may play a role in their continued satisfaction with sterilization.

REFERENCES

Benjamin, L., Rubinstein, L. M., & Kleinkopf, V. Elective sterilization in childless women. *Fertility and Sterility*, 1980, *34*, 116.
Lindenmayer, J. P., Steinberg, M. D., Bjork, D. A., & Pardes, H. Psychiatric aspects of voluntary sterilization in young, childless women. *Journal of Reproductive Medicine*, 1977, *19*, 87.
Rubinstein, L. M., Benjamin, L., & Kleinkopf, V. Menstrual patterns and women's attitudes following sterilization by falope rings. *Fertility and Sterility*, 1979, *31*, 641.

Chapter 12

Women in Swinging

America's Amazon Society?

Lloyd M. Levin

Not long ago, I conducted a market research project on various forms of group interaction and living arrangements. One of these "group interactions" was the life-style currently known as *swinging*. The people I interviewed were different, and the settings changed; but over a number of interviews the story remained substantially the same, and it went something like this:

She was dressed as if she were 25; she looked 35; she admitted to 38 and was actually 47. On the surface, she seemed the typical suburban housewife—complete with two kids, mortgaged home, dog, and husband holding down a middle-level executive position. Unquestionably, she was a real, live example of the female component of the American nuclear family . . . but here she was, openly talking about five years of active participation in a life-style that is anything but traditional.

It seemed that, as for many married people, a certain amount of boredom had entered her and her husband's lives. Part of that boredom was sexual, and her husband dealt with that boredom by "playing the field."

Now, this was back in the days when the print media took swinging under their feature-section wing. Newspapers had discovered a new weapon in their battle for survival with television. Print could offer what television could not report: S-E-X! Sex sold papers, and swinging stories—whether real or romanticized—only whetted the readers' appetites for more.

LLOYD M. LEVIN • Founder, All Together, Inc., an organization providing resources for participants in alternate life-styles, Suite 3612, 405 North Wabash Avenue, Chicago, Illinois 60611.

Her husband was one of these readers. Like Don Quixote, he believed all the romantic fantasies he read. Soon he was enchanted, enthralled, and aroused by all these tales of "wife swapping." He just couldn't wait to whip out his lance and go jousting at all these sexual windmills. He became convinced that the only way to save the failing marriage was to reinject the missing spice, and he proclaimed to his wife that they must enter the swinging life-style. At first she was shocked, but he insisted. Hounded daily, nagged, threatened, and intimidated by her husband, she finally gave in, with a sigh. In the choice between swinging and divorce, she chose swinging.

Thus, they attended a swingers' social: he excited and eager; she reluctant and apprehensive. But the torrid stories of swinging suburbia that so captured the imagination and other sensation seekers like him turned out to be anything but true. The women were not all Sophia Loren; few of the men were even vaguely reminiscent of the well-endowed studs that the feature page promised. Most of the people were as ordinary as the couple themselves. And, as with most of the couples I interviewed, their first meeting with swingers and swinging groups was a disaster. Whatever they were looking for, it just wasn't there. Most of the people they met were a complete disappointment, and the couple left unfulfilled.

Unsatisfying as this first face-to-face meeting was, they went back for more. Finally, somewhere along the line, they "got it off" and were firmly entrenched in the swinging life-style. Of course, five years ago, it was still known as *wife swapping*. As feminism caught hold gradually, it came to be known as *mate swapping* and, of course, *swinging*. But with the trends in America today—with women changing from housewives into corporate executives—and the trends in swinging, we just may see the day when all those "action" stories of the past will be reprinted just as they were first presented, with only the name of the life-style updated with the times. We may look forward to reading steamy exposés of "husband swapping"!

At this point, let me catch you up on my background facts. Regardless of the name, the activity or life-style known as *swinging* involves a married couple who have sex with one or more persons, usually another married couple. As divorce becomes more prevalent, the number of unmarried couples who get into swinging increases. Surprisingly, it is not the young freethinkers who adopt swinging as a way of life; it tends to be the over-35 individual, who has been *previously* married.

What *is* swinging? Let me quote *Psychology Today*'s definition of swingers as a married couple who have sexual interchange with at least three different couples during a 12-month period.

How do people become involved in swinging? Well, the sensational press would have us believe a little fairy tale that their writers invented called the *seduction scene*. The setting is middle-class suburbia. It's Saturday night, and the neighbors are over. As the story goes, the groundwork has been carefully, gradually laid; the conversation has been directed ever closer to the subject of sex, the martinis flow like water, the dancing becomes a little more intimate, the dirty jokes begin to become erotic, and then it's just a matter of time before the situation gets out of hand—or is it *in* hand?

The next morning, the guilt sets in. Some handle it; some can't handle it. Some decide it was really what they were looking for: a total relationship with their closest friends; and a group-type marriage could be the end result—but that's not swinging. The stories tell us that's how it happens, and maybe in some cases it does. The seduction scene is, I believe, what most people consider the major part of swinging.

Why are there such misconceptions? Well, the Eskimos may consider it a gesture of friendship and hospitality to share their wives with their house guests, but the idea has been far from popular in the "civilized" world. In America, no other life-style I have researched brings forth so many negative comments from those outside it. Since swingers face negative opinion on so many fronts, they tend to remain underground rather than "coming out" and voicing the facts of the matter. Swinging causes a lot of anger, even hatred. Why?

Perhaps it's jealousy; perhaps it's a feeling that swinging threatens the whole concept and structure of the sacred American family. The swinger is inimical to the concept of a self-contained, independent, nuclear unit of father–mother–children—because the swinger seeks to expand, rather than to contain. Whatever the cause of the social pressures placed on swingers to disappear, they continue to exist—perhaps even to increase in number. In reality, there seem to be two primary doorways into the swinging world. First, there are what are known as *swinger magazines*. These are publications whose purpose is to provide space for personal advertisements, somewhat like a pen-pal club, except that the desired communication is sexual. Here, in the ad columns, are listed people from every background and location who are interested in meeting "like-minded" others.

Almost invariably, there are pictures, perhaps hundreds of them, of people who are advertising. The photos come complete with descriptions of the bodies, the pertinent organs, and the sexual preferences. All you do is take your pick! Write a letter to the coded box number, in care of the magazine, and enclose the "forwarding fee" (usually a dollar plus postage). Thus, you're on your way to meeting the couple of your dreams. Maybe.

After an exchange of letters, a meeting is arranged on some neutral ground—in order to establish that the pictures were really of the advertisers today, not 10 (or more) years ago. After a period of small talk and what I call *teeth checking* (to see if these, too, are real), the players might move quickly to the field of action: the nearest motel.

The chances of "success" using the personal ad columns are questionable. Several years ago, I interviewed the editor of the then-largest swingers' publication. Like most swingers' magazines, it was directed primarily at couples. However, like most others, it did include ads from singles, couples, threesomes, and moresomes—as long as these people paid for the ad in advance. My editor acquaintance believed that 100% of the single male ads were legitimate and that 85% of the couple ads were for real, but that only 15% of the single female ads were sincere. The rest (85%) of the single females were looking to sell pictures, or even themselves, rather than seeking a true swinger relationship.

Swinger ads are used primarily by new-to-swinging people. Therefore, the content of the ad reflects the fantasized ideas of the "superstud" husband, a role that will change as the couple gets more involved in swinging. Even those ads that include a picture (for "bait") usually display only the female form. Naturally, the people reading the ads are also new to swinging, so the appeal of the ad is directed toward the male, the "boss" of the couple—for now.

The second introductory method is mostly restricted to the larger metropolitan areas and entails the discovery of and a visit to a swingers' bar or other commercial establishment. At the swingers' club, people meet others looking for sexual partners, but at the bar, everything is strictly social. A place where you *meet* others is a *social*, but when it comes to the "action," that's a *party*.

At a party, the rules are very specific. A "no" is a "no"! Unlike the standard singles' pickup bars, where a "no" usually means "sell me," a "no" in swinging means something like "Don't push for it, not now, not at this particular moment."

The rules also define the various forms of swinging. There is *closed* swinging: a one-to-one relationship in private. There is *open* swinging: more than one relationship taking place in the same room, but usually on a one-to-one basis. Finally, there is the *orgy*: sex with more than one person at a time, threesomes, foursomes, moresomes.

And the cardinal rule for all swingers is: *No emotional involvement!*

Okay, that's the nuts and bolts of swinging. But how does all this relate to the concept that swinging is really a female-dominated lifestyle? How does our docile, oppressed, badgered, and used housewife get transformed from a reluctant, unwilling accomplice into an eager, active member of a female-dominated society?

Part of the answer lies in the "rules"; part of the answer lies in biology; and another part lies in psychology. The male is put immediately into a position of having to perform "on demand" regardless of the environment. Therefore, starting almost with the first encounter, the male finds himself in a world of "perform or else." The male who believed himself to be a sexual athlete, who was convinced that his every sexual fantasy would magically come true, now understands what it is to be intimidated sexually. At this point, roles start to change. The woman is better able to handle the situation, even if her heart isn't in it. Then, as time passes, she grows to *like* the sexual attention and begins to emerge as the leader of the couple.

Now, you must remember that this scenario is based on a limited number of interviews. I despise generalizations, and I am sure that there are some swinging associations that do not find the following to be true. But I have heard this theme repeated again and again, so it has some validity, some basis in fact. I am uncertain only of the exact degree of permeation in the swinging society.

You see, for most couples who are into swinging, the reason they got there in the first place was the husband's self-image coupled with unreal expectations of the nature of swinging. Hubby thought of himself as some kind of superstud. Swinging was to give him the unlimited opportunities he needed to realize that romanticized role. The feature section promised it. Gee, golly! He'll be just like a kid in a candy store—or so he thinks.

What really happens is that something goes wrong on the way to the vagina, and nobody in swinging is prepared to talk about it. Before very long, our superstud turns up as a superdud more often than not.

Why? It's certainly not the availability of unlimited, impersonal sex that turns him off; nor is it the sight of his wife having sex with a total stranger that gets to him. What really starts the pattern of impotence and *mental* castration seems to be the discovery the next morning that his poor little mousy, boring, uninteresting wife really enjoyed the evening! She has come to realize that she can outlast any man, anytime, and under *her* terms and conditions!

The female discovers that she has the right and the ability to enjoy sex in a variety of situations, and her demand for sex expands. All her preconditioning about sex being dirty and an unpleasant wifely duty for the happiness of her man has proved to be false. And as her demand for guiltless and enjoyable sexual relationships increases, the male now feels that it intimidates his needs and desire for sex. The result for many males is a form of temporary impotence.

At first, fearful about the causes and consequences, and not yet able to understand the intimidation that comes with "erection on demand," the female does her best to assist her partner. The help comes in the form of trying everything to create the emotional atmosphere and the erotic stimuli necessary for the male to be able to "get it up." While the female may not openly acknowledge, or even be totally aware of, what's happening to her male, instinct and training tell her to do something, anything. The female, for the moment, becomes the martyr. She places herself in front of him, on the altar of erotica, through participation in any type of sexual relationship or activity that might turn him on. In many cases, this means participation in sexual activity with another female. The ritual of lesbian sex supposedly will turn him on, and he will regain his manhood.

The end result of the little drama is that the female realizes that there are other ways to satisfy her newly increased sexual appetite. A male is not always required. It is estimated that among females who have been active in swinging for at least one year, up to 80% have experienced bisexuality, and some become actively bisexual. This activity begins to liberate the female even further, and she becomes less and less dependent on a specific male—or males in general—to fulfill her sexual needs.

Now this is not to say that any large percentage of the women involved in swinging are latent lesbians. Lesbian sex is merely the vehicle by which they cement the understanding that the woman has control of her own sexual well-being, that she has choices, options— and that when it comes down to the nitty-gritty, it is *she*, not he, who holds the reins.

This discovery contributes to the male's uncertainty. The longer the couple stays in swinging, the more probable it is that the woman will take charge of her own sexual life and, by extrapolation, her own life in general. The role relationship—as to who is really the "dominant" partner—is well on the way toward the female's assuming the upper hand. The farther that develops, the more the male's ability to perform is in jeopardy.

The male starts to cover up this role change with excuses for not taking as active a part in the sexual parties. "I've become more selective" is a standard line. What was originally a hot-to-trot, active male becomes a relatively inactive bystander. It seems that a form of emasculation has set in.

As the woman becomes less dependent on her husband for sexual release, suddenly *she* becomes the one who starts to demand that they go to the socials and parties. Suddenly, she's the one to suggest that they hold their own parties. Eventually, she's the one doing the inviting, deciding in advance with whom she plans to have sex. Finally, the changeover is complete, and she is in total control of the couple's social life.

Now that she directs the social side of their lives, the female increases their participation in swinging and decreases their nonswinging involvements. Their friends from yesterday, who are nonswingers, are seldom if ever seen anymore. Swingers, or those interested in becoming swingers, become a larger and more important part of their lives. But here is an interesting aspect: as friendships are developed with other swinging couples—real friendships—sex with those other couples ceases.

Emotional relationships, with sexual interchange, threaten the relationship and even the marriage of the original swinging couple—or so they may feel. As long as they swing together, the bond between them is felt to be relatively stable. When they start to swing alone, or when they become attached to someone else, then the relationship between them cannot hold. There is an axiom among swingers: "If your marriage is strong to begin with, swinging will make it that much stronger. But if your marriage is shaky, swinging may break it apart."

The stratagem for keeping the marriage going is to avoid emotional relationships with others at all costs, especially if those relationships include sex. The easiest way for a couple to stop swinging with another couple is to become real friends with them. Again, it is the wife who decides when that time has come. I could find no evidence about whether emotional involvements stem more from the male or the female, only that the female is usually the one to stop the action.

It is interesting to note some of the obvious signs of role reversal among swingers. Those relatively new to swinging will find that females without a male escort are invited to the parties they attend. As their time "in harness" increases, the parties they attend will include males without a female escort. Where it was once important for the male who believed himself to be a superstud to have a wide field from which to pick and choose, now, since his performance has become questionable, the needs of the woman come to the forefront. Hence the change in gender mix. Among longer-term swingers, a party of only couples does not guarantee sufficient male erections to go around. The extra, unescorted males are essential to ensure the females' satisfaction.

Now it is the female's turn to place the male on the altar of erotica. Just as lesbian sex was a male turn-on, the women find it enjoyable to arrange triads and larger groups with multiple males for each female.

Another striking sign of role reversal occurred regularly as I interviewed more and more of the longer-term swingers. Almost every interview began with the male telling how they got involved in swinging, and ended up with the female taking the narrator's role. I asked what the couple got out of swinging. She answered. What do they think of the people? She answered. How frequently did they go to parties? She answered. And so on. A pattern began to emerge of a society in which women were the ones in control. The swinging female is America's modern Amazon: independent, strong, self-assured, and—dominant!

If this is true, and not just a figment of the interviewer's mind, a question arises as to what can be learned from this "Amazon" arrangement, and where it may be headed. Statistically, women will be in such a majority by the year 2000 that one prominent actuary predicted that we may have to legalize polygamy—there just may not be enough men to go around. But we have seen that in swinging, one man may not be enough to provide for the sexual needs of several women.

While polygamy may be a far-fetched idea today, the possibility of such things as a woman president in the next century is not remote at all. Futurists should be seriously considering what a world dominated by women might be like. Will the decision-making processes, currently controlled by men, change radically? Will such things as approaches to product sales be turned around? (Imagine a tall, blond young *man* draped over the seats of a luxury car. Imagine *men* as the eye-catching models selling soup, nuts, business machines, and so forth.) Will the demand for goods and services be different with the females in control? For example, we might see more pressure applied to research on an effective male "pill." Some of these questions can be tentatively answered by careful observations of the swinging society. Think about it!

While you're thinking, let's get back to our opening interview. There's yet more to consider.

Like many of the people I spoke with, there are a great many swingers—my interviewee included—whose sole interest is in the physical. I asked her what she thought of the commercial club we were in at the time. Her comment: "I think it's a sexual supermarket, where people tour the aisles looking to pick up their late-night snack to take home!"

As our conversation progressed, out came the fact that she had become one of the more sexually active females in her group—to say the least. "The least" turned out to be her estimate that she had had approximately 4,000 encounters over the past five years.

Four thousand! If we were to break it down, that would be an average of three sexual encounters a day, every day, for five years. However, she did not space her activities so neatly.

A party, to her, means as many sexual relationships within one evening as possible. It was usual for her to have sex with 8–10 men in a night, with maybe an occasional female-to-female relationship thrown in. In amazement at her capacity, I asked what she got out of all this unlimited sex.

"When I swing," she replied, "I feel very good about myself. Swinging makes me feel very feminine."

I asked her to explain that feeling.

"Well, look at it this way," she stated. "When we go to a party, there are, say, ten couples involved. The men are good for maybe two or three rounds each, right? But a liberated woman—*sexually* liberated that is—can go on almost forever.

"Now, at every party there are younger women, there are prettier women, better-built women, and maybe even better-performing women than me. Swinging is the most competitive society in the world where a woman is involved, so when I get more than my 'share' in an evening, I've got to feel really super about myself."

Fascinated, I let her continue. "By my lasting abilities and my capacity, I come away realizing that I'm better and more desirable than all the others, for I've gotten more than my share. All in all, unlimited swinging is a real trip for me. The kinds of strokes I get out of swinging add credence to my feelings that I am the most desired woman of the evening. Therefore, how can I *not* feel feminine?" And so stating, she went off into the club looking for her "late-night snack."

But the kinds of strokes she talked about may soon become hollow victories for many who have engaged in the swinging life-style for any length of time. As the female becomes aware of the changes in her role within the couple unit—as she begins to feel her increased strength—she may use that strength to gain some retribution.

If the female has been nursing some deep hurt or hate against her husband, she may flaunt the change of roles with a "get-the-husband" game. In this game, the female goes to great lengths to get even with her man. It may be a sort of diabolical poetic justice in the form of "See, you s.o.b., you got me into this life-style against my wishes. Now I'm having a ball, and you can't even get it up." Her increased freedom allows her to express this old resentment, and she may do everything possible to destroy him, his ego, and his abilities to perform. His business may suffer; if she has a job, she may move up. Once, she was the boring, sexually innocent stay-at-home. Now, it may be his turn to wear that costume. And where she once cringed before the threat of divorce, she may now blithely serve him the separation papers and move in with someone else!

This stage of development is really a crossroads. While a great number of those I interviewed showed little depth or thoughtfulness about their lives and about swinging, there was a segment—maybe a growing segment—for whom swinging had become a growth experience. The female, understanding what happened to her once superstud husband, starts to take stock. She may decide to abandon her now boring mate, who may be reduced to impotence, hardly even able to fit the description of a man.

Alternatively, it seems that if there was really something between them, there may be a new future for them. The female, if she decides to keep her husband, must find a way to build a new foundation on which they can grow together. A new form of communication develops between them, and at this point, the couple may very well discover that swinging was just a door that they had to go *through* to find what they were really looking for.

Someone pointed out to me once that coupling was nothing more than a vehicle for sharing life's loneliness. If that is true, then what our swinging couple *may* have found is the need to share this loneliness with more than only one other person. Many people are desperate for love and yet are afraid to ask for it. They ask, instead, for sex.

In this rebuilding period, a couple's discovery that they can handle a group sexual relationship without tearing each other apart can start them on the way to finding new paths, new horizons. Maybe the discovery that sex by itself, without emotional involvement, is not enough pushes them along to emotional growth. Regardless of what it takes to find that starting place, it is the female, by her actions, who mentally pulls the male back up to a level of equality and gives the couple a chance for a future together.

Could it be that swinging has really pinpointed the fact that for many, the concept of the nuclear family is unworkable? The extended family (father, mother, children, grandparents, cousins, etc., under one roof or within close physical proximity) served a human need for outreach and intimate communication greater than the one-adult-to-one-adult system of the nuclear family. There seems to be a growing need for that greater outreach.

With the mobility of the current American population, combined with the demands of growing businesses that move people away from the extended families, we have become (in the words of the author Vance Packard) a "Nation of Strangers." I don't know if most swingers are uprooted couples, but I do notice more open swinging scenes in cities noted as being heavily populated with first-or second-generation Americans.

The stage is set now for new family models to develop, and as the couple goes through the sexual side of swinging and emerges into the potentials of the group-relationship, freer-woman side of swinging, the possibility that we will see more and more new modes of living increases. We'll leave a thorough discussion of the expanded or extended family for another time and another place. But regardless of one's personal feelings about swinging and swingers, these people may have opened up new avenues toward finding acceptable and workable new ways of living and achieving personal growth. It is true, in many cases, that unlimited sex hurts the relationships of the people involved. It is also true that many have found that swinging adds an important plus to their lives. Yes, some people involved have no capacity for a relationship deeper than unemotional sex, but some have found the ability to search further. Yes, many people have broken up their marriages over swinging, but many believe that their relationships have been strengthened by swinging. Most swingers took pride in telling me that no matter how late the hour, the last sexual encounter was always reserved for each other. Many said it was always the "best" of the evening; all of them said it was the female partner who made it so. Interesting?

Only time will tell what impact swinging as a life-style will have on the nuclear family, but there are certain things that all swingers seem to be in agreement on. Swinging is not the way to solve marital problems, because swinging not only brings problems into focus, it can blow them up out of proportion. Many have suffered and will suffer mentally because of swinging, but mainly because the media "promised them a rose garden."

In the long run, those partners who have only swinging in common will probably break up. Those who really care for each other will find a way to survive—and maybe even to grow. In the longer-term swinging groups, a kind of comradeship can develop between marriage partners, which shows signs of passing on to the next step. For many, that next step could be a group marriage. For many of them, swinging will have been a growth experience.

But no matter what role swinging will play in opening the doors to tomorrow, what comes across loud and clear is that *women* will lead the way. It may be too much to hope for, but wouldn't it be wonderful if, out of all of this, came a world in which there was no place for sexism—only equality?

Discussion of Chapter 12

Extramarital Sex

A Multifaceted Experience

Joann DeLora Sandlin

Lloyd Levin gives us an insightful discussion of swinging based on his interviews with a selected sample of swingers. In most respects, I concur with his conclusions, with one exception which I will discuss below. Before discussing Levin's article, however, it is useful to describe all the forms of consensual extramarital sex. This is necessary for two reasons. First, it should be made clear that the joys and problems of swinging are different in certain respects from those associated with other forms of extramarital sex. Second, as Levin implies, swinging is usually only one phase in the process of searching for the marital form that best meets the needs of a given couple. The process of searching often involves trying one or more of the other forms when swinging does not live up to the ideals sought. Marriages cannot be simply dichotomized as either monogamous or swinging. An understanding of the various forms of nonmonogamous alternatives, the reasons these forms are tried, and the reasons they are abandoned takes us one step further toward an understanding of all marriages, both monogamous and nonmonogamous.

Forms of Consensual Extramarital Sex

In a marriage that is nonmonogamous, the extramarital sexual relationships may be either clandestine or consensual. The implications for a marriage of a clandestine extramarital relationship (an "affair")

Joann DeLora Sandlin, Ph.D. • Professor, Department of Sociology, San Diego State University, San Diego, California 92182.

have been discussed at great length in both popular and professional literature. I will not repeat these discussions here. Instead, my focus is on the phenomenon that has more recently come to public and professional attention—that of consensual extramarital sex, which includes swinging as one type.

Forms of consensual extramarital sex may be characterized by reference to two dimensions: (1) the degree of independence of action of the spouses in their extramarital sexual activities and (2) the degree of emotional involvement with sexual partners outside the marital dyad. (See Figure 1.) The dimension of independence of action may be divided into two categories. The first category is low independence, in which the spouses agree to participate together, at the same time and in the same place, in their extramarital sexual activities. When spouses engage in this form of extramarital sex, it is referred to as *swinging* or *mate swapping*, although these terms may be used somewhat differently by different writers.

The second category of independence of action is high independence. In this form, the spouses agree that each may pursue his or her own extramarital activities independent of the other's activities. When spouses operate independently in their consensual extramarital sex, they have what is generally referred to as an *open marriage*.

The dimension of independence of action has implications for the potential for jealousy within the marital unit, particularly *exclusion jealousy*, or the jealousy that is associated with a feeling of being left out of others' enjoyable activities. The more the members of a marital pair are free to pursue independent outside sexual activities, the more potential there is for one or both persons to develop exclusion jealousy.

The second dimension for categorizing types of consensual extramarital sex is the degree of emotional involvement with sexual partners outside the marital dyad. Outside emotional involvement may range from virtually no involvement at all to an almost complete involvement and commitment. The higher the degree of outside emotional involvement, the more potential there is for one or both members of the marital pair to develop *fear jealousy*, or jealousy based on a fear of losing a loved one (emotionally, legally, or both) to another relationship.

Within the framework of these two dimensions, we can construct a typology of the different forms of consensual extramarital sex. (See Figure 1.) The form with the lowest independence and the lowest degree of outside involvement is sometimes referred to as *hard-core swinging*. In this form, the spouses participate together in an exchange with another couple or in a larger party. The primary motiva-

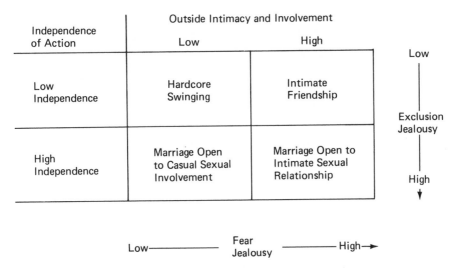

Figure 1. Types of consensual extramarital sexual interaction.

tion is sexual variety with no emotional involvements that might threaten the security of the marital bond. Swinging is generally limited to a very few contacts with the same person, and there is a continual search for new couples or new swinging parties. Contact outside the swinging situation usually does not occur.

A form with low independence but a fairly high degree of outside involvement is called *intimate friendship*. In this form, the spouses participate together and often form friendships with the couples with whom they have sexual exchanges or swing-party contacts. Since swinging relationships may continue for a long period of time, there is no need for a continual search for new partners once compatible relationships have been developed. But the search of swinging couples for this form of relationship is more difficult than it is for transitory relationships, since some degree of social and emotional compatibility between couples is necessary for a long-run friendship.

I would describe a marital arrangement with a high degree of independence of action and a low degree of outside involvement as a *marriage open to casual sexual involvements*. In these situations, each spouse is free to pursue sexual relationships outside the marriage as long as these relationships are characterized by a lack of emotional involvement. Outside relationships are not necessarily limited to "one-night stands" but usually involve very few encounters with the same person. Some persons find this absence of emotional involvement in a sexual relationship quite comfortable and compatible with their objectives in seeking sexual relationships. Other persons may find the relative absence of emotional intimacy a detriment to their enjoyment.

I would describe a marital arrangement with a high degree of independence of action and a high degree of outside involvement as a *marriage open to emotionally intimate sexual relationships*. In these arrangements, each spouse independently may pursue sexual relationships outside the marriage even when these relationships are emotionally intimate "love" relationships. This form of extramarital sex contains two elements valued by many persons—independence and intimacy—but because of these elements, it poses the strongest threat to the marital bond. There are no rules to protect against either exclusion jealousy or fear jealousy. This form of open marriage may become so open that it ceases to function as a marriage.

Swinging as a Phase

The discussion above of forms of extramarital sex permits us to put into perspective the phenomenon of swinging as Levin describes it. I think Levin is correct in implying that swinging, when it occurs in a marriage, is usually only a phase in a relationship that develops and changes through time in the couple's efforts to meet their needs better. Swinging is only a phase because they may discover after a time that it cannot meet all their needs—a conclusion they had previously applied only to monogamy. Thus, they may change the ground rules and try other arrangements. For example, the rule among swingers about no emotional involvement is helpful in preventing attachments that may lead to jealousy or that may threaten the primacy of the marital bond. But this rule introduces other problems while it helps alleviate jealousy. "No emotional involvement" often means limiting swinging to only a few contacts with the same person, a continual search for new partners, and a kind of superficiality and impersonality in swinging relationships that many persons find less than fulfilling. One alternative, as Levin suggests, is including friendship and real emotional intimacy in the sexual exchange. This new form of extramarital sex (intimate friendship) presents its own unique set of advantages and disadvantages. Impersonality is eliminated, but jealousy may be exacerbated. In addition, a couple interested in intimate friendships may find it difficult to locate another couple who can be compatible with them in their emotional and social as well as their sexual needs. A stable, intimate friendship requires some similarities between the couples with respect to income, education, life-style, values, age, and amount of free time. Most importantly, it requires that both the husband and the wife in each couple have a similar degree of sexual and interpersonal attraction to the opposite-sex person in the other couple. It is not unusual for either the husband or the wife to be more interested in an intimate friendship with a given couple than is his or her spouse.

If intimate friendships present problems in locating compatible couples, an open marriage may appear to be a solution. While an open marriage allows for intimacy, variety, and free choice in extramarital relationships, it makes jealousy management more difficult. The two implicit rules for hard-core swinging (spouses participate together, and there is no emotional involvement) are designed to minimize jealousy. A marriage open to emotionally involving outside relationships eliminates these requirements and their disadvantages, but offers no alternatives for jealousy management. For example, it takes a person who is very secure within herself or himself, as well as secure within the marital relationship, to remain home alone while his or her spouse goes away for a romantic weekend with a lover.

Of course, a couple with an open marriage may decide that they will limit emotional involvement with their extramarital partners to help alleviate the kind of jealousy based on the fear of losing the spouse. If they do so, however, they still are faced with the problem of relative impersonality in their extramarital relationships. Or a couple may try to alleviate the kind of jealousy based on a feeling of being excluded by agreeing that each will engage in extramarital sex only at times when the other is similarly involved. This agreement, however, presents knotty problems of timing for all concerned.

Swinging and the Emergence of Women

An important theme running through Levin's article is the emancipation of women and their eventual emergence as the dominant sex as a consequence of swinging. I do not fully support his conclusions in this regard. Generally speaking, the sexuality of females is more repressed than that of males in this society. In swinging, this difference is minimized, and both sexes are accepted, to a large degree, as sexual beings. This acceptance of her sexuality may be an exhilarating and freeing experience for a woman who has been taught from her earliest years that she should be "nice" and somewhat reluctant sexually. I agree with Levin that a woman may realize a sexual equality in swinging that she may not have felt before. But this is not dominance.

Swinging couples often notice that most women are capable of having more orgasms in a given time period than are most men. Knowledge of this fact does not inevitably lead to female ascendance to a position of total power. Also, many women who swing discover that sexual interaction with other women is quite pleasurable and satisfying. Discovery of this new joy, however, does not necessarily free them from seeking out men as a source of sexual, as well as other, pleasures.

While women may discover in swinging (if they never did so previously) that they are sexual beings who are capable of many orgasms with either male or female partners, men also may make some liberating discoveries. A man may realize that he does not need to have multiple orgasms to be an unquestioned success at a swinging party—in fact, he does not even need an erect penis. An imaginative use of tongue, fingers, or a vibrator will probably bring him more social acclaim.

These sexually liberating discoveries for men and women may result from swinging experiences, or they may simply be the result of experiences or knowledge acquired in other contexts. I see them possibly as leading to a little more equality between men and women, at least in the sexual sphere of their lives. Capacity for orgasms, however, does not appear to me to guarantee dominance or to determine all of one's interpersonal relationships. Even if it is true, as Levin claims, that the swinging experience results in the woman's emergence as the sexually dominant member of the marital pair, this sexual superiority does not necessarily effect a dominance in all other spheres of life. After some years of marriage, a complex interdependence usually develops. For example, the wife often depends on her husband for all or a large part of her financial support, as well as assistance in parenting their children and managing a household. Her greater capacity for orgasms will not automatically change this interdependence.

Monogamy versus Extramarital Sex

In leaving the security of a traditional monogamous marriage, many couples are searching for expanded opportunities for personal growth, for self-expression, and for developing intimacy—as well as for sexual variety. At the same time, they want to retain the emotional security they find in their marital relationship. Most encounter a dilemma when they discover that the forms of extramarital sex that give them the most potential for growth, self-expression, and intimacy are also the ones that leave them the most open to jealousies and emotional insecurities. Some couples are able to work out an arrangement that balances their unique combination of needs fairly well. Others, after a time, may choose to return to the relatively secure haven of monogamy and to forgo their pursuit of expanded horizons.

No one structure, either monogamous or nonmonogamous, provides the ideal solution for all persons. Therefore, we can expect that each couple will continue to search for the form of relationship that will best suit their particular needs and preferences. Part of this search may include swinging. Levin's article is important in helping us to understand some of the ramifications of this phenomenon and its impact on the participants.

Chapter 13

Wife Beating

A Product of Sociosexual Development

Del Martin

From a national survey of 2,143 couples (Straus, 1977), it is estimated that, of the 47 million couples living together in 1975, 1.7 million had faced a spouse wielding a knife or a gun, well over 2 million had been beaten up by a marital partner, and approximately 2.5 million had engaged in violence with a high risk of injury.

Because they do not have the physical strength that men do, women are more often the victims of marital violence. When it comes to murder, however, men are almost as often the victims as women. In desperation to put a stop to a beating, a woman may pick up the nearest object to defend herself. That object may turn out to be a lethal weapon.

Richard Gelles (1972) called the marriage license "a hitting license" (p. 153). In his research he found that numerous incidents of violence between married partners were regarded by them as being "normal," routine, and generally accepted behavior. Gelles's study was limited to legally married couples. However, the shared home, not the marriage vow, seems to be the key element, since violence also occurs among couples who live together without benefit of marriage. But even more significant are the male–female, dominant–submissive roles played out in these relationships.

Historical Roots of Wife Beating

From my own review of the history of marriage, I would call wife beating a "custom" that has prevailed since the emergence of the mo-

Del Martin • Commissioner, California Commission on Crime Control and Violence Prevention, Sacramento, California 95827.

nogamous pairing marriage. In earlier, primitive, "promiscuous" societies, women were the only discernible parents; as such, they were highly regarded and were a great power in the clans.

According to Frederick Engels (1948), their downfall came with the transition from polygamy and group marriage, when the "mother right" was overthrown and replaced by the "father right." The strictest fidelity was demanded of the woman to guarantee and authenticate the husband's identity as father. While polygamy and infidelity remained men's privileges, "purity" was demanded of the wife to protect her husband's "honor."

The word *family*, derived from the Roman word *familia*, signifies the totality of slaves belonging to an individual. The husband–owner had absolute power of life and death over the wife–slave, who "belonged to him." Wives, as private property, were bought and sold like livestock. The practice of bride capture (Brownmiller, 1975), in which a man abducted the woman forcibly and raped her and thereby staked claim to her body, was an acceptable form of mating in England in the fifteenth century. In medieval times, according to Elizabeth Gould Davis (1971), women were burned at the stake for such heinous crimes as talking back, scolding or nagging, refusing to have intercourse, and miscarrying (even though the miscarriage was caused by a kick or a blow from the husband). A discarded wife was often sold into prostitution, and when legal reform came in the 1880s, prohibition of the practice applied only to wives who were under 16 years of age. The law was also changed to permit a wife who had been habitually beaten by her husband to the point of "endangering her life" to separate from him, though not to divorce him.

In our own country, a husband was allowed to whip his wife so long as the switch he used was no bigger than his thumb (Calvert, 1975). But this rule of thumb was disavowed in 1874, when the Supreme Court of North Carolina stated that "the husband has no right to chastise his wife under any circumstances." The court added, however, "If no permanent injury has been inflicted, nor malice, cruelty nor dangerous violence shown by the husband, it is better to draw the curtain, shut out the public gaze, and leave the parties to forget and forgive." This qualifying statement, unfortunately, has become the basis on which our legal system deals with wife-abuse complaints. Unless there is severe injury, police, prosecutors, and judges tend to leave the parties "to forget and forgive." The danger of escalating violence and of possible murder is overlooked. The victim's definition of what constitutes "malice," "cruelty," or "dangerous violence" differs significantly from that of law enforcement.

Too numerous to mention here are the atrocities, still being committed in the name of church and state, against women and wives, indicating how deeply entrenched sexual inequality (at the least) and woman hating (at the extreme) are in human history.

The Marriage Contract

Barbara Hirsch (1973) described marriage as a contract entered into by three parties: the husband, the wife, and the state. The power in the relationship is not divided equally. The state maintains controlling interest, the husband has the authority in the home, and the wife serves at the pleasure of both. The state's exclusive jurisdiction over the marriage status has a tremendous effect on husband–wife behavior.

The marriage contract is unlike most contracts. Lenore Weitzman (1974) pointed out:

> Its provisions are unwritten, its penalties are unspecified, and the terms of the contract are typically unknown to the 'contracting' parties. Prospective spouses are neither informed of the terms of the contract nor are they allowed any options about these terms. (p. 1170)

Implicit in the unwritten contract is the early English common law (Blackstone, 1765/1966):

> By marriage, the husband and wife are one person in law. . . . The very being or legal existence of the woman is suspended during the marriage, or at least is incorporated and consolidated into that of the husband, under whose wing, protection, and cover she performs everything. (p. 442)

In marriage, the woman loses her personhood: she is identified in terms of her husband. Legally, he is the head of the household and is responsible for supporting the family; she is the subordinate and is responsible for housework and child care. With few exceptions, the wife takes her husband's name and his domicile and becomes his legal dependent. She must literally "love, honor, and *obey*"—or suffer the consequences. Her labor is a duty to be performed without value or compensation. In many states, the husband has exclusive authority over "community" property (DeCrow, 1974), including all of the wife's earnings, and can dissipate the family assets without the wife's prior knowledge or consent. The wages earned by the husband belong to *him*, and the wife is totally dependent on his whim or generosity.

The expectations that women have about marriage differ significantly from the reality of the marriage contract. In a study conducted in Chile by Hernán San Martín (1975) on the reasons that women and men marry, the women's chief motive stemmed from the desire to get out from under parental control and to be free. They also married because of the consequences of not marrying. The men's reasons for marrying were more in keeping with the interests of the state: marriage should incorporate fatherhood and provide the man with a "companion" to do the housework, to take care of his sexual needs, and to look after the children.

Jessie Bernard (1972, p. 17) said that "two separate marriages" exist: his and hers. For centuries, men have railed against marriage as a trap set for them by scheming women to gain protection and security, Bernard said, but in reality, it seems to work in the opposite way: "Men have cursed it, aimed barbed witticisms at it, denigrated it, bemoaned it—and never ceased to want and need it or profit from it." Research shows that marriage has positive effects on a man's mental health, his career and earning power, his longevity, his happiness, and his comfort. Women, on the other hand, do not fare as well. The bride who was catered to before marriage becomes the caterer after marriage. She must actively accommodate herself to suit her husband's expectations. Often, she reshapes, adapts, adjusts, or represses her personality to keep the marriage intact. Many women make fulltime careers of protecting the self-image of their husbands, for failure of the marriage in patriarchal society means the wife's personal failure as a woman.

SEX-ROLE STEREOTYPING

The roles of "wife" and "husband" did not grow out of biological realities or necessity; they were arbitrarily set to preserve the patriarchy. Concepts of masculinity (strong, active, rational, aggressive, authoritarian) and femininity (submissive, passive, dependent, weak, masochistic) were adopted by men, who seized power in the family and in society with the advent of monogamous marriage. The roles were mandated by the unwritten marriage contract and were incorporated into the culture by church and state.

Jean Baker Miller (1976) wrote that dominant groups usually define acceptable roles for subordinates, which typically involve providing services that no dominant group prefers to perform for itself. Functions that a dominant group prefers to perform are carefully guarded and closed to subordinates, who are usually said to be unable to perform them because of "innate defects or deficiencies of mind or body, therefore immutable and impossible of change or development" (pp. 6–7).

An apt illustration is the 1944 Florida Supreme Court decision (DeCrow, 1974) that describes a woman's legal status:

> A woman's responsibilities and faculties remain intact from age of maturity until she finds her mate; whereupon incompetency seizes her and she

needs protection in an extreme degree. Upon the advent of widowhood she is reinvested with all her capabilities which had been dormant during marriage, only to lose them again upon remarriage. (p. 169)

Miller also pointed out that if subordinates adopt the characteristics assigned to them, they are considered "well-adjusted." This is the means by which the dominant group legitimizes the unequal relationship; incorporates it into the prevailing cultural values, morality, and social structure; and thereby obscures the true nature of the relationship—that is, the existence of inequality.

The Broverman, Broverman, Clarkson, Rosenkrantz, and Vogel study (1969), in which professional therapists were asked to describe typical male and female behavior as well as that of "normal, adult behavior" (sex unspecified), is a classic example of this technique. Not surprisingly, the therapists described male and female behavior in stereotypical terms and equated the normal adult with commonly accepted male characteristics. Ruth Pancoast and Lynda Weston (1974) pointed out that men thus experience no dichotomy between adulthood and manhood, because society says the two are identical. But the woman who tries to be a healthy adult does so at the expense of being "feminine," and the woman who adjusts to her "normal" role does so at the expense of being a healthy adult. Society then has constructed a no-win situation for women.

In other words, if a therapist believes, as Freud did, that all women are born with an innate streak of masochistic self-destructiveness, any and all clinical experience that the therapist has with women will confirm that bias. If the therapist believes that a battered wife or a rape victim somehow precipitated the crime against her, her words and actions—even her dreams—will be interpreted to support that theory. Naomi Weisstein (1970) said that the problem with a discipline that rests its findings on "insight, sensitivity, and intuition is that it confirms for all time the biases that one started with" (p. 210).

Theories of victimology tend to excuse the battering husband from responsibility for his brutal acts, since the victim is seen as somehow provoking the violence for her own masochistic needs. According to Stephen Schafer (1968), the victim-precipitation theory requires the victim "to do nothing to provoke others" and to attempt actively to prevent a crime in order to escape responsibility. But Andrea Dworkin (1974) pointed out that "even a woman who strives for passivity sometimes does something. That she acts at all provokes abuse" (p. 48). Again the wife–victim is caught in the double bind.

Donald Morlan (1977) suggested that we "recognize that virtually all men are angry at women; that a man who batters is acting out in an extreme form what most men feel, at least part of the time." He attributes men's anger toward women to the repression of emotion in men, to limitation of intimacy to relationships with women, and to the socialization of men to be powerful. He warned, "Given the few number of men who really get to exercise power and the fact that we are all socialized to be powerful, there are a lot of us walking around who are pent-up volcanoes" ready to explode (pp. 15–18). Together, he says, we need to break down the impossible image of masculinity that dooms men to feelings of frustration and rage and puts women in the role of men's projection targets.

THEORIES OF MALE AGGRESSION AND SEXUALITY

Considering the long history of brutality against women and the mandated dominant–submissive roles of men and women in marriage, it is not surprising that many people believe there is a correlation between the physical abuse of wives and sexual arousal and/or pleasure. Anthony Storr (1970), for instance, not only regards male aggression as innate and instinctive, but also believes it to be a normal component of sexuality. He stated, "It is only when intense aggressiveness exists between two individuals that love can arise. Even sex itself does not seem to overcome aggression" (p. 39). He built part of his case on the Kinsey findings that anger and sexual arousal produce very similar physiological changes in the body and that it is not uncommon for one response suddenly to change into the other. That is why quarreling husbands and wives often end up in bed together and why some fights end in orgasm, Storr wrote.

"A touch of ruthlessness" in men is admired, Storr claimed, and the stability of the family and the sexual happiness of the couple depend on the dominance of the male. Aggression, he contended, is an important element of male sexuality because of the primitive necessity of male pursuit and penetration of the female: "The idea of being seized and borne off by a ruthless male who will wreak his sexual will upon his helpless victim has a universal appeal to the female sex," he declared. A little "fear of the more dominant male reinforces rather than inhibits erotic arousal in females." Storr criticized the church for teaching men to conceive of love in terms of self-sacrifice and gentleness, making them too restricted to enjoy "the full splendor of sexuality." If aggressiveness is inhibited, he wrote, "their wives cannot fully respond to them, and they themselves fail to gain complete sexual satisfaction" (pp. 66–71).

With the emphasis on male "conquest," sexual intercourse becomes a vital source of a man's self-esteem, and, Storr warned, rejection by a lover can therefore have extremely grave effects. Rejection can result in extreme rage from a husband who feels insecure about his "masculinity." Storr went on to say that a man who is not masterful and who fears women may become impotent.

J. C. Rheingold (1964) concurred:

> A woman can, under certain circumstances, make a man impotent. Expression of reproach, derogatory remarks, indications of disinterest, or expressions of exaggerated anxiety may have a castrative effect on a sensitive man and lead to lasting disturbance.

Wolfgang Lederer (1968, p. 283) pointed out another possible link between sexual insecurity and male violence. He wrote that some wife beaters "are potent only with a woman defective or somehow inferior." And P. Evans (1973) stated:

> The best aphrodisiac in the world . . . is the palm of a masculine hand applied to the cheek of a recalcitrant woman. . . . violence *is* sexy. . . . there is an erotic shock in a good slap. It establishes the first pleasurable principles of man over a woman. There is a satisfying *humiliation* in that. . . . the sensual masochism in a girl's makeup, however slight, is undeniable. (pp. 208, 226–227)

These theories reflect a general assumption that *male* sexuality and security are the stakes being played for. They concern themselves with the grave effects of sexual dissatisfaction in the male. But what of the woman and *her* sexual fulfillment? Phyllis Lyon, codirector of the National Sex Forum, an educational organization that has developed the sexual attitude restructuring (SAR) process, described for me (Martin, 1976) the bias surrounding female sexuality in our culture:

> Historically, women have been seen as nonsexual, existing only as receptacles for the pleasure of their husbands. Prior to World War I it was not ladylike for a woman to gain pleasure from sex, and more than one woman went to the doctor for relief of her unseemly feelings. Consequently, most women were raised to be sexy, not sexual. (p. 68)

"Historically, too, men were told they must be masterful in the bedroom," Lyon added. "Husbands were supposed to be skilled lovers who take total initiative in all sexual relations" (p. 68). Young men were encouraged to engage in premarital sex in order to gain experience and to learn technique. The partners they used for their education were "loose" women or prostitutes—beneath contempt as compared with the virginal maidens they expected to marry.

Thus, with the historical emphasis on the man as the master sexually, and the traditional association between sexual intercourse and the conquest of the weaker sex by the stronger, it is no wonder that sexual pleasure has been confused in some men's minds with physical strength and, by extension, with physical pain. Many men—and some women—have expressed their belief that a wife–victim who stays with a battering husband must somehow "enjoy" it.

According to Gelles (1972), the second most likely room in the house to be a scene of violence is the bedroom. J. J. Gayford (1975) found that half of the 100 battered wives in his study expressed satisfaction with their sex life, despite their husband's violence. For one-fourth, sexual relations had never been satisfactory, and one-tenth reported a deterioration of the sexual relationship. Fifteen women claimed that their husbands seemed to get some sexual excitement from the violence, but Gayford pointed out that the evidence for this perception stemmed from the fact that their husbands wanted sexual intercourse soon after the violent episode. Gayford stated, however, that we cannot exclude the fact that sexual intercourse in such instances can be an act of reconciliation rather than of sadism. According to Lenore Walker (1977), who has developed a three-phase cycle theory of marital violence, the period following the acute battering incident is one of "calm, loving respite." This is probably the only time in the marriage that the woman feels any closeness to or intimacy with her husband, which she may confuse with sexual satisfaction. Further probing into the couple's sex life, Walker told me, indicated that it is not really satisfactory to the woman.

Rather than suggest that a woman stays in a violent home because she somehow gets some emotional or sexual satisfaction out of being beaten, we should be asking what it is about the institution of marriage and society that keeps a woman trapped in a violent home. A woman stays because she has no place else to go, because she is financially dependent on her assailant, because he has threatened to kill her or the children if she leaves, because fear is paralyzing, because her self-confidence has been destroyed by her husband's denigrating behavior, because law-enforcement and social-service agencies have been ineffective in offering her protection or a roof over her head. By its inability or reluctance to apprehend the battering husband, society gives permission for or tacit approval of his violent behavior, yet blames the woman for being victimized.

RAPE WITHIN MARRIAGE

Marital rape frequently occurs in a battering relationship. A study of more than 400 battered women conducted by the Colorado Battered Women Research Center in Denver (Thyfault, 1980; Walker, 1979) indicated that 59% had been forced to have sex, and for 49% it had happened more than once. A total of 41% had been forced to perform unusual sex acts. The women were tied up, threatened with a gun, beaten or otherwise intimidated to act out the sexual fantasies of their batterers. The acts included insertion of objects into their vaginas, engaging in group sex, having sex with animals, and partaking in bondage and other sadomasochistic activities.

While rape is a common, acknowledged form of wife abuse, most states explicitly exempt husbands in their rape statutes. By early common law a husband had "sexual title" to his wife, the absolute right to have sex with her—even if it was against her will or if it meant sexual violence. As of January 1, 1980, in 44 states a woman is barred from charging rape where she is married and living with her husband/assailant ("Marital Rape Exemption," 1980). The exceptions are New Jersey, Oregon, Nebraska, Delaware, California, and Florida. South Dakota amended its statute to strike the marital rape exception, but the following year it repealed the amendment.

New Jersey changed its law after a precedent-setting case (Martin, 1976) in which the Essex County Grand Jury indicted a 27-year-old New Brunswick man for raping his estranged wife. The defendant was charged with rape, assault, illegal entry (having been previously ordered by the court to stay away from his wife), and impairing the morals of his children (having allegedly forced the young children to watch as he beat and raped their mother). When the original charges were brought the judge refused to refer the matter to the grand jury, since common law gives the husband absolute right to have intercourse with his wife. Joseph P. Lordi, the prosecutor in the case, opposed the judge's decision, taking the position that a wife is an independent spirit and not the chattel of her husband, and that the husband should be held responsible for his criminal acts whether they involve his wife or a third person.

In ten states women who are separated from their husbands can bring charges against them for rape. In another eighteen states charges may be brought under certain conditions. Some require that the separation be under court order; others merely require a petition for annulment, divorce, separation, or separate maintenance. Presumably, sixteen states still operate under the old common law which protects the husband's conjugal rights until the divorce is final. In these states, even though the woman has separated from her husband and established her own domicile, technically she is still married to him and he is still entitled access to her person.

Marital rape was used successfully in the defense of a wife who had killed her husband (White, 1977). In a defense argument, attorney Mark Weiss challenged Michigan law, arguing that a wife should not be forced to submit to her husband's sexual demands. On the witness stand, the wife testified that her husband had come home and said,

"We're going to have sex *my* way!" She went on to say, "I knew he meant we were going to have oral sex. I got undressed and he threw a butcher knife at me and missed." She stabbed her husband five times with a paring knife, killing him. The prosecutor, Andrew Telek, charged the woman with second-degree murder and claimed during the course of the trial that all the husband was "looking for was a little satisfaction." A change in Michigan's rape laws, which presently permit a wife/victim to bring charges of rape against her husband only after she has filed a petition for divorce or separation, is pending in the state legislature.

Legislators, who are mostly men and who persistently refuse to recognize rape in marriage as a crime, argue that vindictive wives may bring false charges against their husbands. But the fact remains that the rules of evidence place the burden of proof on the complainant. If husbands were no longer exempted from rape laws, there probably would not be any great increase in prosecutions. This has been the experience of the states which have lifted the husband exemption.

Adherents of law reform see it more as a deterrent or educational tool—a declaration by the state that sexual assault of wives will no longer be tolerated. As the law now stands in 44 states a man can rape his wife with impunity and with state approval.

THE EROTICIZATION OF DOMINANT–SUBMISSIVE ROLES

Ellen Morgan (1975, p. 1) protested "the violence that has been done to women specifically as sexual persons—to that dimension of them which is their sexual identity or selfhood and their sexual integrity." She went on to say:

> We cannot just dismiss the old Freudian notions of female passivity, submissiveness, etc., because some of our own deep sexual feelings are mixed up with these qualities, however unhappy that fact may make us. . . . Nor will we be able to justify our struggle for equality by compartmentalizing, asserting that our "nighttime" sexual nature must be passive and submissive, but our "daytime" selves are not. We are too aware that our sexual identities are not separable from the rest of our psyches. (p. 3)

Morgan cited as an example a young college student who confessed to her that she was unhappy because her boyfriend was not taking responsibility for her, shaping her life with a "firm but gentle" dominance that would make her feel cared for, protected, and "feminine." In a burst of rather painful honesty, she exclaimed, "I wish that my boyfriend would *master* me!" (p. 4).

Another woman admitted to her, "I have rape fantasies, but it doesn't mean anything in terms of who I am or what I'm like" (p. 8).

These remarks triggered Morgan into analyzing the sexual games that men and women play, the sexual signaling, and what she calls "chivalrese" and "rolese." She found that many of her women friends, who were characteristically assertive and independent beings, were nonetheless involved in erotic patterns of male domination–female submission. Morgan began to realize that a person's sexuality may be "organized," and that how it is organized may be "different from, alien to, and distressingly inconsistent" with the individual's personal identity. She saw that some women's sexuality seemed organized by the sex stereotype that links maleness to dominance and violence, even though in the deepest core of these women's beings, they held diametrically opposed values, and even though their fantasies did not dictate their conduct.

Judith Long Laws and Pepper Schwartz (1977) stated, "What is internalized through primary socialization retains much of its subjective reality, even when later learning overlays and contradicts it" (p. 9). Thus, it would appear that even though the women have shed some of the shackles of sex-role stereotyping in terms of personality, the old patterns remain when they relate to men sexually.

Morgan observed that men and women are taught that they are vastly different from each other and then "are trained to exhibit those supposed differences in order to be attractive to each other." The "differences" accentuated in a patriarchal culture, of course, support a system of male sexual dominance.

> In the pubertal years, [this conditioning] leads straight to the connection of sex-role—instead of actual sexuality—with eroticism. Our developing female and male bodies are the real base of the attraction we feel for each other, of course, but we are so conditioned to the notion that femaleness and maleness are essentially composed of the qualities we have been taught to regard as feminine or masculine [that only those who] display "appropriate" sex-role behavior are perceived as sexy and appealing. (pp. 13–14)

Young women are given the message of the power of sexual surrender, that women who reach erotic gratification are demure and passive and that male dominance and female submission are erotic.

> But the emotional quality of the girl's response to powerlessness is likely to be ambivalence, since at the same time she feels rebellious against male dominance, she finds it erotic; her male partners will be confused at her ambivalence to their actions, but will probably conclude that she really wants to be dominated and treated chivalrously, and she will probably arrive at the same conclusion. (p. 18)

For the woman is conditioned, along with the male, to see herself as his prey.

Laws and Schwartz (1977) agreed that the first component of sexual identity rests on female and male sex-role categories, which they have termed "a collection of prescriptions" for femininity and masculinity that are carried over into the realm of sexual behavior: "The understanding of sexual identity requires an appreciation of both biological givens and social realities. A common error is to assume that biological facts determine social realities" (p. 27).

Shere Hite (1976) pointed out that the glorification of the male "sex drive" has often been justified as a kind of natural law of the jungle, but that available information does not justify such conclusions. Lester Kirkendall (1958), for example, said that we must learn to distinguish between *sexual capacity, sexual performance,* and *sexual drive,* which he defined as what you can do, what you do do, and what you *want* to do. Kirkendall explained that while capacity may have a biological base, sex drive "seems to be very largely a psychologically conditioned component" and is more a function of desires than "needs."

Hite argued that a man's physical "urge" is a desire for further stimulation of the penis or for orgasm and *not* an "instinctive" need to penetrate a woman's vagina. She claimed that there is no reason that masturbation could not provide him with an equally strong orgasm, though she admitted that the *psychological* satisfaction may not be the same. The point is that there is no *physically* demanding male sex drive that forces men to pressure and intimidate women into having intercourse when they don't want it.

Sexuality as conquest is a learned behavior pattern—a pattern that implies the use of force. Thus, it is not surprising that some women have internalized, romanticized, and eroticized fantasies of being overpowered by the proverbial knight in shining armor. A woman struggling to identify and validate her own personhood must become conscious of the dichotomy between such erotic patterns and the nonsexual part of her personality, Morgan said. If she is to attain an egalitarian relationship, which is sexually and personally satisfying—and violence-free—her erotic patterns must be changed to correspond with her personal values.

INFANT PHYSICAL AFFECTION AND ADULT VIOLENCE

James W. Prescott (1975) has contended that major causes of adult violence are the deprivation of physical affection when the adults were children and the repression of female sexuality. He has also claimed that while we relate the biological with the social or cultural influences on violent behavior, we must also examine philosophical–religious value systems that determine the morality of sensory pleasure.

Laboratory experiments with animals (Suomi & Harlow, 1972) show that there is a reciprocal relationship between pleasure and violence, in that the presence of one inhibits the other. "When the brain's pleasure circuits are 'on,' the violence circuits are 'off,' and vice versa," Prescott wrote (p. 11). Monkeys allowed to develop social relationships through sight, hearing, and smell but not through touching or movement became pathologically violent.

Likewise, it has been found among human beings that lack of tender, loving care or somatic–sensory deprivation in early childhood creates a predisposition toward violence-seeking behavior later in life. Prescott stated that body contact *and* movement, or lack thereof, have a tremendous effect on the development of the pleasure systems of the brain and psychosexual functioning. That is why babies should be picked up and carried, and never left to cry themselves to sleep. Prescott sees the use of alcohol and drugs as compensation for lack of touching and the reason some people become hostile and aggressive when they drink. He also sees rape as derived from male deprivation by the mother.

But, Prescott has warned, we must not blame the mother, as we have been prone to do in the past. While nurturance by the mother is necessary in very early stages, the father in our society plays the most significant role in structuring the family. It is he who sets the tone or regulates family activity. If the father is affectionate, the mother is likely to be; if he is not, she is not likely to be affectionate either.

Brandt F. Steele and C. B. Pollock, psychiatrists at the University of Colorado who studied child abuse in three generations of families, found that parents who abused their children were invariably deprived of physical affection during childhood. They also found that their sex life was extremely poor and that almost without exception the women who abused their children had never experienced orgasm.

Prescott tested his hypothesis that deprivation of physical pleasure results in physical violence by examining cross-cultural studies of child-rearing practices, sexual behaviors, and physical violence. He found that societies that lavish affection on infants have low religious activity and less crime and violence among adults. He also found that societies in which there is low infant indulgence are more likely to practice slavery and polygyny and to display fear of an aggressive god. Societies that punish premarital and extramarital sex are likely to engage in wife purchasing, to worship a high god in human morality, to practice slavery, and to have a high incidence of crime and violence.

From these studies, Prescott contended that the "origins of the fundamental reciprocal relationship between physical violence and physical pleasure can be traced to philosophical dualism and to the theology of body/soul relationship." The Judeo-Christian concept of sex—saving the soul, seeing the body as an impediment to that objective, and equating men with spirit and women with evil (sex)—has had a deep and negative influence on American society, which is certainly violence-prone.

CONCLUSION

The batterer and his victim are no different from the rest of us, except perhaps that they act out to an extreme the battle of the sexes that permeates all of Western society. Marital violence, in one form or another, occurs in more than half of American homes. By its numbers, it cannot be viewed as a personal aberration that can be solved by counseling. Most therapists admit that the best they have accomplished is to reduce but not eliminate the violence. The legal and social-service systems have also proved inadequate. The only real protection that wife–victims receive is through the network of shelters—safe places—provided by grass-roots women's groups that have developed an "underground railway" whereby women who are refugees from their own homes can escape to another state.

If we really wish to eliminate violence in our society, we must first recognize that the home is where it begins. We must look behind those closed doors and examine the ways in which we rear our children and socialize them to conform to ill-fitting and destructive roles; we must change our attitudes about sex and learn to accept and respect female sexuality; we must begin to "parent" children and share responsibilities for the family; and we must put more emphasis on human relationships rather than corporate gain.

If marriage is to survive, it must become an egalitarian relationship in which both partners have mutual respect and responsibility. Couples should be allowed to draw up their own marriage contracts to fit their individual needs and life-styles. The rigid values of monogamy, chastity, and virginity to protect the "father right" and the mores that denigrate women as sexual objects rather than recognizing them as sexual beings have helped to produce physical violence. It is time we called a truce.

REFERENCES

Bernard, J. *The future of marriage*. New York: Bantam, 1972.

Blackstone, W. *Commentaries on the law of England*. Dobbs Ferry, N.Y.: Oceana, 1966. (Originally published, 1765.)

Broverman, I. K., Broverman, D. M., Clarkson, F. E., Rosenkrantz, P. S., & Vogel, S. R. Sex role stereotypes and clinical judgments of mental health. *Journal of Consulting and Clinical Psychiatry*, 1970, 34(1), 1–7.

Brownmiller, S. *Against our will*. New York: Simon & Schuster, 1975.

Calvert, R. Criminal and civil liability in husband–wife assaults. In S. K. Steinmetz & M. Straus (Eds.), *Violence in the family*. New York: Dodd, Mead, 1975, pp. 88–91.

Davis, E. G. *The first sex*. New York: Putnam, 1971.

DeCrow, K. *Sexist justice*. New York: Random House, 1974.

Dworkin, A. *Woman-hating*. New York: Dutton, 1974.

Engels, F. *The origin of family, private property and the state*. Moscow: Progress, 1948.

Evans, P. Do pugilists have more fun? *Cosmopolitan*, May 1973, pp. 208; 226–227.

Gayford, J. J. Battered wives. *Medical Science Law*, 1975, *15*, 240.

Gelles, R. *The violent home*. Beverly Hills, Calif.: Sage, 1972.

Hirsch, B. *Divorce: What a woman needs to know*. New York: Bantam, 1973.

Hite, S. *The Hite report*. New York: MacMillan, 1976.

Kirkendall, L. Towards a clarification of the concept of male sex drive. *Journal of Marriage and Family Living*, 1958, *20*, 367–372.

Laws, J. L., & Schwartz, P. *Sexual scripts: The social construction of female sexuality*. Hinsdale, Ill.: Dryden Press, 1977.

Lederer, W. *The fear of women*. New York: Harcourt Brace Jovanovich, 1968.

Marital rape exemption. *National Center on Women and Family Law Newsletter*, April 1980, pp. 6–8.

Martin, D. *Battered wives*. San Francisco: Glide Publications, 1976.

Miller, J. B. *Toward a new psychology of women*. Boston: Beacon Press, 1976.

Morgan, E. *The erotization of male dominance/female submission*. Pittsburgh: Know, 1975.

Morlan, D. Why are men angry at women? In *The Battered Women Conference Report*. New York: American Friends Service Committee, 1977, pp. 15–18.

Pancoast, R. D., & Weston, L. M. Feminist psychotherapy: A method for fighting social control of women. In position statement of the Feminist Counseling Collective, Washington, D.C., February 1974, p. 7.

Prescott, J. W. Body pleasure and the origins of violence. *Bulletin of the Atomic Scientists*, November 1975, pp. 1–12.

Rheingold, J. C. *The fear of being a woman*. New York: Grune & Stratton, 1964.

San Martín, H. Machismo: Latin America's myth-cult of male supremacy. *UNESCO Courier*, March 1975, pp. 28–32.

Schafer, S. *The victim and his criminal*. New York: Random House, 1968.

Storr, A. *Human aggression*. New York: Bantam, 1970.

Straus, M. Normative and behavioral aspects of violence between spouses: Preliminary data on a nationally representative U.S.A. sample. Paper, VA-2, University of New Hampshire, March 15, 1977.

Suomi, S. J., & Harlow, H. F. Social rehabilitation of isolate-reared monkeys. *Developmental Psychology*, 1972, *6*, 487–496.

Thyfault, R. *Sexual abuse in the battering relationship*. Paper presented at annual meeting of the Rocky Mountain Psychological Association, Tucson, Arizona, April 11, 1980.

Walker, L. E. *The battered women syndrome revisited*. Paper presented at American Psychological Association annual meeting, San Francisco, August 29, 1977.

Walker, L. E. *The battered woman*. New York: Harper & Row, 1979, pp. 107–126.

Weisstein, N. "Kinder, Kuche, Kirche" as scientific law: Psychology constructs the female. In R. Morgan (Ed.), *Sisterhood is powerful*. New York: Random House, 1970, pp. 208–210.

Weitzman, L. Legal regulations of marriage: Tradition and change. *California Law Review*, 1974, *62*, pp. 1169–1288.

White, K. Rape within marriage. In *Violence against women*, a pamphlet of reproduced news articles. Portland, Ore.: Rape Relief Hotline, 1977.

Psychoanalytic Reflections on the "Beaten Wife Syndrome"

Harold P. Blum

The problem of wife beating, so clearly outlined and documented in Del Martin's paper, is a complex issue, with many dimensions. The very title of the paper points to both social and sexual determinants, and many other determinants are mentioned. The paper demonstrates that civilization has not progressed in its treatment of and attitudes toward women in many areas even in relatively recent times. Women were often romantically exalted and idealized as mothers, while they were actually disadvantaged. Women were kept socially and economically dependent, often deprived of full legal status and protection, educational opportunity, and direct political expression. If they were the power behind the throne, that power was usually exercised by proxy and vicariously. Martin emphasizes that even in areas of contemporary society, women are still subjugated and are subject not only to discrimination and disparagement, but to physical assault.

At the same time, the position of women in Western civilizations has definitely improved and even now is in the process of further major alteration. The modern woman lives a social, sexual, and maternal role drastically altered from that of her grandmother and great-grandmother. Modern medicine and family planning have removed the masochistic expectation of death or disease from childbearing and the martyrdom of the endless rearing of an uncontrolled number of sickly children. Economic freedom of action and social mobility are present as never before, and the very independence of modern women doubtless is related to the high current divorce rate.

Harold P. Blum, M.D. ● Clinical Professor, Department of Psychiatry, New York University, New York, New York 10003.

Why then, does a woman remain in a situation where she is chronically mistreated and sometimes brutally beaten? Does she get emotional release or sexual satisfaction from the beating and the contempt? Martin disregards possible masochistic inclinations and indicates that the woman may feel in "bondage," trapped out of fear for herself or her children, financial insecurity, and loss of self-respect and confidence. No doubt powerful concerns about her own safety and that of her children are operative; some women are thwarted and immobilized by external circumstances beyond their control. The couple may be isolated from extended family and friends; this isolation intensifies the problems of seeking help, as well as control of and escape from aggressive behavior. Many forms of "wife beating" occur in subcultures that sanction such assault, but the problem cuts across social, educational, and economic lines, and also, like child abuse, is not limited to any specific category of psychiatric disturbance. Drug abuse, particularly alcoholism, is a common facilitating factor, which may diminish impulse control and frustration tolerance and may impair judgment. Yet neither alcoholism, indigence, ignorance, or any other single concomitant problem categorizes either the beating or the beaten spouse.

The assault on the wife may be relatively unprovoked, and the mistreatment may be rationalized or justified in terms of her fantasied misbehavior. Even where some degree of provocation or of unconscious complicity in the evocation of violence is present, and this often occurs, the attack may be far more serious than was sought or sanctioned. The violence itself may tend to evoke escalating regression, counterattack, and retribution in a vicious cycle. The effort to appease or or to placate the assailant may continue after the assault, along with fear of identifying the abusive partner, ascribing injuries to accidents, and escaping immediate punitive reactions but inviting future spouse assault. The victim's suffering in silence may indirectly perpetuate the violent pattern.

The serious traumatic effect of severe physical injury from violent assault has to be considered. The physical trauma is inevitably associated with psychological trauma, and the psychological sequelae may be crippling apart from and in addition to enduring damage to physical health. A crippling dependence may be psychological, social, and physical. Repeated assault on self-esteem, respect, and confidence; fear of the partner's rage and one's own fury; traumatic neurosis; and the terror of helplessness and repeated trauma—these and other consequences of physical abuse may serve to undermine personality organization and to induce regression. Trauma may lead to pathological alteration of the personality. Psychic intimidation, torment, and terror transcend concrete external and internal injuries, which may heal. The threat of revelation or separation may incite "massive retaliation" and deadly violence by the spouse. Each case is unique and requires individual evaluation, though various characteristics of battered wives may eventually be outlined. A depression-prone woman, for example, may engage in self-blame, and assume that she is responsible for her spouse's assaults.

It is also apparent to the psychoanalyst that many women and men create their own hell on earth and seek their own form of misery. The analyst would not be content with a good girl–bad guy or victim–villain explanation of such marriages. Sadomasochistic relationships abound, and women are not only victims of circumstances, but partners in provocation and punishment. This does not mean that an injured woman has necessarily sought her mistreatment or that she hankers for humiliation, but guilt, masochism, passivity, deficient judgment, defective reality testing, and many other psychological factors are very important. The need for punishment or masochistic gratification may be disguised, subtle, and outside awareness. Psychological forces are no less potent than social and cultural pressures, and in the long run, personality resources are crucial to mature marriage, motherhood, and social adaptation. It follows that women with the requisite personality strength are unlikely to marry or to remain married to violent men and that they tend to avoid men who abuse women and children, alcohol and drugs, etc.

There are guilt-ridden individuals who are gluttons for punishment and masochistic characters who derive hidden gratification from pain and humiliation. Masochistic women are far more likely to remain attached to abusive husbands or lovers and to repeat patterns of victimization with new partners. The masochistic woman is also identified with the sadistic partner and may live out beating fantasies, which stem from her own childhood, in the current family situation. The masochistic pattern can often be inferred from the choice of partners and from provocations, the repetitive enactments of specific forms of exciting abuse, the frequent initiation or association of assault and sexual excitement, the sexual form of the assault as in rape, and, when available, the masochistic coloring and content of the woman's fantasies. However, masochism does not account for all cases or causes. It is itself a complex personality constellation with many determinants and in no way condones or excuses the physical or psychological abuse of a woman—or anyone. It is important for the treating physician and the psychotherapist to be aware of the healthy as well as the pathological personality trends, and to recognize that assault activates sado-masochistic tendencies and fantasies of punishment. As in child abuse, the victim may come to believe it's her "fault," regardless of actual provocation, if the beating confirms masochistic degradation, self-re-proach, and self-hatred.

Some families are violence-prone. Marital battles are either com-bined with or alternate with child abuse. Women are by no means either all heroines or all witches, but some women are very disturbed individuals living in distressing circumstances without needed emo-tional support and ego assistance. Conscious fantasies of child abuse are not uncommon, and abusive acts by mothers indicate that women can also physically assault and psychologically insult relatively help-less victims, that is, children. They can also assault and even murder husbands or others, so that aggression and sadism are not purely sex-linked phenomena. It is possible that masochistic tendencies are more common in women than in men and that they may more readily inter-nalize aggression, but aggressive proclivities are universally found in *Homo sapiens*, so that one can accurately speak of sadomasochism. Both sexes seem to be amply, if not equally, endowed with aggressive po-tential, which may be directed externally or internally at the object or the self and usually at both.

I should like to draw attention to the importance of internal con-trols, self-regulation, and sublimation of aggressive and sadomasoch-istic tendencies. Without such regulation and tamed transmutation of primitive drives, human beings would be dominated by their drives and passions. These regulatory processes are greatly influenced by early rearing and identification. Like other primate females, women who have not experienced adequate mothering are likely to be impaired in maternal qualities and at risk for child abuse. The mechanism of iden-tification, with the aggressor and/or with the victim, is a very impor-tant but not an exclusive factor in both wife beating and child abuse. The child who is the beaten victim may be the punitive parent of the next generation or the willing victim of a spouse or partner who rep-resents the original abusive parent. The child may predominantly identify with an abused, self-effacing, or self-punitive parent and may perpetuate the masochistic relationship in adult life. The girl who has identified with a martyred mother or who was reared with ideals of self-sacrifice may be liable to resign herself to acceptance of mistreat-ment. Her own ideals as a woman, her convictions and controls, will enormously influence her choice of mate, her marital relationship, and her maternal attitudes and function. The prevalence of familial vio-lence and of sadomasochistic behavior throughout society is indicative of the power of the instinctual drives and the primitive passions in humanity; it is also a manifestation of the fragility of self-regulation and of identification with impulsive, threatening, punitive figures without consistent values of concern about and consideration of others.

Chapter 14

The Prostitute as a Victim

JENNIFER JAMES

INTRODUCTION

Prostitution is often referred to as a "victimless crime" or a "crime without a complainant." These terms are used to characterize crimes, such as vagrancy, gambling, pornography, and prostitution, wherein, typically, none of the involved citizens files a complaint with the police. Because the prostitute and her customer are involved in a mutually agreed-upon relationship, neither party feels any need for the services or interference of the authorities—in contrast to the relationship between a burglar and his home-owner victim, where the latter is quite clearly an involuntary participant in the interaction. Those who refer to the prostitute as a victim do so in a nonlegal sense. She is seen as a victim because of her life-style, her "immorality," or her "degradation."

Many of those who view prostitutes as the victims of prostitution base their judgments on assumptions about the individual psychology—or pathology—of prostitutes. As Stein (1974) said about her attitude at the beginning of her study of call girls,

> I kept looking for signs that the women were really miserable or neurotic
> or self-destructive. I wanted them to be that way. I think I wanted call girls
> to be "sick" because I believed that anybody—at least any woman—who
> sold sexual access ought to be sick. (pp. 21–22)

The plethora of myths about prostitutes, prostitution, and the effects of prostitution on its practitioners is an inevitable result of prostitution's illegality. Prostitutes are labeled criminals and are forced to lead undercover lives that are far removed from and inaccessible to "re-

JENNIFER JAMES, PH.D. • Associate Professor, Department of Psychiatry and Behavioral Sciences, University of Washington Medical School, Seattle, Washington 98195.

spectable" members of society. Aside from the customers with whom the prostitute conducts her business—men who usually are far more interested in their own immediate needs and desires than in investigating the life-style of the prostitute, who may have a considerable psychological investment in maintaining their fantasies about prostitutes, and who, in any case, are unlikely to broadcast widely their experiences since they are committing an illegal act by patronizing a prostitute—the only members of "respectable" society who ordinarily have much contact with prostitutes are police officers and other employees of the criminal justice system. In other words, police and jail records have been until recently our only source of "hard data" on prostitutes and prostitution—a very limited source of information, and one that raises an interesting possibility. Rather than being the victims of prostitution itself, prostitutes may be the victims of the laws against prostitution and their enforcement.

DISCRIMINATORY LAW ENFORCEMENT

Violations of the prostitution statutes account for approximately 30% of most women's jail populations. Convicted prostitutes serve long jail sentences compared with other misdemeanants, such as shoplifters or those involved in larceny or assault. The judicial attitude represented by those sentencing patterns has no justification with reference to the traditional legal concerns of danger to person or property loss. Nor does the large number of women arrested for prostitution (34,226 in 1973, according to the Uniform Crime Reports of 1974) indicate the commitment of the criminal justice system to an effective, realistic campaign to eliminate prostitution. Each act of prostitution, after all, requires at least two participants: a seller *and* a buyer. Despite this incontrovertible fact, the arrest rate for customers is only 2 per every 8 prostitutes (Uniform Crime Reports, 1975). It has been estimated by Kinsey and others that about 20% of the male population has some contact with prostitutes. There are obviously many more customers than prostitutes, and yet the prostitutes seem to be singled out to bear virtually the entire weight of legal reprisals. Since the prostitution laws in almost every state are neutral on their face, holding the prostitute and the customer equally culpable, the above figures prove that prostitutes are the victims of discriminatory law enforcement.

CLASS DISCRIMINATION

The traditional justification for discriminatory enforcement of prostitution laws was stated by Davis (1937):

The professional prostitute being a social outcast may be periodically punished without disturbing the usual course of society; no one misses her
while she is serving out her term—no one, at least, about whom society
has any concern. The man [customer], however, is something more than
partner in an immoral act; he discharges important social and business
relations. . . . He cannot be imprisoned without deranging society. (p.
752)

This argument assumes a class difference between prostitutes and their
customers: customers are middle- or upper-class "pillars of society";
prostitutes are lower-class "lumpenproletariat." While we may doubt
whether law enforcement should discriminate on the basis of class, the
characterization of customers as middle class implied by Davis is accurate: most customers are middle-class, married, white professionals
or businessmen who live in the suburbs. The class of prostitutes,
however, is not as easily categorized. In one study (James, 1976b)[1]
including 136 streetwalkers, for example, 64% of these subjects reported their childhood family's income as middle- or upper-class. It is
social mobility, as effected by societal application of the *deviant* label,
that makes this common assumption of "prostitute = lower class"
nearly absolute in fact. As Davis further stated, "The harlot's return is
not primarily a reward for abstinence, labor, or rent. It is primarily a
reward for loss of social standing." Benjamin and Masters (1964) also
noted that "The economic rewards of prostitution are normally far
greater than those of most other female occupations" (p. 93), in large
part because the prostitute is paid not only for providing a service but
also for incurring a loss of social status. The statistics on prostitutes'
class standing as measured by income, education, etc., are not at issue
here. We are merely pointing out that, through "working the streets"
as a prostitute, a woman becomes defined by the larger society as
lower-class and thus gains all of the liabilities appertaining to that
social status. No parallel social process exists to label customers as deviant, and their higher-class status is therefore not affected by their
illegal participation in prostitution.

The accepted class status of customers as opposed to that accorded
to prostitutes tends to protect these men from the possibility of involvement in the criminal justice system. Judging by the arrest statis-

[1]My research (1974–1977) has also included a sample of 240 female offenders, 136 of
whom have been identified as prostitutes. This research was funded by the National
Institute on Drug Abuse, No. DA0091801, "Female Criminal Involvement and Narcot-
ics Addiction."

Current research includes a sample of 100 female juvenile prostitutes (1977–1979)
and one of 100 male juvenile prostitutes (1979–1982). This research is being funded by
the National Institute of Mental Health, MH29968, "Entrance into Juvenile Prostitution."

tics, the majority of customers seem to be either invisible to the police
or else above the law. The latter is, of course, more likely, especially
since "Agencies of social control do not operate with impunity; they
must protect themselves from public reprisal and antipathy" (Kirk,
1973, p. 24). Any attempt to routinely arrest, process, and label a large
proportion of a politically powerful class (middle-class white males, in
this case) can lead only to "organizational strain and trouble" (Chambliss, 1969, p. 21). Harassment and labeling of social outcasts, on the
other hand, has always been considered a reasonable way to gain public approval and support. It has been reported that 70% of the women
who are now inmates in American prisons were initially arrested for
prostitution, a percentage that indicates the possible importance of
prostitution law enforcement as a labeling device and of the jail experience as an introduction to other crime:

> The adolescent girl who is labeled a sex offender for promiscuity . . . may
> initially experience a conflict about her identity. Intimate association with
> sophisticated deviants [in jail], however, may provide an incentive to learn
> the hustler role . . . and thus resolve the status anxiety by gaining prestige
> through association with deviants, and later, experimentation in the de-
> viant role. (Davis, 1971, p. 305)

Finally, in considering the possible class differential between
prostitutes and their customers, it must be remembered that women
in this society traditionally have no class standing of their own: they
are regarded as belonging to the class of their closest male associate
(father, brother, husband, lover, etc.). The illegal, "deviant" status of
prostitution means that the circle of those with whom a prostitute can
form close associations is arbitrarily limited to a very small number of
men, virtually all of whom are—or are considered—lower-class. (This
point will be amplified later in this chapter, when we discuss the relationships between prostitutes and pimps.)

NATURE OF LAWS

A second justification for the discriminatory enforcement of prostitution laws is implicit in the nature of the laws themselves. The control of overt prostitution is achieved in the United States through two
main types of laws: laws against loitering with the intent to commit
an act of prostitution and laws against offering or agreeing to an act
of prostitution. The most common enforcement procedures involve the
use of police officers as decoys. The officer behaves as he assumes a
customer would behave and, when approached by a suspected prostitute, elicits evidence of intent. The prostitute is arrested if she men-
tions money and sexual service in her verbal exchange with the officer.

These arrest techniques frequently involve the officer in the possible use of entrapment and questionable sexual exchanges. Some jurisdictions use civilian agents who complete acts of sexual intercourse before the arrest is made. These agents view themselves as protecting society by committing immoral acts for moral reasons. The use of female agents to solicit and arrest customers is rare because this use would require a violation of appropriate behavior for women and an "unfair" use of female sexuality to entrap men. In most states, customers are rarely, if ever, arrested. A woman who has once been convicted of offering or agreeing, regardless of the circumstances, is subject to future arrests under loitering statutes as a "known prostitute." (A *known prostitute* is a woman who has been convicted of an act of prostitution within the past year.) If she is seen in the area "known to be inhabited by prostitutes," she may also be arrested for loitering. Loitering is a statutory violation frequently used by enforcement agencies to control individuals labeled as deviants.

Obviously, it is easier to arrest prostitutes—at least, streetwalkers[2]—than to arrest their customers. The location of the streetwalker's place of business in itself makes her an obvious target. Men may walk the streets freely wherever and whenever they wish; a woman downtown late at night without a male escort is *ipso facto* suspect. George R. Cole (1972) reported that a police expert, in delineating for police officers the "subjects who should be subjected to field interrogations," included "unescorted women or young girls in public places, particularly at night in such places as cafes, bars, bus and train depots, or street corners" (p. 97). Unescorted men or young boys in public places were not included in this list of suspect persons. Moreover, it is considered acceptable behavior for men to initiate conversations—including conversations with overt or covert sexual content—with female passersby. This last point leads us to a discussion of *why* prostitutes have been made the victims of discriminatory law enforcement, aside from the argument of what is most convenient for the police.

Customers

In this society, there are some behaviors that are considered acceptable for men but not for women, for example, standing on a street-

---

[2]Attempts are occasionally made to arrest women who work in houses or massage–sauna parlors, but the arrest figures on these women are less than 5% of the total. Their prostitution is at least partially hidden by the offering of other, more legitimate services. Subtle prostitutes found on all social levels (e.g., call girls and conventioneers) are rarely arrested because they cause no direct affront to the public. Their sexuality is not explicit in their behavior.

corner alone at night or starting up sexual conversations with strangers. Prostitutes are women who are simultaneously rewarded and punished for choosing to earn their living through patterns of behavior that are unacceptable for members of their sex. In other words, prostitutes are the victims of sex-role stereotyping. The sexual needs of customers are loosely defined as normal, with the exception of those of a small percentage of "freaks" or perverts. In fact, the customers of prostitutes, and their activities as such, have enjoyed a long tradition of "normality." Even during periods when intensive official attempts to end the business of prostitution were under way—see, for example, descriptions by Anderson (1974) of Chicago, 1910–1915, and by Holmes (1972) of nationwide efforts at about the same time—customers' needs were accepted as inevitable. At most, the men were chided for risking venereal disease and implored to practice self-control. Today, men who purchase the services of prostitutes are still considered normal (nondeviant), even though their actions may be seen as unpalatable, or even immoral, according to the personal standards of the observer. Customers of prostitutes are, of course, acting outside the law, but where the law and the accepted male sex role come into conflict, the norms of sexual role-playing overshadow the power of the law to label deviance. Men are expected to have a wide variety of sexual needs and to actively seek fulfillment of those needs. As part of that search, men are allowed to purchase illegally the sexual services of women with relative impunity, as arrest statistics demonstrate.

A review of the acceptability of men's reasons for visiting prostitutes can be given only as an impression of common attitudes. Quantity of sexual partners has long been a praised accomplishment for men in many social groups. Although some restraint may be considered important after marriage, the attitude clearly is that a man who has been with many women has positive status. The epithets *Don Juan* and *stud* do not carry the connotation that *whore* and *promiscuous* do for women. The male "need" for sexual variety, a common subject in the commercial media and in sexual-joking behavior, and the desire for sex without emotional involvement are both frequently expressed as common, acceptable male sexual behavior, while they are both strongly rejected for women. Men with these desires and "needs," as well as traveling salesmen, convention attenders, participants in stag parties, etc., are all considered "natural" customers of prostitutes. The provision of sexual services to males by women is, in contrast, clearly labeled deviant. Males break few social rules in patronizing a prostitute; females break almost all the rules of their sex role in becoming prostitutes. Streetwalkers, in particular, place themselves at the wrong end of the whore–madonna spectrum: they accept money for sex, they are promiscuous, they are not in love with their customers, they are not subtle, and they engage in "abnormal" or deviant sex acts—acts that "respectable" women are not expected to accept (e.g., anal intercourse). As mentioned earlier, even the streetwalker's place of business is a violation of her sex role.

Most importantly, however, the independent, promiscuous, overt sexuality of the prostitute challenges the traditional assumption that female sexuality is entirely dependent on—and awakened only by—male sexuality. As Davis (1937) stated, "Women are either part of the family system, or they are prostitutes, members of a caste set apart." Unregulated sexuality is accepted from males; from females, however, whose sexual stability is the *sine qua non* of our family concept, ultrafamilial sex threatens the basic structures of society. So threatening is the idea of female sexual independence that we have laws defining juvenile women who engage in sexual intercourse without official permission as deviants "in danger of falling into habits of vice." Because women and their sexuality are tied so closely to the family structure—a long-term relationship based on a complexity of economic, emotional, and sexual expectations that are dictated by law and custom—sexual interactions between male and female social equals are commonly more-or-less channeled and controlled by these social expectations. Prostitutes are not considered the social equals of their customers, however. As we have seen, customers are primarily middle- or upper-class, and prostitutes are considered lower-class. Customers do not usually see prostitutes as being potential members of that section of womanhood to whom they may have to relate according to the prescribed roles of the family system, and these customers are therefore able to interact with the prostitutes in a much freer way. Gagnon and Simon (1973) stated that

> Since many of the organizing constraints on sexual activity are related to maintenance of the family and its future, the contact with the prostitute is significant, because it allows sexual expression without such controls on behavior. (p. 230)

It is true, of course, that the female sex role followed by nondeviant, nonprostitute women also consists in large part of barter transactions:

> Non-deviant male and female expectations concerning how women use [their] sexuality, and the exploitation of sexuality to achieve gain otherwise unavailable all add up to a routine exchange of sexual favors for pay. . . . The distinction between prostitution and the mundane characteristics of the female sex role simply are not as distinct as one might hope. (Rosenblum, 1975, p. 182)

The point we are making here is that the less overtly pragmatic sexual transactions that a man enters into with a nonprostitute are likely to involve or lead to a variety of consequences that may be legally, "morally," or emotionally binding. Moreover, the variety of sexual services a man can obtain from a nondeviant woman is likely to be smaller than that possible with a prostitute; and has in a sense recognized her as his social equal and thus must "pay" more (e.g., a house, a car, and clothes) for the same sexual service.

When the effects of sex-role stereotyping are taken into account, we can see that the perceived difference in class between the prostitute and her customers has a larger function than simply protecting the latter from social and legal labeling. One aspect of this function, for example, is that "many a client [customer] is sexually neutral or impotent with his wife and erotic or potent with a woman he can safely degrade—usually a prostitute" (Esselstyn, 1968, p. 130). This supposed inferiority of the prostitute may be a matter of her presumed lower-class status alone, or it may include recognition of her "deviant" label: some men desire the excitement of sexual relations in an illegal, or "I'm OK, you're deviant," situation (James, 1976c).

More importantly, however, the perceived interclass nature of prostitution is an expression of the middle-class man's need for liberation from the sex-role stereotyping of his class. The accepted range of male sexual behavior in our society is considerably wider than the accepted behavior conventions of the middle class—and especially of middle-class women. Women defined as lower-class, then, and particularly those who have been "set apart" by the label *deviant*, must serve as substitutes for the middle-class women so firmly restricted by their class-related sex-role proscriptions. Prostitution allows men "to regress to an 'Id' state of complete freedom from all restraints of civilization and acculturation" (Winick & Kinsie, 1971, p. 97). They move briefly into the deviant subculture, secure in their class-guaranteed ability to return to "normality." As noted by Gagnon and Simon (1973),

> The frequency of contacts with prostitutes by males at conventions and in other situations that are separated from the home suggests the loosening of social controls that are [sic] necessary for such contacts to take place. (p. 231)

The more highly restricted female sex role contains almost none of the sexual motivations and behaviors allowed to the male; nor does it allow a woman to serve as a professional accompanist for those men who would rent her participation in sexual activities. Rather than stating, then, that the prostitute is a deviant human being and that the prostitute's customer is a normal human being, it is actually more exact—and more telling—to say that a prostitute is a deviant *woman* and her customer is a normal *man*.

The puritan aspect of middle-class society means that the full acting out of the male sex role by middle-class males requires the existence of prostitution. As a result, the male need for purchased female sexual service is, and has long been, accepted as inevitable and therefore not to be punished. To have laws against prostitution almost seems to imply that some aspects of the male sex role itself are intolerable—or at least dangerously at odds with the conventions of middle-class society. Women are daily jailed, stigmatized, and exiled from "decent" society for their ability to recognize and deal with this conflict between male sexual needs and male social ideals.

ECONOMIC DISCRIMINATION

Far from being limited to the traditionally "private" sector of sexual behaviors, sex-role stereotyping has a pervasive influence in many public aspects of our society, including the economic system. Money-making options are still quite limited for women—especially for unskilled or low-skilled women. Recognition of this basic sex inequality in our economic structure helps us to see prostitution as a viable occupational choice for some women, rather than as a symptom of the immorality or the deviance of individuals. There is evidence that some women, in choosing the occupation of prostitution, are reacting to their victimization by this sex-based economic inequality. Pomeroy (1965), for example, studied 175 prostitutes, up to 93% of whom were motivated by economic factors; he noted that "the gross income from prostitution is usually larger than could be expected from any other type of unskilled labor" (p. 175). Benjamin and Masters (1964) were also aware of this sex-based economic differential and its relationship to prostitution: "The economic rewards of prostitution are normally far greater than those of most other female occupations" (p. 93). According to Esselstyn (1968), "Women are attracted to prostitution in contemporary America because the income is high and because it affords an opportunity to earn more, buy more, and live better than would be possible by any other plausible alternative" (p. 129). Davis (1937) summed up the economic pull of prostitution: "Purely from the angle of economic return, the hard question is not why so many women become prostitutes, but why so few of them do" (p. 750).

Some researchers claim to find an abnormal, perhaps even a neurotic, materialism among prostitutes. Jackman, O'Toole, and Geis (1967), for example, stated that

> The rationalization by prostitutes violating social taboos against commercial sex behavior takes the form of exaggerating other values, particularly those of financial success, and for some the unselfish assumption of the financial burden of people dependent upon them. (p. 138)

However, as Greenwald (1970) more accurately pointed out:

> Economic factors helped to mold the entire society, the family structure, and therefore the very personalities of these girls [call girls]. . . . the girls were caught up in the worship of material success. (p. 200)

In what way is the economic motivation of these women different from that of men who strive to attain a position on the executive level so that they can afford the "good life" and support the people dependent on them? The majority of Americans, it would seem, share the desire for financial success. Prostitutes are women who, usually with good cause, see prostitution as their only means for moving from a $3,000- to $6,000-a-year income to the gracious living possible with $50,000 a year. It is important to note that this view of prostitutes contradicts the traditional stereotype of prostitutes as wretched creatures forced into prostitution by extreme economic deprivation. In one recent study of 136 streetwalkers (James, 1976a), 8.4% of the subjects claimed to have started prostitution because of economic necessity, while 56.5% were motivated by a desire for money and material goods—a desire that, because of sex-based economic discrimination, they saw no other way to fulfill than by prostitution. A typical comment by a street-walker in that study referred to "the excitement of buying whatever you wanted without asking anybody . . . of having big sums of money that you never had before." Once accustomed to a higher income, as another subject of that study noted, "It would be pretty hard to go back to less money."

A person's choice of occupation is not limited solely by external realities. One's self-image plays an important part in one's perception of viable alternatives. If a man believes himself to have a "poor head for math," he will probably not be able to visualize himself attaining great success as a physicist. Women as a whole suffer from an especially narrow self-image in terms of occupational choices—because of sex-role stereotyping. Traditionally, women's roles have been those of wife and mother, both of which are exclusively biological and service roles. The emphasis on service carries over into the definition of "new" traditional women's roles, such as teaching children, serving food or drink, and secretarial work. The importance of physical appearance of many of these occupations reinforces women's self-image as physical–biological objects, limited to the confines of their sex-role stereotype at work as well as at home. As Rosenblum argued (1975), "Prostitution utilizes the same attributes characteristic of the female sex role, and uses those attributes towards the same ends" (p. 169). In other words, prostitution is a very natural extension of the female sex role into the occupational arena.

Some researchers (e.g., Esselstyn, 1968) believe that certain occupations lead women easily into prostitution. These occupations are those that adhere most closely to the traditional female service role, often emphasizing physical appearance as well as service. Clinard (1959) commented that "Quasi-prostituting experiences, such as those of a waitress who, after hours, accepts favors from customers in return for sexual intercourse, may lead to prostitution" (p. 228). It is not unusual for a woman who is required by her employer to flirt with customers and to "be sexy" to find that the men with whom she must interact in business transactions relate to her as a sexual object or a potential sex partner. Once she has been cast in this role of sex object, she may decide to make the best of a negative situation by accepting the "favors"—or the money—that men are eager to give her for playing out the implications of the role. Again, these low-status service occupations are among the few occupational alternatives available to unskilled or low-skilled women.

INDEPENDENCE AND EXCITEMENT

Another possibility excluded by the traditional female sex role is financial independence. In a sense, then, a financially independent woman is a deviant woman. These roles are beginning to shift and broaden now, but there are still virtually no occupations available to unskilled or low-skilled women that allow the independence or provide the adventure of prostitution. Rosenblum (1975) stated that the "specific precipitating factors" that cause women to choose prostitution as a profession "can be identified simply as independence and money" (p. 177). Data from the recent study (James, 1976a) mentioned earlier support the assertion that independence is highly valued by many of the women who choose prostitution. When asked, "Why did you leave home?" the largest category of responses by the subjects in that study was "desire for independence," and the second largest category was "dispute with family," which may also imply a desire for independence from the strictures of family life. Another question in that study—"What are the advantages of being a prostitute?"—also revealed the value that independence has for these women. Although the economic motivation overwhelmed all other categories in the first responses, in the second responses independence had first place. The search for an independent life-style can lead a young woman into a situation where she sees prostitution as her only alternative: "It [her entrance into prostitution] was actually caused because I ran away [when I was] too young to get a job. So I either had the alternative to go back home or to prostitute. So there was no way I was going to go back home, and so I turned out [became a prostitute]." Davis (1971), Benjamin and Masters (1964), and Esselstyn (1968) also specifically mentioned independence as a motivating factor in the choice of prostitution.

For many women, the "fast life" of prostitution represents more than simply economic independence unobtainable within the conventions of the "straight" world's female sex role. The life-style of the prostitution subculture has itself proved very attractive to a large number of women over the years. "Fondness for dancing and restaurant life" and the "tendency to vagabondage" comprise over one-fourth of the "immediate causes of prostitution" listed by Kemp (1936, p. 190). In tabulating the factors in becoming prostitutes of three groups of prostitutes, Pomeroy (1965, p. 184) found 3%–19% influenced by their perception of prostitution as "an easy life," 12%–24% by the "fun and excitement" they found in the "fast life," and 14%–38% by the fact that prostitution enabled them to meet "interesting people." Gray, in a study examining "why particular women enter prostitution" (1973), reported that "many of the respondents . . . felt intrigued by the description [by prostitutes] of prostitution which appeared exciting and glamorous. . . . the initial attraction for the girls in this study was social as well as material" (pp. 410–411). Benjamin and Masters (1964) stated that the life-style inherent in identification with the prostitution subculture continues to be a strong attraction after women have committed themselves to the profession: "There is an abundance of evidence that on the conscious level it is the *excitement* of the prostitute's life, more than any other single factor, which works to frustrate rehabilitation efforts" (p. 107). Following are some excerpts from interviews with streetwalkers (from James, 1976a) illustrating these attractions of prostitution:

> "The glamour side . . . being able to be in with the in crowd. . . . you really feel kind of good because you meet people who say, I wish I was like you—have diamond rings, a pocketful of money, and go out and drink." "To see if I can get away with it before I get caught: a game, like." "You don't have certain hours you have to work. You can go to work when you want, leave when you want. . . . you don't have a boss hanging over you, you're independent." "It's really kind of fun. . . . it's a challenge."

I believe that the above discussion provides a substantial explanation of why some women choose prostitution rather than the economic dependence of the traditional wife's occupational role—as defined by the female sex role—even when both options are available to them. Neither marriage nor extralegal monogamy provides or allows for the economic independence, the excitement, the adventure, or the social life available through prostitution. The basic fact of sexual objectification (exchanging sexual services for financial support) may be the same in either case, but for many women, prostitution obviously has benefits that outweigh the privileges—and the limitations—of "respectable" women's roles. Winick and Kinsie (1971, p. 75) referred to a rehabilitation program for prostitutes in Japan in the 1950s that included such traditional women's activities as arts and crafts and homemaking. The program failed, the authors reported, because the prostitutes were simply not interested. As Greenwald discovered (1970), most prostitutes feel "overt hatred of routine, confining jobs" (p. 202). The traditional female occupations—including that of housewife—can be seen as among the most "routine, confining jobs" in this society, and thus they present limited temptation to women who value the relative freedom of the "fast life." To sum up this section of our discussion, prostitution is one way for women to reject their victimization by our sex-biased economic system by choosing an independent and exciting, albeit "deviant," occupational life-style.

Pimps

Thus far, we have examined prostitutes as the victims of discriminatory law enforcement, sex-role stereotyping, and economic discrimination. Now we will take a look at prostitutes as victims of those who are traditionally assumed to be their primary oppressors: pimps. A common myth in this society pictures prostitutes as defeated women cowering under the coercion of brutal pimps. Kemp (1936), for example, stated that "In many cases friendship with a pimp may be considered the immediate cause of a woman's becoming a harlot. It is the man who leads her on" (p. 214). However, "friendship" and "leading on" are not necessarily coercive, and Kemp earlier (p. 190) stated that the influence of a pimp was the "immediate cause of prostitution" for only 8.3% of prostitutes. Gray (1973, p. 412) found that the influence of pimps, when it was a factor, "was generally minimal." Data from the James (1976a) study showed a somewhat larger role for pimps in recruiting women for prostitution. It should be noted, however, that the influence of "girlfriends" was more than equal to the influence of pimps, that more than twice as many women reported choosing prostitution solely on their own initiative, and that my field experience has led me to agree with Gray that the pressure applied by pimps in recruiting women is generally minimal. One woman described her entrance into prostitution this way: "The only reason I got started was because of my old man's suggestion, because otherwise I don't think—maybe I would have, later. I liked the money; it was easy money."

Women in this society are socialized to feel that they need a man to take care of them, to "take care of business," to "complete" them, to love them, to make a home with them; this is part of the traditional female sex role. Prostitutes are no exception to this rule. "Well, everybody wants a man," said one streetwalker. "You can get lonesome," explained another; "even though they laugh and say, if you're with that many men how can you get lonesome. But believe it or not, it's just like getting up at eight o'clock in the morning, going to work, and coming home at five o'clock in the evening; it's just something you do to survive and that's it. There's no feelings involved." For many of these women, a relationship with a pimp means "just knowing that you have somebody there all the time, not just for protection, just someone you can go to." Because of their involvement in a deviant life-style, however, prostitutes must share their lives with men who understand the dynamics and values of their deviant subculture—men who will accept their violations of the traditional female sex role. Any man who lives with a prostitute will be called a pimp, although usually the only factors that distinguish a prostitute–pimp relationship from that of a "normal" marriage relationship, aside from the illegality of both roles, are the woman's status as sole breadwinner and, often, the man's overt maintenance of two or more similar relationships simultaneously. It has become obvious that physical male abuse of females in marital relationships is common. As is true throughout society, women's socialized need for men is reinforced by the fact that a woman's status is determined by that of her man. The prostitute who can achieve a relationship with a "high-class" pimp has a higher standing in the subculture of prostitution. This rise in status pays important dividends in her interactions with other members of the subculture: "If you have a pimp, other guys on the street, they kind of leave you alone." Thus confounding the scenario of the coercive pimp, one can often find prostitutes actively seeking to attach themselves to those pimps whose patronage they feel will be most beneficial.

Of course, not all prostitute–pimp relationships are desirable models of human social interaction. Some pimps are physically abusive, just as some husbands are. Perhaps prostitutes who experience abuse from their pimps are in a better position than nonworking wives with abusive husbands, in that prostitutes are financially more independent. On the other hand, prostitutes—whether they are married to their pimps or not—are likely to be taken less seriously by authorities, such as police, to whom they turn for help. This lack of respect and concern on the part of law-enforcement personnel toward prostitutes also prevents prostitutes from seeking legal help when they are abused or assaulted by customers, which is not an uncommon occurrence. Faced with the attitude that she was "asking for it," or at least, "had it coming to her," a prostitute who reports abuse from a customer or her pimp to the police is liable to feel more victimized by the discrimination of the legal system than by the violence of individual men (James, 1973).

Review of Theories

There is yet another way of looking at prostitutes as victims. Rather than seeing them as simply victims of prostitution itself and of societal reactions to prostitution, one can ask whether prostitutes are women with histories of victim experience that influenced them in their choice of occupation and life-style. We have seen that prostitution is an aspect of, not a contradiction to, the female sex role as it exists in this society; and yet the choice to become a prostitute is obviously heavily loaded with negative valuations, according to the judgment of the majority culture. What, then, determines which individual women will act out the prostitution components of the female sex role? What factors enable certain women to accept the deviant status conferred on them by their choice of prostitution? Scores of researchers, theorists, and moralists have published their opinions on what is "wrong" with prostitutes, individually and as a class. At the end of the last century, for example, Lombros (1898) cited physiological abnormalities and deficiencies as the cause of all female crime, including prostitution. Another researcher (Kemp), as late as 1936, stated that "from 30 to 50 percent of all prostitutes must be classed as feeble-minded." More recently, these discredited theories have been replaced by psychological evaluations of prostitutes, which are more modern sounding, if not necessarily more valid. "Latent homosexuality" has been seen as a mainspring of prostitutes' motivation by some (e.g., Greenwald, 1970; Maerov, 1965; Hollander, 1961). Since homosexuality, like prostitution, is popularly considered deviance, the temptation to put all the "bad eggs" in one theoretical basket is perhaps understandable. There are no hard data, however, linking homosexuality—whether latent or overt—with female prostitution. Some researchers believe that many prostitutes have an oedipal fixation. Winick and Kinsie (1971, p. 83), for example, see prostitution as atonement for guilt produced by incestuous fantasies. This theory is impossible to disprove, since we cannot accurately measure the incidence of incestuous fantasies. On the other hand, it is impossible to prove their theory, or to prove that it applies more to prostitution than to other occupations. "Money is heavily loaded with all kinds of psychological conflicts. In our civilization, among many other things. . . it symbolizes the will to power and the ensuing unconscious guilt of having taken the father's place,"

Choisy stated (1961, p. 1). Perhaps every woman, prostitute and business executive alike, who desires economic independence is acting out oedipal fantasies. It seems unlikely, however, that many women are motivated solely or primarily by such a tenuous subconscious factor in making their occupational choice. Again, the literature provides virtually no hard data to justify including this theory among the significant prostitute-motivating factors.

The myth that women become prostitutes because they are "oversexed" has been countered by the discovery that most prostitutes see their sexual activities with customers as purely business and usually get no sexual pleasure from them. Unfortunately, an opposite myth also exists, that of "the invariably frigid prostitute" (Maerov, 1965, p. 692). Responding to this myth, Pomeroy (1965) reported that the 175 prostitutes he studied "were more sexually responsive in their personal lives than were women who were not prostitutes" (p. 183). As noted earlier, emphasis on physical appearance is an important aspect of the female sex role: "Movies, television, popular literature and, particularly, advertising make it seem that the cardinal sin a woman can commit is to be unattractive" (Greenwald, 1970, p. 201). Some researchers believe, with Greenwald, that prostitutes are motivated by the need to prove their attractiveness through sexual contact with many men. Taking the theory a step further, Winick and Kinsie (1971) stated that

> . . . many prostitutes apprehended by the police tend to be overweight and short. They often have poor teeth, minor blemishes, untidy hair, and are otherwise careless about their personal appearance. Docility and indifference are common. This leads one to conclude that such women may feel inadequate to compete in more traditional activities and thus more readily accept a vocation that involves the sale of something they may not value highly. (p. 35)

Winick and Kinsie did not seem to consider the fact that a large percentage of the prostitutes apprehended by the police are "hypes"—drug addicts working as prostitutes to support their habit—who form a special, lower class in the hierarchy of the "fast life." In any case, since it is demonstrably true that the majority of unattractive women do not become prostitutes, and since it is a matter of personal opinion what percentage of prostitutes are unattractive, the importance of the Winick and Kinsie statement quoted above lies in its assumption that women's "traditional activities" are those that emphasize physical appearance. This assumption is very pervasive throughout society and is a major influence on women in the development of self-image—and self-image is always a factor in the individual's choice of occupation. Perhaps we could find women who became prostitutes because their "attractiveness" rating was not high enough for them to gain employment as receptionists or cocktail waitresses. On the other hand, prostitutes generally make more money than waitresses or receptionists, regardless of physical appearance, and we are inclined to believe that the economic motivation is statistically far more important than the psychological one presented by Greenwald and by Winick and Kinsie. The last of these common psychological theories about prostitutes pictures them as using their profession to act out their hostility toward men. If we look at this theory objectively, it would seem equally valid, except for the illegality of prostitution, to suggest that some women become elementary-school teachers in order to act out their hostility toward children. Perhaps this motivation is real for some women, both teachers and prostitutes, but documentation is very scarce.

Moving on from theories based on psychological evaluation, we will now consider some theories based on hard data about prostitutes' lives—data obtained from prostitutes themselves. The James (1977) study and a few other recent studies indicate that the factors that enable some women to accept the deviant status inherent in prostitution can be tentatively identified as exposure to the prostitution life-style, certain patterns in child–parent relationships, and perhaps patterns of negative sexual experiences that lead to the development of a self-concept that includes a high degree of sexual self-objectification. The latter two of these three factors can be seen as evidence that prostitutes are women with histories of victimization.

CHILD–PARENT RELATIONSHIPS

Parental abuse or neglect is widely considered a typical childhood experience of women who become prostitutes. Kemp (1936), Choisy (1961), Maerov (1965), Jackman et al. (1967), Esselstyn (1968), Greenwald (1970), Davis (1971), and Gray (1973) all mention unsatisfactory relationships with parents as a fact of life for these women. Whether the condition is simple neglect by absence or outright physical or psychological abuse, the result is generally considered alienation of the child from the parents and a consequent inability—greater or lesser, depending on the circumstances—on the part of the child to be adequately socialized to the conventional mores of "respectable" society. Data from the James (1977) study seem to reaffirm the prevalence of parental abuse–neglect experience among prostitutes. The mean age at which the women in that study left home permanently was 16.25 years. As previously mentioned, "dispute with family" was one of the major reasons given by these women for leaving home, and physical and emotional abuse was also a significant factor in separating many of them from their families. Of the 136 prostitutes in the James study, 65.4% had lived apart from their families for some period prior to moving out permanently, and 70.4% reported the absence from the family of one or more parents—most often the father—during the subject's childhood. Neglect, rather than abuse, was the pattern for the majority of James's subjects, although abuse was reported by a significant number. Some typical comments about relations with parents were

> "We had a lack-of-communication problem, me and my parents, for a long time. I didn't even know how to approach them. I was scared to talk to them, because every time I did something wrong, they'd yell at me." "My mom didn't let us go out with boys. We were at home and always working. If anyone called up, we got cursed out and then a beating." "I felt isolated, and that's why I ran away. I just felt that my mother didn't care." "My stepfather, it's been negative since he's been around. . . . He hits me till I'm all stiff."

One apparent area of neglect on the part of parents of women in this study was sex education. Compared to the 31%–34% found by other researchers (e.g., Wittels, 1961; Sorensen, 1973) among normal female populations, only 15.4% of these prostitutes had learned about sex from their parents.

SEXUAL HISTORY

This lack of parental guidance may help to explain why many prostitutes apparently are sexually active at an earlier age than the majority of women in the United States. A full 91.9% of the prostitutes in the James (1977) study, for example, were nonvirgins by the age of 18 (including 23% who had experienced intercourse by the age of 13 or younger), compared with 74.9% of the black subjects and 19.9% of the white subjects studied by Kantner and Zelnick (1972). Although information on sexual experiences prior to first intercourse was not elicited through the questionnaires used in the James study, extensive interviews of the subjects in that study revealed a pattern similar to the one found by Davis (1971) in her study of 30 prostitutes: "The 'technical virginity' pattern typical of the middle-class female was not in evidence here. First sexual contacts typically involved sexual intercourse" (p. 301). More than one-third of the subjects in the James study reported that they had no further sexual relationship with their first intercourse partner, while other studies have found 10%–15% of their sample in this category (e.g., Eastman, 1972). That the superficial, non-emotionally-charged nature of the first sexual intercourse of many of these women initiated a series of such encounters is supported by the fact that the mean number of private (not-for-profit) sexual partners of subjects in the James study was 23. Making this figure even more significant is the fact that the mean number of persons with whom these subjects felt they had developed a "significant relationship" was only 5.

Societal reactions to juvenile female sexual activity may be an influence on some women's entrance into prostitution, especially for those young women who are more sexually active and less discreet than the majority of their peers, as seems to be the case with many prostitutes. "At what number of lovers is a girl supposed to lose the status of a decent person?" asked Choisy (1961). Carns (1973) explained: "A woman's decision to enter coitus . . . implies that she is creating for herself a sexual status which will have a relatively pervasive distribution . . . she will be evaluated downwardly. Such is the nature of the male bond" (p. 680). Girls learn society's moral valuation of their sexuality early. For example, in discussing her childhood sex education, one streetwalker stated, "I think the basic theme of the whole thing was that it was a dirty thing but that it was a duty for a woman to perform, and if you fooled around, you were a prostitute." Female promiscuity, real or imputed, virtually guarantees loss of status in the majority culture: "I got pregnant and kicked out of the house and school." "I was accused of being promiscuous while I was still a virgin. They did that because I used to run around with a lot of guys." The labeling implied by such loss of status may be an important step in the process by which a woman comes to identify with, and thus begins to see as a viable alternative, a deviant life-style such as prostitution. For its youthful victims, the labeling impact of such status loss must strongly affect the development of an adult self-image. These women may attempt to rebuild their self-image by moving into a subculture where the wider society's negative labeling of them will not impede their efforts toward a higher status—although that status itself will be perceived as negative by the wider society.

However negative the long-term effects of juvenile promiscuity on a woman's social status, the short-term effects of contranormative juvenile sexual activity may often appear quite positive to the young woman involved. Young women suffering from parental abuse or neglect, a common pattern for prostitutes, may be especially susceptible to the advantages of what Greenwald (1970) called "early rewarded sex—that is, . . . engaging in some form of sexual activity with an adult for which they were rewarded. [These women] discovered at an early age that they could get some measure of affection, of interest, by giving sexual gratification" (p. 167). This type of positive sexual reinforcement, particularly when coupled with the cultural stereotype of women as primarily sexual beings, may cause some women to perceive their sexuality as their primary means for gaining status: "Sex as a status tool is exploited to gain male attention" (Davis, 1971, p. 304). Since all women in our culture must somehow come to terms with the fact that their personal value is often considered inseparable from their sexual value, it is not uncommon for female adolescents to use "sex as a status tool" through makeup, flirting, dating, petting, etc. Prostitutes, however, more often skip over the usual preintercourse sociosexual activities in favor of an active and more-or-less promiscuous intercourse pattern. Victimization results when "there is a 'drift into deviance,' with promiscuity initially used as a status tool, but later becoming defined by the individual as having consequences for the foreclosure of alternative career routes" (Davis, 1971, p. 300).

INCEST AND RAPE

There is some evidence (e.g., James, 1977) that prostitutes are women who have also been the victims of less subtle negative sexual experiences. Specifically, the James study showed that prostitutes are disproportionately victimized by incest and rape compared with normal female populations. The only study populations with father-incest rates comparable to James's are those selected from the specialized samples of police reports or the case loads of child-protection agencies (e.g., DeFrancis, 1969). The effect of incest on the child involved is virtually unknown. Some researchers (e.g., Jaffe, 1975) prefer not to comment: "Little is known of the physical and emotional effects of incest" (p. 691). Ferracuti (1972) stated that "it is hardly proved that participation in incest . . . results in psychological disturbances" (p. 179). He noted, however, that "Frequently [victims of incest] become sexually promiscuous after the end of the incestuous conduct." De Francis (1969) found guilt, shame, and loss of self-esteem to be the usual reactions of child victims of sex offenses. He also found that these feelings often led to disruptive, rebellious behavior, and that some older (i.e., adolescent) victims later became prostitutes. Sexual abuse "continued over a long period of time," as is usual with incest, was found by Gagnon (1965, p. 192) to be "extremely disorganizing in its impact" on the victim. Weiner (1964) echoed Ferracuti in stating that "girls who begin incest in adolescence frequently become promiscuous following termination of the incest" (p. 137). In an earlier James study (1971), including 20 adolescent prostitutes, a full 65% of these young subjects had been the victims of coerced sexual intercourse, with 84.7% of these experiences occurring while the subject–victim was aged 15 or younger. Over half (57.4%) of James's later prostitute population had also been raped, and 36.2% of the women in this sample were multiple rape victims.

It is not possible, of course, to conclude that because certain study populations of "deviant" women were disproportionately victims of rape and incest, these sex-related abuses were therefore the cause of deviance. On the other hand, the overly frequent victimization of these women, particularly in youth and childhood, is a fact—just as their status as deviants is a fact—and should not be lightly dismissed. We realize that incidences of sexual victimization such as incest do not occur in a social vacuum and are virtually always surrounded by a complexity of causal, mitigating, or aggravating factors. In fact, a large proportion of the available research on incest—like the majority of studies of other, more common types of sexual experience—focuses primarily on the family background of the victim–subject. Study of the *causes* of sexual behaviors and experiences should not be our only concern, however. What we want to emphasize here is the importance of evaluating the *effects* of certain sexual patterns and experiences on the life of the individual. A simultaneous evaluation of cause and effect would be the ideal, but such as evaluation is beyond the scope of this chapter. We second DeFrancis (1969) in his assertion that

> . . . it would be valuable to conduct a longitudinal study to determine more accurately what the long-term effects are on a child victim of sexual abuse. There are many conjectures which should be tested. Does exposure to sexual abuse lead to prostitution, as so often asserted? Does it lead to delinquency; to promiscuous behavior; to confusion of sexual identity; or to marital problems? We know that serious family dislocations, impairment of interfamily relationships and emotional disturbance are some of the immediate consequences of sexual abuse, but how permanent or far reaching is this impact? (p. 225)

We would offer another conjecture on the effect of sexual abuse: early, traumatic sexual self-objectification may be one factor influencing some women toward entrance into prostitution or other "deviant" life-styles. Sexual self-objectification is experienced by all women in this society to some degree because of the simultaneous cultural adoration and vilification of the female body and its sexuality (the familiar madonna–whore spectrum). It seems possible, however, that to be used sexually at an early age in a way that produces guilt, shame, and loss of self-esteem on the part of the victim would be likely to lessen one's resistance to viewing oneself as a salable commodity. The relationship between early sexual history—especially incidences of sexual victimization—and adult deviance needs, and deserves, further study.

CONCLUSION

There is no obvious victim in a typical act of prostitution. Willing seller meets willing buyer, and both parties receive some gratification from the encounter: money, on the one hand, and sexual and/or psychological satisfaction on the other. It is when we examine the entrance of women into prostitution and when we review the enforcement of antiprostitution laws that we find elements of victimization coming into focus. Because prostitution is an expression of deviance from the traditional female sex role and therefore entails ostracism from the status and privileges of respectability, entrance into the profession is typically preceded and facilitated by an inadequate parent–child relationship and the development of a negative or sexually objectified self-image. These personal factors are then compounded by sex-role stereotyping and sex-based economic discrimination. Only widespread changes in sociosexual attitudes will effect changes in these patterns of victimization and their relationship to prostitution. In regard to the victimization of prostitutes by discriminatory law enforcement, however, change is more readily possible.

Most other countries have stopped trying to end prostitution and instead have made various less abusive legal arrangements for its regulation. In West Germany, for example, prostitution is considered a social necessity, and the government supports the building of pimp-free prostitution hostels where prostitutes can live and work in comfortable rooms with access to shopping centers, recreational facilities, and mandatory health inspection. The Netherlands uses zoning laws to prevent street solicitation's offending the general public. A total of 100 member nations of the United Nations have eliminated the crime of prostitution and have abandoned experiments in regulation (United Nations, 1951). The criminal laws in those countries seek instead to control public solicitation and to discourage the pimps and procurers who live off the earnings of prostitutes.

We view decriminalization as the least abusive method of dealing with prostitution in the United States. Decriminalization differs from legalization in that instead of creating more legal involvement, it removes prostitution from the criminal code entirely. An ideal approach would be to put all sexual behavior in private between consenting adults outside the purview of the law, but this ideal must be balanced by the reality of public expediency. Failing the ideal, then, options for controls would depend on communities' concern about the overtness of sexual activities, the possible disease problems, business and zoning regulations, and age of consent. Taxation, health, and age requirements can be approached in a number of ways. The least abusive to the individual woman would be a small-business license with a health-card requirement. A prostitute would obtain a license much as a masseuse does; her place of business would have to conform with zoning requirements; she would be required to report her income, be of age, and keep her health card current. Violations would mean the revocation of the license and would be handled by a nonpolice agency. Regulations such as the above would, of course, still limit personal freedom in a purely private area. The nonlicensed prostitute could still be prosecuted, although hers would be a civil citation rather than a criminal one. Decriminalization, with some restrictions, is regarded as a provisional solution to the victimization of prostitutes by the criminal justice system only while efforts are made to change the more fundamental causes of prostitution itself. As long as we retain our traditional sex-role expectations, however, we will have prostitution. As long as women are socialized into the traditional female role and see their alternatives limited by that role, prostitution will remain an attractive occupational option for many women. It is within the power of our legislatures to lessen the victimization of prostitutes as prostitutes, but to eliminate the victimization of prostitutes as women will be a longer, far more difficult struggle.

REFERENCES

Anderson, A. Prostitution and social justice. *Social Service Review*, 1974, *48*(2), 203.
Benjamin, H., & Masters, R. *Prostitution and morality*. New York: Julien Press, 1964.
Carns, D. Talking about sex: Notes on first coitus and the double sexual standard. *Journal of Marriage and the Family*, 1973, *35*, 677–688.
Chambliss, W. *Crime and the legal process*. New York: McGraw-Hill, 1969.
Choisy, M. Psychoanalysis of the prostitute. New York: Philosophical Library, 1961.
Clinard, M. Sociology of deviant behavior. New York: Rinehart and Company, 1959.
Cole, G. Criminal justice: Law and politics. New York: Duxbury Press, 1972.
Davis, K. The sociology of prostitution. *American Sociological Review*, 1937, *2*, 744–755.
Davis, N. The prostitute: Developing a deviant identity. In J. Henslin (Ed.), *Studies in the sociology of sex*. New York: Appleton-Century-Crofts, 1971, pp. 297–322.
DeFrancis, V. Protecting the child victims of sex crimes committed by adults. American Humane Association, Children's Division, *Final report*. Denver: 1969, p. 215.
Eastman, W. First intercourse: Some statistics on who, where, when, and why. *Sexual Behavior*, 1972, *2*, 22–27.
Esselstyn, T. C. Prostitution in the United States. *Annals of the American Academy of Political and Social Science*, 1968, *376*, 123–135.
Ferracuti, F. Incest between father and daughter. In H. Resnik & E. Wolfgang (Eds.), *Sexual behaviors: Social, clinical, and legal aspects*. Boston: Little, Brown, 1972, pp. 159–183.
Gagnon, J. Female child victims of sex offenses. *Social Problems*, 1965, *13*, 176–192.
Gagnon, J., & Simon, W. *Sexual conduct*. Chicago: Aldine, 1973.
Gray, D. Turning-out: A study of teen-age prostitution. *Urban Life and Culture*, 1973, *1*, 401–425.
Greenwald, H. *The elegant prostitute*. New York: Ballantine, 1970.
Hollander, M. Prostitution, the body and human relatedness. *International Journal of Psychoanalysis*, 1961, *42*, 404–413.
Holmes, K. Reflections by gaslight: Prostitution in another age. *Issues in Criminology*, 1972, *7*(1), 83.

Jackman, N., O'Toole, R., & Geis, G. The self-image of the prostitute. In J. Gagnon & W. Simon (Eds.), *Sexual deviance*. New York: Harper & Row, 1967, pp. 133–146.

Jaffe, A., Dynneson, L., & Ten Bensel, R. Sexual abuse of children. *American Journal of Disabled Children*, 1975, *129*, 689–692.

James, J. A formal analysis of prostitution. *Final report to the Division of Research*, State of Washington Department of Social and Health Services, Olympia, Wash., 1971.

James, J. The prostitute–pimp relationship. *Medical Aspects of Human Sexuality*, 1973, *7*, 147–160.

James, J. Motivations for entrance into prostitution. In L. Crites (Ed.), *The female offender: A comprehensive anthology*. University, Ala.: University of Alabama Press, 1976. (a)

James, J. Normal men and deviant women. Unpublished manuscript, 1976. (b)

James, J., & Meyerding, J. Early sexual experience in prostitution. *The American Journal of Psychiatry*, 1977, *134*(12), 1381–1385.

Kantner, J., & Zelnick, M. Sexual experience of young unmarried women in the United States. *Family Planning Perspectives*, 1972, *4*, 9–18.

Kemp, T. *Prostitution: An investigation of its causes, especially with regard to hereditary factors*. Copenhagen: Levin and Munksgaard, 1936.

Kinsey, A., Pomeroy, W., Martin, C., & Gebhard, P. *Sexual behavior in the human female*. Philadelphia: Saunders, 1953.

Kirk, S. Clients as outsiders: Theoretical approaches to deviance. *Social Work*, 1972, *17*, 24.

Lombroso, C. *The female offender*. New York: D. Appleton and Company, 1898.

Maerov, A. Prostitution: A survey and review of 20 cases. *Psychiatric Quarterly*, 1965, *39*, 675–701.

Pomeroy, W. Some aspects of prostitution. *Journal of Sex Research*, 1965, *3*, 177–187.

Rosenblum, K. Female deviance and the female sex role: A preliminary investigation. *British Journal of Sociology*, 1975, *25* (June), 69–85.

Sorensen, R. *Adolescent sexuality in contemporary America*. New York: World, 1973.

Stein, M. *Lovers, friends and slaves*. New York: Putnam, 1974.

Uniform Crime Reports. *Crime in the United States*. Washington, D.C.: U.S. Government Printing Office, 1974, 1975.

United Nations. International Convention for the Suppression of the White Slave Traffic. New York: United Nations Publishing, 1951.

Weiner, I. On incest: A survey. *Excerpta Criminologica*, 1964, *4*, 137–155.

Winick, C., & Kinsie, P. *The lively commerce*. New York: New American Library, 1971.

Wittels, F. *Sex habits of American women*. New York: Eton, 1951.

Legal Victim or Social Victim?

Lois Lee

Dr. Jennifer James presents a comprehensive review of current research in the area of prostitution. In addition, she provides a social–
psychological evaluation of the prostitute. Dr. James is one of the first
social scientists to study prostitution with a high regard for the individual prostitute. She clearly depicts the victimization of the prostitute
by the laws, by law enforcement, and by societal attitudes.

Dr. James provides a framework in which prostitution may best
be understood. She states, "Prostitution is, in reality, an institutional,
if illegal, occupational choice like any other." While other researchers
have concluded that prostitution is a result of pathology, Dr. James
has presented a view of the prostitute within the larger socioeconomic
system.

Limitations of Dr. James's studies include the geographical restrictions of her research. For instance, in Los Angeles, 66% of prostitution arrests occur on the street, 22% are massage-parlor and sex-
club arrests, and 11% of arrests are made in hotels, compared with
James's studies, which suggest that massage parlors comprise less than
5%. Dr. James's findings suggest that prostitutes frequently come from
broken homes and have been subjected to incestuous relationships.
Dr. James's studies fail, however, to compare these findings with
studies on nonprostitute women. If, in fact, the experiences of prostitutes are significantly different from those of nonprostitutes, are we to
assume that these experiences are the cause of women's entering prostitution and, if so, how?

Despite these limitations, Dr. James integrates both the objective
and subjective views of her research findings. Children of the Night,

---

Lois Lee, Ph.D. • Founder, Children of the Night, a social service program for teenage
prostitutes, Beverly Hills, California 90211.

as an organization that works intensively with prostitutes, cannot endorse Dr. James's suggestion that "prostitution is one way for women to reject their victimization by our sex-biased economic system by choosing an independent and exciting occupational life-style." In fact, prostitutes fall prey to our sex-biased economic system by choosing a *dependent but* exciting life-style consistent with strict female socialization processes, in that women give up virginity or sex in return for being taken care of by a more responsible individual.

My own study of 500 street prostitutes in Los Angeles indicated that the female prostitute buys into the female sex-role socialization and expectation patterns much more than do other groups of women and, in some instances, much as did the 18-year-old female of 1950. When asked where they wanted to be in five years, prostitutes overwhelmingly responded, "I'm just working to save up enough money so me and my ol' man can buy a house and have a baby." Note that pimps exploit this middle-class value of deferred gratification in order to encourage young women to work as prostitutes. Rarely, if ever, does this dream become a reality. To excuse the pimp as satisfying a legitimate female need for a man or companion dictated by the larger society is to overlook the pimp's conscious manipulation of larger socially acceptable values and ideologies. For instance, pimps rarely participate in sexual activity with the prostitute. The pimp denies both love and sex, a denial that reinforces the prostitute's low self-image. In fact, most prostitutes are not allowed to return home until they have reached the quota established for them by their pimp. Then why does a prostitute remain with a pimp? Because these men, representative of "square" society, not only reject prostitutes but never allow them to forget what they have been. While this statement may sound simplistic, it is in fact a very complicated problem derivative of larger social issues.

On some points Dr. James falls prey to the naive assumptions of most researchers that if you ask a subject a question, she or he will tell you the truth. Our field experience in ongoing daily contact with Los Angeles prostitutes indicates that prostitutes do not know themselves why they became prostitutes.

While Dr. James has completed essential and well-documented research on prostitution, we still need to reach out to the prostitutes themselves to gain a better understanding of their life situation. Emphasis in further research should be directed toward what to do now, not how they got there.

Chapter 15

Women—Victims of the VD Rip-Off

Edward M. Brecher

There was once a young man named Wilbur who drove a Mercedes-Benz and had VD. Wilbur enjoyed having sexual intercourse with young women, especially young women with whom he hadn't had intercourse before. One week, while he had VD, he enjoyed sexual intercourse with seven of them:

Sunday	Alice
Monday	Betty
Tuesday	Connie
Wednesday	Doris
Thursday	Edna
Friday	Frances
Saturday	Greta

Alice was one of those old-fashioned girls who still hadn't switched to the pill or an IUD to keep from getting pregnant. She continued to use the same vaginal contraceptive cream her mother had always used. The chemicals in that old-fashioned cream kill not only sperm cells but also the germs that cause syphilis and gonorrhea. That's why Alice's mother never got VD. And that's why Alice, even though she had intercourse with Wilbur, didn't catch his infection.

Betty was superhygienic. As soon as she was through having intercourse with Wilbur, she went to the bathroom and douched her vagina thoroughly, adding to the warm water the same medicated douche powder her mother had always used. That's why Betty didn't catch VD either.

Connie had a generous friend named Bob who had come back

Edward M. Brecher ● Journalist/Author: *An Analysis of Human Sexual Response*, *The Sex Researchers*, and *Love, Sex, and Aging*, West Cornwall, Connecticut 06796.

from Japan last year with several hundred tablets of Penigin, a foaming vaginal tablet that prevents VD and is sold in many countries. Bob divided his Penigin supply among his women friends, including Connie. Connie slipped a Penigin tablet into her vagina, and after a few minutes, she had intercourse with Wilbur; so she didn't catch Wilbur's VD either.

Doris was a very prudent woman. "You've got to wear a condom," she told Wilbur. "But I don't have a condom," Wilbur replied happily. "I do," said Doris, taking one out of her purse and rolling it down over Wilbur's erect penis. So Doris didn't get VD.

Edna was a $50-dollar-an-hour New York call girl. She used the standard methods of VD prevention that have been used for decades by well-turned-out prostitutes. These highly effective methods are never mentioned in sex education courses or in programs about VD on radio and television. I shall describe them in practical detail below, for I believe that women who have sex for fun are at least as entitled as prostitutes to know how to protect themselves from VD. Thanks to following "the call-girl ritual," Edna didn't catch Wilbur's VD either.

Frances was a very lucky woman. After conscientiously shopping around, she had found a gynecologist she could trust, and with whom she could talk frankly about her sexual activities and problems. "Every time my husband goes out of town," she told him, "I screw around and then worry myself sick about VD. Any suggestions?"

"Take two of these tablets every time you screw around," her gynecologist replied, "and give your husband some to take when he screws around." Frances took two of the tablets after her night with Wilbur, so she didn't get VD either.

Greta also consulted her doctor about how not to catch VD. "I'm shocked and disgusted with you," he replied. "A nice girl like you shouldn't be thinking about such filthy things. Don't you know that VD germs can spread all through your body? They can cause pelvic inflammatory disease so you may have to have your uterus taken out. They can make you sterile or damage your unborn baby. Shame on you, coming in here with a filthy, immoral request like that. What kind of quack do you think I am? I'm a respectable doctor; I'm willing to cure VD infections, but I don't give sluts a license to go around being immoral without fear of the consequences. Chastity is the only reliable safeguard."

That's why Greta got VD.

All six women who escaped VD in this parable had one important thing in common: they refused to rely on the misleading advice given in sex education courses, by U.S. government agencies, and through

We don't want people wandering around with VD, so we set up clinics to cure infections *after* they have occurred. But we do want people to fear VD, in the hope that fear will keep them chaste. Hence, methods of preventing VD are kept hush-hush, so we won't be guilty of selling "a ticket to sin without fear of divine retribution." (In California, for example, it was a criminal offense until 1971 for anyone to give anyone else any VD preventive.) The fear of syphilis and gonorrhea will function, many people hope, as "God's little helper" in the war against nonmarital sex.

Few doctors are willing to provide prophylactic information except in special circumstances. For example, suppose you are assaulted and raped tonight and are carried beaten and bruised to a hospital emergency room. The physician there won't turn up his nose and tell you, "Go away and don't come back until you notice symptoms of infection; I won't help you until symptoms appear." With the full approval of the U.S. Public Health Service and of other voices of authority, he will immediately make available to you at least two methods of prophylaxis: he will thoroughly douche your vagina with a suitable antiseptic, and he will give you some tablets or an injection to prevent VD. Why must a woman be raped in order to receive prompt and adequate protection?

Many physicians and some VD clinics also make an exception to the "no-prophylaxis" rule for certain *husbands*. A husband comes in and says, "Doc, I was out with a broad last night and I'm worried about VD. Can you fix me up before I go home to my wife?"

Many private physicians faced with such a request accede, for a well-to-do white husband who pays his bills promptly is a welcome patient. They aren't protecting just the sinning husband, these doctors explain, but also his innocent wife. They are acting as priests and not as doctors. They are using their medical authority—their power to give or withhold prompt preventive treatment—to buttress their personal views of sexual morality. As a result, single women, single men, and not-so-innocent wives—indeed, the young, the poor, the black, and the female—are deprived of the prompt protection available to at least some husbands.

Clearly, our present national VD policy leaves women far more vulnerable to VD than men. A man who follows the conventional media advice and sees a physician at the first sign of genital infection is reasonably well protected. About three weeks after exposure to syphilis, he is very likely to notice a sore, called a *chancre*, on his penis. A few days after exposure to gonorrhea, he will have a burning sensation when he urinates, and a day or two after that he will notice a creamy discharge from his urethra (urinary passage). If he sees his physician the mass media. That misleading advice can be summed up in two familiar statements:

1. See your doctor or a VD clinic at the first sign of a genital in fection.
2. Have a routine laboratory test for both syphilis and gonorrhea from time to time.

Because women (and men, too) have been relying on this grossly inadequate advice, gonorrhea today is at an all-time high and syphili is on the increase. Don't play that losing game. Don't wait until yo have caught VD. Protect yourself at the time of exposure or as soo thereafter as possible. The methods recommended by the governmen and by medical authorities are essentially *curative*: they permit you body to become a battleground for germs and antibiotics *after* the germ have gained entry, multiplied prodigiously, and spread widely. Th best methods are *prophylactic*, that is, preventive. Some prophylacti methods keep VD germs out of your body altogether; others promptl attack and destroy the germs while they are still few in number, an while they are still localized on surfaces (such as the lining of the va gina) where they do no harm.

Killing both syphilis and gonorrhea germs is absurdly easy; the are among the most fragile of all living organisms. Moderate heat kil them; drying kills them; many antiseptics kill them; so do a wide rang of antibiotics. Indeed, plain soap and water kill them. Unlike mo other germs, syphilis and gonorrhea germs cannot survive outside th shelter of the human body. They can be transmitted from person t person only by the most intimate personal contacts, which is wha makes them *venereal* infections.

But after these germs have entered a new victim and multiplie there for a few days (gonorrhea) or weeks (syphilis), they are no longe defenseless. They invade the body tissues, finding lurking places an sanctuaries that are hard to reach, like an enemy hidden in caves an trenches. They are now beyond the reach of antiseptics, and muc larger doses of antibiotics are needed to wipe them out. Obviously the time to attack them is either during or just after their transfer from one human body to another.

If VD prevention is so easy, you will ask, why doesn't the U.S Public Health Service tell us how to use prophylaxis? Why don't ou physicians tell us? Why isn't prophylactic information included in se education courses? Why aren't prophylactic products advertised in th mass media?

The answer is absurdly simple. Ours is still a puritanical society or visits a VD clinic promptly, he will be quickly cured by a dose of penicillin or some other antibiotic—and no harm done.

For a woman, the same advice may lead to altogether different consequences. She, too, develops a chancre three weeks or so after exposure to syphilis, but in the vast majority of cases, the chancre is hidden inside her genitals and goes wholly unnoticed. The germs of syphilis continue to spread throughout her body day after day, perhaps doing substantial harm. Not until she reaches at least the secondary stage of syphilis, when additional symptoms occur, does she become aware that anything is wrong. And even the secondary stage can be difficult to diagnose.

The course of gonorrhea in women is much the same. Unless the gonorrhea germs happen to invade her urethra as well as her vagina, she will notice no burning while urinating. Indeed, in four cases out of five, according to a recent estimate, she will notice no symptoms sufficient to warn her of her peril. In a regrettably high proportion of cases, her first warning will be a very serious condition known as PID (pelvic inflammatory disease), indicating that the gonorrhea germs have attacked her fallopian tubes and uterus. Sterility and the need for a hysterectomy are common effects of PID. By preventing venereal infection at the time of exposure or as soon thereafter as possible, these very serious risks are minimized.

The contrast between VD prophylaxis and VD cure is very similar to that between contraception and abortion. No sensible woman ignores contraceptive precautions and relies instead on having an abortion after she becomes pregnant. Yet this is, in effect, the advice she receives about VD: wait until you body is riddled with VD germs and then visit a physician or a VD clinic.

This does not mean that you must take anti-VD precautions every time you have sexual intercourse. On the contrary, precautions are necessary for most men and women only on relatively rare, special occasions.

Suppose you are married and that both you and your husband have sexual relations outside your marriage a few times a year. It is necessary for each of you to take VD precautions on those rare occasions when you engage in *extramarital* relations.

The same is true if you are single, divorced, or widowed and maintain a continuing and relatively exclusive relationship with one lover. Precautions are necessary only for the outside contacts you or your lover may have.

If you are married or have a continuing relationship and, in addition, if either of you has a continuing relationship with one other person, precautions are needed only for sex outside the triad. The same principle holds even if you belong to a commune in which sex is freely shared. A sexually transmitted disease will spread like wildfire in such a group. But all that is necessary to prevent it is that each member take suitable precautions against infection during sexual contacts *outside* the group.

Here an interesting problem arises. Mary and John meet for the first time on Saturday night at a rock concert or a church social; later they have sex. This is obviously a casual contact for which VD prophylaxis is prudent. A week or two later, however, Mary and John begin living together. They become engaged and then marry. At what point can they safely abandon prophylaxis? The answer is simple: whenever they decided to have most of their sex with one another and agree to take precautions whenever they have sex outside their relationship.

The entire country could have become VD-free a generation or two ago if our national VD policy had not been hamstrung by moralistic taboos. It could have been accomplished this year if the same taboos had not continued. I propose that we do it ourselves during the coming year, without waiting for our laggard leaders in the U.S. Public Health Service and in the medical profession. The first group of anti-VD procedures I shall describe are the ones used by New York City's top-quality call girls. They are among the oldest methods, and also among the best. They require no drugs whatever, and no equipment beyond a good light, a wash bowl, a bar of soap, and a washcloth. In addition to minimizing the risk of syphilis and gonorrhea, they also afford some real protection against a wide range of other sexually transmitted diseases such as trichomoniasis, moniliasis (*Candida albicans*), and herpes infections.

The method of VD self-protection that a call girl uses has to be good. Thus, before a well-turned-out call girl goes to bed with a man, she takes him to the bathroom, fills the washbowl with warm water, soaps it up a little, and then, using a well-soaped washcloth, she thoroughly cleanses the shaft of his penis and the surrounding area. The soap and water kill some germs that may be lurking on the surface of the penis, and they wash away others. Like washing your hands before dinner, washing a man's penis before it enters your vagina is one of those simple sanitary measures you should have learned—but didn't—at your mother's knee.

As the call girl washes the penis, she inspects it under a good light. She looks for two signs of VD. One is a chancre or other sore on the shaft or nearby, the first sign of syphilis. Even if a sore isn't a chancre, it may be a sign of some other sexually transmittable infection. Her inspection is thorough: she lifts up the penis and examines the underside and the creases at the groin. If the man is not circumcised, she retracts his foreskin all the way and checks the surface thus exposed. Next she grasps the penis firmly with her fingers and pulls the loose skin up and down the shaft a few times, much as if she were masturbating or "milking" it. Then, drawing the loose skin down toward the root of the penis with one hand, she uses the fingertips of the other hand to spread the tiny lips at the entry to the urinary passage and looks to see whether she has milked out a creamy discharge—the first sign of gonorrhea. (The discharge may be due to a minor infection rather than gonorrhea, but it is a warning signal.) This procedure is the one traditionally used in the armed forces (where it is known as the *short-arm inspection*) to spot VD. Only after her customer has passed this inspection does the call girl take him to bed.

The short-arm inspection of the male by the female (or by another male in homosexual encounters) is highly effective if conscientiously carried out, for relatively few men are infectious without a visible chancre or discharge. The reverse, however, is far from true: the signs of VD in the female are often so well hidden that even a skilled gynecologist is likely to miss them during a visual examination.

After the sexual encounter is concluded, another safeguard ritual takes place. Once again, the call girl leads her client to the bathroom, and once again she thoroughly washes his whole genital area with a soapy washcloth. This is in part for his protection and a courtesy to him, but it also helps protect the next call girl he visits and thus helps curb·the spread of VD throughout the call-girl subculture.

An intelligent customer at this point in the ritual proceeds to urinate: the flow of urine down the urethra can wash out stray germs. Furthermore, the acidity of the urine as it passes makes it less likely that gonorrhea germs will survive and multiply. Indeed, some very cautious men drink a glass of water or a can of beer before having intercourse with a call girl, to make sure they will have a vigorous urinary jet on tap afterward. Women are wise to urinate promptly after intercourse for the same reason.

Another safeguard, which concludes the call-girl ritual, is commonly known as the *American bidet*. Women who have traveled abroad, especially in France, are familiar with the bidet, a basin similar to a toilet bowl, with hot and cold running water, built low so that a woman or a man can straddle it and sit in or just above the water. Fancy bidets have, in addition, a fountain that squirts up onto the genitals. A French woman jumps out of bed after sex and rushes to the bidet without a moment's delay to wash out her vagina thoroughly; she does this for protection against VD, to lessen the likelihood of pregnancy, and as a simple hygienic measure. American puritanism has blocked the introduction of the bidet into the United States, though we pride ourselves on our modern plumbing and sparkling tiled bathrooms. Fortunately, bidets are beginning to come into style in upper-class American homes, and any good plumber can tell you what the department of health regulations and the cost of installation are.

Lacking a bidet, the New York City call girl uses her regular washbowl instead. She fills it with warm, soapy water, then turns her back to it and boosts herself up so that she straddles it. Thus strategically stationed, she proceeds to wash her vagina and vulva (the external portion of her genitals) thoroughly with a soapy washcloth.

These call-girl rituals—the washing of the penis before sex, the short-arm inspection, prompt urination, and the American bidet after sex—are not 100% effective. But they are effective enough so that a very busy call girl, serving hundreds of men a year, has little fear of syphilis or gonorrhea.

Throughout the past century or more, males have sought (and found) effective methods of protecting themselves and the prostitutes with whom they sometimes consort from VD. But men have kept these safeguards secret from their sweethearts, sisters, wives, and daughters, lest "respectable" women also engage in sexual intercourse without fear of venereal infection.

In much the same way, men attempted until quite recently to keep methods of preventing pregnancy a closely guarded secret. Not until 1968 did the U.S. Supreme Court declare anti-birth-control laws unconstitutional. The veil of secrecy surrounding safe methods of abortion has also been torn away. But women are still kept ignorant of the simple, safe, and effective methods that prostitutes have long used— and that other women can use—to safeguard both themselves and their sexual partners from VD.

For hundreds of years, conscientious men have protected both themselves and their sexual partners by wearing condoms. But most condoms limit male (and, to a certain extent, also female) enjoyment. So men have found other means to block the transfer of VD germs.

One such barrier was announced in Germany late in the nineteenth century by Professor Albert Ludwig Siegmund Neisser (1855–1916), the man who discovered the gonorrhea germ. Neisser recommended that prostitutes anoint their genitals with petroleum jelly (now sold under the trade name Vaseline). The woman would be protected by "the mechanical nature of the fatty layer," which traps the germs (Neisser, 1919). Neisser also proposed that disinfectant chemicals capable of killing VD germs be added to the jelly.

Since then, knowledgeable prostitutes in many parts of the world have used such medicated vaginal ointments and jellies. So have millions of "respectable" women in the United States and other countries. They, however, use the vaginal products for *contraception*. The fact that such products may also prevent VD has been kept secret from them.

Contraceptive creams, jellies, and foams sold under such familiar brand names as Ortho-Creme Contraceptive Cream, Ortho-Gynol Contraceptive Jelly, Delfen Contraceptive Cream, Delfen Contraception Foam, Emko Vaginal Foam Contraceptive, Preceptin Contraceptive Gel, Koromex Contraceptive Cream, and many more are all based on Neisser's two principles: a barrier that traps the sperm cells and chemicals (used in some but not all of these products) that simultaneously kill the spirochetes that cause syphilis and the gonococci that cause gonorrhea. Thus, a woman who happens by good fortune to use the right vaginal product to avoid pregnancy is also unwittingly protecting herself from VD.

English physicians knew all this at least as early as 1920, but they kept it a secret. An American authority on VD, Dr. Evan Thomas (brother of the socialist leader Norman Thomas) dramatically rediscovered the secret during the 1930s.

Thomas was the head of the Bellevue VD clinic in New York City, then the world's largest. Reviewing his clinic's records, Thomas noted the almost total absence of VD in women who used what was then the most popular vaginal contraceptive jelly. He wondered if this jelly could prevent VD in the same manner as a condom. A simple laboratory experiment confirmed Thomas's hunch: microscopic examination revealed dead spirochetes when the germs were exposed to the contraceptive jelly.

Thomas promptly transmitted this astonishing news to the maker of the contraceptive jelly. Here, at long last, was a way for women to safeguard themselves from VD. But company executives, to Thomas's amazement and distress, were not interested.

In retrospect, a variety of reasons can be conjectured for one company's refusal to market a VD prophylaxis for women. But why have *all* American companies failed to market such products?

We venture to suggest a reason. The companies are run by men, who don't *want* their women to have such protection available at the corner drugstore. In 1963, the research director of a major contraceptive company tested his company's vaginal creams and jellies and found that they killed spirochetes and gonococci. Nothing came of this discovery either.

Meanwhile, other countries forged ahead. In the 1950s, the Japanese developed Penigin, a small tablet to be inserted into the vagina a few minutes before sexual intercourse. When exposed to the moisture in the vagina, the tablet foams, and the foam contains small amounts of an antibiotic capable of killing both syphilis and gonorrhea germs. Tested in Japanese brothels, Penigin tablets proved highly effective. They are now marketed in many countries—but not in the United States. The FDA forbids their manufacture and sale here because they have not been tested for safety and efficacy within our borders. And neither U.S. government agencies nor private companies have been willing to invest in such tests.

Another product, C-Film, is of great interest. It is a film impregnated with a chemical that kills sperm cells. Introduced into the vagina, it promptly dissolves, forming a barrier. Men and women who have used C-Film report that they cannot detect its presence during sexual intercourse. It is on sale in several countries, but not here.

Why not develop for American use a modified form of C-Film containing a chemical that kills germs as well as sperm cells? Again, our cultural puritanism stands in the way.

Fortunately, there are exceptions. Two men who deserve an award for their contribution to women's liberation are Dr. John C. Cutler, of the University of Pittsburgh Graduate School of Public Health, and Dr. R. C. Arnold, of the Missouri Crippled Children's Service.

Back in the 1940s, Drs. Arnold and Cutler were engaged in prophylactic research at the Venereal Disease Research Laboratory (VDRL) of the U.S. Public Health Service. Most VDRL projects were concerned with methods of male prophylaxis. These men developed instead a douche preparation for use by women after sexual intercourse. It contained a chemical to kill VD germs and a "spreading agent" to encourage its spread through the vaginal tract. Tried out in a Guatemalan brothel, the Arnold–Cutler douche provided a high level of protection against VD, and the prostitutes liked to use it.

But in 1950, under President Harry S. Truman, U.S. government policy beat a retreat. All VD prophylaxis research was abandoned abruptly, and no account of the Guatemalan study was ever published in English. Drs. Arnold and Cutler, and others at the VDRL, abandoned VD research. Today Drs. Cutler and Arnold are back in the VD field. Their goal is a vaginal product effective both for VD prophylaxis and for contraception. Their project began at the University of Pittsburgh Graduate School of Public Health, where a team assembled by Dr. Cutler launched laboratory tests of many vaginal creams, jellies, foams, suppositories, and douche preparations. All the products are safe (as evidenced by FDA clearance and by use through the years by large numbers of women) and are readily available in drugstores without a prescription. This availability frees women from dependence on moralistic physicians who may refuse to prescribe VD prophylaxis.

A number of these contraceptive products also killed syphilis and gonorrhea germs in the Pittsburgh laboratory tests. Some also killed trichomonad bacteria and moniliasis yeasts. The Cutler team selected Conceptrol Birth Control Cream for the first tests on human subjects. It is a vaginal cream made by the Ortho Pharmaceutical Corporation and is also marketed under the brand name Delfen Contraceptive Cream. It is conveniently packaged in single-dose kits with a disposable applicator for introducing the cream into the vagina. A Conceptrol pack can be carried like a condom, in purse or pocket, by women and men alike.

Neisser's early study and the Japanese Penigin research suggest that VD germs can on rare occasions lodge in the urethra (the urinary passage). To minimize this risk, Neisser suggested that women smear a little of the prophylactic substance over the entrance of the urethra, too.

Another product warrants mention—a vaginal oil called Progonasyl, developed by Frank Bickenheuser, a patent medicine entrepreneur in Tulsa, Oklahoma. It is based on Professor Neisser's principle of a barrier plus an antiseptic. Bickenheuser started with an oil that forms an emulsion, or gel, when exposed to vaginal moisture. To this, he added an organic iodide antiseptic. After preliminary laboratory tests, it was confirmed that Progonasyl kills syphilis and gonorrhea germs. Bickenheuser offered a supply to four Tulsa physicians.

The physicians first gave some to women arrested for prostitution. Many of them had gonorrhea. The physicians reported that when the women returned to the streets, "the males with whom they had contact did not become infected."

But could Progonasyl also protect women who had intercourse with infected men? The physicians carefully planned an experiment with four female and two male volunteers. The men had had gonorrhea for 7 to 10 days and were at the peak of infectiousness for others. Each of the men had intercourse with two of the women. Before intercourse, however, a teaspoonful of Progonasyl was introduced into each vagina. The women were then locked up in an apartment for 10 days, under continuous surveillance to make sure they had no access to medication: "On the tenth day, clinical and microscopic examinations were made and the vaginal smears were examined by each physician and were found negative. Later examinations similarly showed the absence of gonococcus and gonorrhea."

A second experiment, with a control, was conducted with two women and one man. This man, too, was in the dripping stage of gonorrhea. One of the women with whom he had intercourse did not use Progonasyl and came down on the fourth day with a severe case of gonorrhea (which the physicians, of course, promptly cured). The other woman used Progonasyl and escaped infection.

Such a demonstration, you might suppose, would have been hailed across the country. Instead, the silence was deafening. Far from being honored for his contributions to VD prophylaxis, Frank Bickenheuser heard himself denounced from the pulpit of his own parish church for having contributed to the breakdown of moral chastity.

Skeptics may dismiss this Progonasyl study as out-of-date (it took place in 1933) and too small-scale. But consider a test of Progonasyl (Edwards & Fox, 1974) involving 324 women and their estimated 25,000 male partners, which was run in Nevada in 1971. In that year, 163 prostitutes in a Nevada brothel agreed to use Progonasyl under the supervision of Dr. William M. Edwards, Jr., Chief of the Bureau of Preventive Medicine in the Nevada State Health Division. In charge of operations was a young VD specialist, Richard S. Fox. Each of the 163 prostitutes was given a supply of Progonasyl and told to insert half a teaspoon or a teaspoonful into her vagina each day, before entertaining her first customer. She was also told to wait at least three minutes so that the medicated oil would have time to coat the vagina. An additional 161 prostitutes in the same brothels served as controls, using no vaginal prophylaxis. "Each of the prostitutes in this study averaged at least five sexual partners each working day," Edwards and Fox reported. "Several prostitutes in this study averaged twenty sexual partners per day." The oil was inserted into the vagina only once a day, regardless of the number of men a woman entertained.

Men who resort to brothels, of course, are rather more likely than men in general to bring syphilis or gonorrhea with them. During the Nevada field trial of Progonasyl, the prostitutes who used the prophylactic oil entertained an estimated 25,000 men. When 259 laboratory cultures for gonorrhea were run on the 163 women, only 1 of the cultures was positive. The 1 infected woman may have neglected to use the Progonasyl on one crucial occasion.

Among the 161 prostitutes who did not use Progonasyl, the gonorrhea rates per 100 cultures and per 1,000 customers were 13 times as high. Progonasyl cut the gonorrhea rate by 93 percent—or by 100 percent, if the single Progonasyl user's infection was caused by negligence.

This 1971 Nevada field trial, like the 1938 Oklahoma experiments, should have made front-page headlines. Edwards and Fox should have been featured on TV news programs. But the Nevada field trials of Progonasyl, like the Oklahoma experiments a third of a century earlier, made scarcely a ripple. Physicians and public health clinics today, as in the past, are willing to cure VD but not to help women prevent it.

Progonasyl, incidentally, has remained on the market continuously since the 1930s. It is currently marketed by the Saron Pharmacal Corporation of St. Petersburg, Florida. But don't bother to ask for it at your corner drugstore; it is available only by prescription. Moreover, it cannot be advertised or labeled for the prevention of VD; that would be a violation of FDA regulations. Instead it is labeled for the *treatment* of vaginal infections.

Conceptrol, Progonasyl, and the other such preparations are, of course, intended for genital intercourse. There is no reason that they cannot also be used for anal intercourse. Better yet would be a medicated form of KY Jelly, a lubricant already popular for use during anal contacts, homosexual and heterosexual. No such medicated lubricant is currently available.

Let us here add a word about homosexual VD. Both syphilis and gonorrhea are readily transmitted during male homosexual contacts. In theory, VD can also be transmitted from female to female during lesbian contacts; the best available evidence, however, indicates that such transmission is relatively rare, partly because lesbians tend to have fewer sexual partners than male homosexuals, and partly because lesbian relations with an infected woman are somewhat less likely to transmit infection (especially gonorrhea) than is heterosexual intercourse. When women who participate in lesbian activities do go to a physician or a clinic with VD, it often turns out that they acquired it during a heterosexual encounter. But a woman who is seriously worried about VD after a lesbian contact should find an understanding physician as soon as possible and ask for antibiotic prophylaxis.

What about douching after intercourse as a means of preventing VD? For almost a century, the French have been convinced that douching provides effective prophylaxis. The Guatemalan studies in the 1940s confirmed this view. Some physicians warn against douching for any purpose, and some leaders of the women's movement agree. Excessively frequent douching, excessively strong solutions, and the use of excessive force to drive in the solution should certainly be avoided. But at least part of the medical opposition to douching appears to have a moralistic rather than a scientific source. It stems from the old tradition that children, and females generally, should leave their genitals alone—shouldn't even look at them, much less keep them clean.

So far as we can determine, no scientific study of douching to prevent VD has been conducted since 1950. The most that can be said is that some douches now on the market kill VD germs in laboratory tests. Federal research agencies should resume the douching studies discontinued in 1950 and should take immediate steps to encourage such studies by the manufacturers of douche preparations.

Finally, what of the condom? Contrary to a widespread impression, condoms remain enormously popular in the United States today, both for contraception and for VD prophylaxis. U.S. production now exceeds 500 million condoms a year, enough to supply every male in the country over the age of 14 with seven or eight a year. Condoms can protect against VD during anal as well as genital intercourse. Without condoms, this country would have vastly more VD and unwanted pregnancies. Moreover, this popularity has been achieved and maintained with only a trickle of advertising and promotion. It has persisted even though sex education courses rarely mention the condom, and some even warn against it. Sales are also limited by many state laws forbidding condom advertising, sales to minors, distribution except through drugstores, and display in drugstores as feminine hygiene products are displayed. I urge the immediate repeal of all such restrictive laws. I also urge a nationwide campaign to explain to male and female high-school students, and to the general public, the value of the condom for VD prophylaxis, as well as for contraception. If you have a high school student in your family, launch your own campaign.

There are many different kinds of condoms currently available, such as the lubricated condom and the "skin" (a sheath made of animal membrane that many users say interferes less with sexual enjoyment). These and other unconventional kinds of condoms are available at most drugstores and sex or family-planning centers.

Traditionally, it is the male who buys condoms. There is no reason, however, that a woman should not buy them, carry them in her purse, and insist that any male who wants to have sex with her wear one to protect her from pregnancy and to protect both of them from VD. Many European prostitutes insist on their customers' wearing condoms during fellatio as well as during genital intercourse.

In the spring of 1971, the Los Angeles *Free Press* and other "underground" Southern California newspapers carried a remarkable advertisement:

> Venereal disease is preventable. The Committee to Eradicate Syphilis (C.E.S. Inc.) is asking your help to prove it. If you are very sexually active, aged 21 to 50, and sincere in your interest, please call 870-8693.

At the same time, passersby at a half-dozen Los Angeles street corners were given handbills that carried the same invitation in more detail:

> A new drug that may be taken orally has become available which may promise to prevent Syphilis and Gonorrhea if taken around the time of

sexual exposure. The Committee is asking you to assist us in evaluating this method of preventing venereal disease. The survey will last for at least a period of six months.

From among those who volunteered, 115 men and women were accepted as participants in a prophylactic field trial. The 115 were selected from among the most promiscuous people in the United States. More than half of them had caught gonorrhea at least once during the six months preceding the field trial; 20 had gonorrhea on the day they applied and had to be cured before admission to the program. The gonorrhea rate among these volunteers exceeded 100 infections per 100 participants per year.

Each volunteer was given a supply of doxycycline, an antibiotic in common use, and was told to swallow two tablets either immediately before or immediately after each casual sexual encounter. They were assured that they could come back for more tablets whenever their supply ran low. In return, the volunteers promised to come in every two months for physical examination, syphilis blood tests, and laboratory gonorrhea cultures. They also promised to record each sexual encounter in a diary.

In all, 5,221 casual sexual encounters were noted in the diaries. In the absence of the tablets, dozens of gonorrheal infections would no doubt have occurred. In fact, there were only two infections, and in both cases, the participants confessed that they had neglected to take their tablets on at least one critical occasion. So for those who took the tablets as directed, the gonorrhea rate was zero. The tablets proved 100% effective.

The syphilis rate was also zero, even though three participants were known to have had sexual relations with partners having infectious syphilis; the actual number of contacts with syphilitic partners was no doubt much greater.

The Los Angeles field trial was almost wholly ignored, not only by the mass media and the medical profession but also by the health departments whose job supposedly is to protect us from gonorrhea and syphilis.

At least a half-dozen other antibiotics are probably also effective in preventing VD. But no one has yet bothered to test them. Why do doctors make the distinction between prescribing before and prescribing after you have sex with an infected partner? I have asked scores of physicians and have been given four explanations.

A few physicians state that they make the distinction on moral grounds. They are opposed to patients' having sex with people to whom they are not married. Fear of VD, they believe, is one of the things that keep patients chaste. The only solution I know is to find another doctor, one more concerned with safeguarding your health than with supervising your sex life.

I personally believe that physicians who take this allegedly moral stance are in fact violating a deep moral principle. The refusal to prevent VD permits infection to spread unchecked through the country year after year. I also believe it is *your* moral duty to take prophylactic precautions, to protect not only yourself and your loved ones but also the hundreds of others who may acquire your VD infection over the next 20 years.

If I were a physician, I would feel deeply distressed if I failed to vaccinate a child in my care against diphtheria or polio if, as a result, he or she fell ill with one of these diseases. I think physicians should feel equally distressed when they refuse to help patients in their care to safeguard themselves against VD when, as a result, some of those patients get VD.

Most physicians today explain that antibiotics should not be taken at the time of exposure because of the hazardous side effects: "You may even drop dead from penicillin."

This year, an estimated 2.5 million Americans will receive massive injections of penicillin to cure VD. If present rates continue, more than 50 million Americans will receive those massive antibiotic injections over the next 20 years, and there will be as much gonorrhea 20 years hence as there is today. Using penicillin merely to cure VD after symptoms appear is the best way to *increase* the number of patients needing antibiotics, and therefore suffering side effects. But the present policy does assure a steady or rising market for the antibiotic manufacturers.

The side-effect argument is limited, strangely enough, to VD prophylaxis. If a physician diagnoses a fresh case of tuberculosis, he will not wait until the patient's spouse and children get tuberculosis before providing TB prophylaxis for the family. Similarly, if a patient is going to travel in a country with a high rate of malaria, a doctor will provide malaria prophylaxis. The drugs used for these forms of prophylaxis are somewhat more dangerous than penicillin, but the physician reasons that the potential benefits far outweigh the hazard.

Children who contract rheumatic fever are unhesitatingly placed on daily doses of penicillin for 10 or 20 years to prevent recurrences. The physician knows that there is a penicillin risk, but he also knows that rheumatic fever patients who are not protected by antibiotics are likely to become "cardiac cripples" at an early age and perhaps die of rheumatic heart disease.

Patients can also be crippled by syphilis and gonorrhea—and can die from them—yet prophylaxis is withheld. So the suspicion arises that what purports to be a medical argument (i.e., the danger of side effects) is in fact a moral argument in disguise. VD is immoral; rheumatic fever is not.

This suspicion grows stronger when we consider the strange case of infant gonorrhea. Half a century ago, countless babies went blind as the result of contracting gonorrhea of the eye from their infected mothers during birth. Today, almost every state requires by law that the eyes of each newborn baby be protected by eye drops containing either a silver salt or penicillin. As a result, gonorrheal blindness is today a very rare condition. The eye drops produce side effects in some cases—and on rare occasions, serious side effects. No physician, however, waits until the baby has shown symptoms of a gonorrhea infection before putting drops in its eyes. And nobody protests gonorrhea prophylaxis for babies—since they, after all, are innocent of sexual intercourse.

There is a risk of side effects from penicillin and other antibiotics. For that reason, no antibiotic should be taken unless there is a good reason to take it. Protecting yourself, your loved ones, and all of your and their future sexual contacts from VD is a very good reason indeed.

Doctors also say, "VD is becoming resistant to antibiotics." You may also have heard that GIs a few years ago brought back from Vietnam "superstrains" of VD that cannot be cured by penicillin. If you ask for antibiotics to protect yourself from VD, your doctor is quite likely to refuse on the grounds that the drugs may contribute to the rise of such superstrains.

Let's note first that this argument is raised only when patients want protection from infection for a nonmarital sexual encounter. If a physician is accidentally exposed to infection himself while treating an infected patient, he will not withhold penicillin on the grounds that it may contribute to an increase in resistance, nor will he fear side effects.

Let's look at the facts. First, many people mistakenly think, as a result of all the "resistant-strains" propaganda, that if they take penicillin, *they* will become resistant, so that penicillin will not work if they later need it. This is simply wrong. It is not the patient but the germs that may become more resistant.

Next, with respect to syphilis, this argument is completely false. Syphilis was very sensitive to penicillin when it was first used more than 30 years ago; it remains precisely as sensitive today. The same amount of penicillin will cure syphilis today as it did 30 years ago. Deliberate efforts to produce a resistant strain in the laboratory have failed. No strain of syphilis resistant to penicillin (or to any other antibiotic) has ever been isolated anywhere in the world, including Vietnam.

The "masking syphilis" argument is the fourth explanation that your physician may give for refusing to prescribe antibiotics to protect you from VD. That is, the drug may merely "mask" the early symptoms of syphilis without preventing a syphilis infection. The germs, according to this theory, may continue to survive and multiply in your body, doing vast harm, without your getting an early warning that you are infected.

To give this explanation to a woman is ridiculous. Four women out of five, as we noted earlier, have no early-warning symptoms of either syphilis or gonorrhea sufficent to send them to a doctor for treatment. Their only hope is to prevent infection *before* it spreads through their bodies. Waiting for symptoms means, for many women, waiting until the damage has been done.

But that isn't all. Dr. R. W. Babione and his U.S. Navy associates proved way back in 1952 that small doses of penicillin do not mask the early symptoms of syphilis. They prevent some cases of syphilis altogether. In a few cases, they may delay a bit the appearance of early syphilis symptoms, but they do not alter or mask those symptoms. Several studies made since 1952 have confirmed Babione's findings. Yet, despite all the scientific evidence, some doctors go right on using the masking-syphilis argument to explain their unwillingness to protect you from VD. Once again, they are making the old moral argument in a medical disguise.

Perhaps your physician will come up with a fifth argument against using antibiotics to prevent VD. If so, I hope you'll let me know. These are the only arguments that the scores of physicians whom I have interviewed have been able to think up. Of all the methods to prevent VD now available, which should you choose? This is very much like the question of which form of contraception you should use. The answers are also quite similar.

Millions of women prefer the pill to prevent unwanted pregnancy. They know there is some danger of side effects, but since they do not personally experience these side effects to an unacceptable degree, they conclude that the advantages of the pill outweigh the risks. Such women can similarly choose the anti-VD pill because of its several advantages. It is simultaneously effective against oral and anal as well as vaginal gonorrhea infections, and it is the easiest and least messy way to protect yourself. It may also prove most effective, though this is not yet certain.

Other women are afraid of the pill's side effects and therefore rely on vaginal contraception or the condom to prevent unwanted pregnancy. Such women can similarly rely on vaginal prophylaxis or the condom to prevent VD.

Finally, no matter what method of contraception you rely on, including IUDs or surgical sterilization, you should review once more the short-arm inspection and the soap-and-water methods of preventing VD. These methods are quite effective. They involve no drugs or chemicals, and therefore no side effects. They are well worth using along with *any* method of contraception, and also with other methods of preventing VD.

REFERENCES

Babione, R. W., Hedgecock, L. E., & Ray, J. P. Navy experience with the oral use of penicillin as a prophylaxis. *U.S. Armed Forces Medical Journal*, 1952, *3*, 973–990.

Edwards, W. M., & Fox, R. S. *Progonasyl as an anti-V.D. prophylactic.* Paper presented at the First National Conference in Methods of Venereal Disease Prevention, Chicago, November 16–17, 1974.

Neisser, A. Is it really impossible to make prostitution harmless as far as infection is concerned? In W. J. Robinson (Ed.), *Sexual truths versus sexual lies, misconceptions and exaggerations.* New York: Eugenics Publishing Co., 1919, pp. 261–274.

Prophylaxis of Sexually Transmitted Diseases

An Overview

KING K. HOLMES

The only two really reliable methods for protecting yourself from sexually transmissible diseases (STD) are limiting sexual exposures—for example, by having one sex partner at a time (i.e., "serial monogamy")—and using a condom. Of the 10 leading sexually transmitted diseases (STD), only crab lice cannot be prevented by using a condom—provided the condom is used properly. The condom also will not prevent the spread of herpes, syphilis, or other causes of genital ulcers from the male to the female if the ulcers are located at the base of the penis, where they would not be covered by a condom. A third useful method of avoiding the spread of STD is to wait for one week after sex with a casual sex partner before resuming sex with your regular sex partner (postexposure abstinence), because symptoms of gonorrhea and herpes usually appear within a week, even in women. The longer you can wait before resuming sex, the better are your chances that you don't have VD, if no symptoms occur. Many other methods of prevention that are often advocated are of unproved or limited benefit and may do more harm than good to the individual user by creating a false sense of security.

The main thing to realize is that while gonorrhea and syphilis are bad, that's not where the action is in sexually transmitted diseases for most people today. For example, in college students, genital herpes

KING K. HOLMES, M.D., PH.D. ● Professor, Department of Medicine, Adjunct Professor, Department of Microbiology, Immunology, and Epidemiology; Head, Division of Infectious Diseases, USPHS Hospital, Seattle, Washington 98114.

simplex virus and Chlamydia infections are 5–10 times as common as gonorrhea, and syphilis is extremely rare. Furthermore, gonorrhea and syphilis are relatively easy to diagnose and treat; but herpes is almost untreatable and Chlamydia is almost undiagnosable—which is why these two are so common.

Let's take a look at some of the other methods advocated for preventing VD:

The Call-Girl Ritual. What I prefer to call *exploratory foreplay* will disclose herpes or syphilis sores, or a discharge from the penis caused by gonorrhea or Chlamydia. However, probably only one-third of women who get herpes, gonorrhea, or Chlamydia infections get them from a man with symptoms or signs; the rest get them from men who have an asymptomatic infection. It is an axiom in STD control that it is the asymptomatic carrier who spreads most infections.

Vaginal Contraceptive Creams. It's true that one study showed that women using a contraceptive cream called Conceptrol with intercourse had less gonorrhea than women using no contraceptive cream—but only for the first six months of the study. During the second six months, the women using the cream did not have a significantly lower rate of infection, so that by the end of the study, there was no significant difference between the two groups. There were 3.35 infections per 100 patient months among women using the cream versus 5.82 infections per 100 patient months among women not using the cream. The authors thought the women assigned to cream use stopped using it after six months (Cutler *et al.*, 1977). Furthermore, since the no-prophylaxis group did not use a placebo vaginal cream, any differences that had occurred between the groups would be inconclusive. Even if the contraceptive cream worked to prevent gonorrhea, there's no way of knowing if it would prevent any of the other STDs. Even though the same contraceptive cream is active in the test tube against herpes virus, in a recent study this cream was shown to have *no* effect, when compared with placebo, in treating genital herpes simplex virus infection in patients (Vontver *et al.*, 1979). Thus, activity in the test tube does not necessarily mean effectiveness in the patient.

Douching, Washing, and Urinating. Hygiene is commendable, but there is no evidence that it will prevent STD. In fact, a recent study of U.S. Navy men in which I was involved (Hooper, *et al.*, 1978) showed the same risk of gonorrhea in men who washed and urinated right after sex as in those who did not.

Use of Penicillin on the Vagina (e.g., Penigin). No one recommends topical penicillin today, even for proven infection, because when penicillin is put on skin or mucous membrane, the chances of causing an allergic reaction are very high—higher than with an injection. When investigators tried to study Penigin in prostitutes in the Far East, the study failed because the prostitutes wouldn't use it.

Progonasyl. No one will get the Nobel Prize for Progonasyl. The study of Progonasyl in Nevada prostitutes showed mainly that the prostitutes found that the drug stained their underclothing and stopped using it. The microbiological tests for gonorrhea were so poor and the willingness of the prostitutes to continue using Progonasyl was so low that the study results were uninterpretable. If the preparation was so good, why don't the prostitutes in Nevada use it now?

Antibiotics by Mouth. I have supervised two studies that showed that the prophylactic administration of long-acting tetracyclines after intercourse reduces the risk of gonorrhea. The first study (Harrison *et al.*, 1979) showed that tetracycline, taken after intercourse with prostitutes, prevented infection with strains of gonorrhea that were highly sensitive to tetracycline but allowed the occurrence of infection with tetracycline-resistant strains. Thus, if everyone used tetracycline prophylaxis, soon we would have only tetracycline-resistant gonorrhea. This should be of special concern to women, since tetracycline is now the best drug available to treat severe gonorrhea infection (e.g., infection of the fallopian tubes) in women. Thus, one must weigh the benefit to the individual who takes tetracycline prophylaxis versus the hazard to the community of the increased resistance of gonococci to tetracycline. In fact, the use of penicillin by mouth for prophylaxis for gonorrhea in prostitutes in the Philippines probably is one factor which led in 1976 to the sudden appearance in that country of gonorrhea strains that are completely resistant to penicillin. These strains now cause half of all the gonorrhea in the Philippines and have spread to many other countries of the world. This concern about community hazard is not puritanically limited to gonorrhea prophylaxis. As the editorial that followed our publication (Sack, 1979) pointed out, equal concern exists about the use of tetracycline prophylaxis to prevent diarrhea due to intestinal infection in travelers.

I go along with Ed Brecher on one point. I agree that conservative sexual ethics have stifled research on VD prophylaxis and the use of prophylaxis. Whether you pejoratively call such ethics "moralism," or you endorse conservative "morality," my own research on VD prophylaxis has been held back by such attitudes. Interestingly enough, it has not been the U.S. Public Health Service, nor exclusively the male establishment, that objected most vocally, and it has not been solely for reasons of puritanical moralism. The USPHS and the U.S. Navy actually helped conduct the shipboard prophylaxis study (Hooper *et al.*, 1978; Harrison *et al.*, 1979) but the naval line officers later asked us to stop the study, in part because of a provocative and childish article concerning the study that appeared on the front page of the *Los Angeles Times* and led to subsequent complaints from the wives of men on the ship. A study of gonorrhea prophylaxis in homosexual men, which we have just finished, ran into opposition from concerned homosexual physicians in the community, who essentially felt that the prophylaxis was more dangerous than gonorrhea, even in this exceptionally high-risk population. Finally, and most discouraging to me, although we have found that 27% of female sexual assault victims in Seattle developed a sexually transmitted infection that was probably attributable to the assault (i.e., not present on first examination, but present on follow-up examination), we have been unable to obtain funding to evaluate methods to prevent STD in this high-risk population of women. Thus, we have had difficulties in studying VD prophylaxis in men and have as yet been unable to obtain support for such studies in women.

I disagree to some extent with Mr. Brecher on other points. Mr. Brecher's uncritical endorsement of unproven methods of prophylaxis is most disturbing. What most concerns me is that by telling people that they can avoid VD by using partially effective, or useless, methods, they will get a false sense of security and will then get burned. It is important to assess realistically the limitations of the methods available today for STD prophylaxis. Although the chances of acquiring any single STD through a casual sexual encounter are small, and one would like to be reassuring, the cumulative chances of getting *any* STD are not small. My perspective is colored by the dozens of patients I see monthly, particularly those with genital herpes, who had a casual sexual encounter without a condom and were not so lucky. I don't know whether doctors in private practice will more readily give prophylaxis to men than to women to reduce the risk of STD following a casual sexual exposure; but in public clinics, the reverse has been true for years with respect to prophylaxis for gonorrhea in people exposed to gonorrhea, partly because the risks of gonorrhea are greater in women.

It is interesting that in general, women seem far more interested than men in STD prophylaxis and seem more willing to do something about it. I am not aware of an in-depth psychological study of why this is so, and I hesitate to speculate. One hypothesis I would like to see tested is that those most interested in self-protection think of themselves as being controlled by events and by others, rather than as being in control themselves. If so, the development of more effective methods of STD prophylaxis may give users more of a sense of independence and control in their sex lives—in a manner analogous to the control afforded by more effective contraception. As effective and acceptable methods of STD prophylaxis become available, they will probably be used most extensively by women—perhaps in conjunction with contraceptive care. I am frequently asked, "If a gonorrhea vaccine becomes available, who would use it?" One likely use would be in women, since they are more likely than men to develop serious complications of gonorrhea. Although research on vaccines for gonorrhea, herpes, and other STDs is proceeding rapidly, there is no vaccine on the immediate horizon for any STD, with the exception of hepatitis B virus vaccine, which was licensed for use in the United States in the fall of 1981.

References

Cutler, J. C., et al. Vaginal contraceptives as prophylaxis against gonorrhea and other sexually transmitted diseases. Advances in Planned Parenthood, 1977, 12, 45–56.

Harrison, W. O., Hooper, R. R., Wiesner, P. J., Campbell, A. F., Karney, W. W., Reynolds, G. H., Jones, O. G., & Holmes, K. K. Minocycline given after exposure for the prevention of gonorrhea. New England Journal of Medicine, 1979, 300, 1074–1078.

Hooper, R. R., Reynolds, G. H., Jones, O. G., Zaidi, A., Wiesner, P. J., Lattimer, K. P., Lester, A., Campbell, A. F., Harrison, W. O., Karney, W. W., & Holmes, K. K. Cohort study of venereal disease: I. The risk of gonorrhea transition from infected women to men. American Journal of Epidemiology, 1978, 108, 134–144.

Sack, R. B. Prophylactic antibiotics: The individual versus the community. New England Journal of Medicine, 1979, 300, 1107–1108.

Vontver, L. A., Reeves, W. C., Ratray, M., Corey, L., Remington, M. A., Tolentino, E., Schweid, A., & Holmes, K. K. Clinical course and diagnosis of genital herpes simplex virus infection and evaluation of topical surfactant therapy. American Journal of Obstetrics and Gynecology, 1979, 133, 548–554.

Index